Visit our website

to find out about other books from Churchill Livingstone and other Harcourt Health Sciences imprints

Register free at
www.harcourt-international.com

and you will get

- the latest information on new books, journals and electronic products in your chosen subject areas

- the choice of e-mail or post alerts or both, when there are any new books in your chosen areas

- news of special offers and promotions

- information about products from all Harcourt Health Sciences imprints including Baillière Tindall, Churchill Livingstone, Mosby and W. B. Saunders

You will also find an easily searchable catalogue, online ordering, information on our extensive list of journals...and much more!

Visit the Harcourt Health Sciences website today!

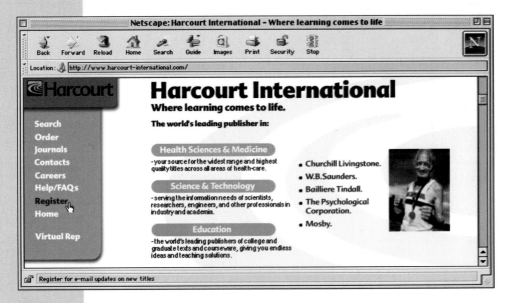

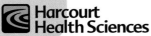

Dermatology Nursing

This book is dedicated to all the people suffering from chronic skin conditions whom we have met and nursed and are the inspiration for our dedication to dermatology nursing; and to our husbands, John and Paul, without whose love and support the book would not have been possible.

For Churchill Livingstone:

Commissioning Editor: Sarena Wolfaard
Head of Project Management: Ewan Halley
Project Development Manager: Katrina Mather
Project Manager: Jane Shanks
Design Direction: George Ajayi

Dermatology Nursing

A Practical Guide

Edited by

Esther Hughes BN RGN RM
Senior Staff Nurse, Dermatology Department, Queen Margaret Hospital,
Dunfermline, UK

Julie Van Onselen RGN RSCN DipN BA(Hons) ENB N25 998
Clinical Nurse Adviser, Medical Department, Leo Pharmaceuticals, Buckinghamshire;
Clinical Nurse Specialist, Department of Dermatology, Stoke Mandeville Hospital, Aylesbury, UK

Foreword by

Steven Ersser PhD BSc(Hon) RGN CertTHEd
Head of Nursing Development, School of Nursing and Midwifery, University of Southampton, UK;
Chair, Advisory Group, International Skin Care Nursing Group

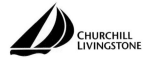
CHURCHILL
LIVINGSTONE

EDINBURGH LONDON NEW YORK PHILADELPHIA ST LOUIS SYDNEY TORONTO 2001

CHURCHILL LIVINGSTONE
An imprint of Harcourt Publishers Limited

© Harcourt Publishers Limited 2001

 is a registered trademark of Harcourt Publishers Limited

First published 2001

ISBN 0 443 06209 9

British Library Cataloguing in Publication Data
A catalogue record for this book is available from the British Library

Library of Congress Cataloging in Publication Data
A catalog record for this book is available from the Library of Congress

Note
Medical knowledge is constantly changing. As new information becomes available, changes in treatment, procedures, equipment and the use of drugs become necessary. The editors, contributors and the publishers have taken care to ensure that the information given in this text is accurate and up to date. However, readers are strongly advised to confirm that the information, especially with regard to drug usage, complies with the latest legislation and standards of practice.

The
publisher's
policy is to use
**paper manufactured
from sustainable forests**

Printed in China

Contents

Contributors

Lynette Boardman MSc MRPharms
Formerly Pharmacist, St John's Institute of
Dermatology, St Thomas' Hospital, London, UK

Mandy Boston RGN ENB N25
Dermatology Sister, Dermatology Treatment
Area, OPD, Harrogate District Hospital,
Harrogate, UK

Rebecca Davis BSc(Hons) RGN ENB N25
Dermatology Nurse Practitioner, Dermatology
Department, Whipscross Hospital, London, UK

Jacqueline Denyer RGN RSCN RHV
Clinical Nurse Specialist for Epidermolysis
Bullosa, Great Ormond Street Hospital for
Children NHS Trust, Great Ormond Street,
London, UK

Christine Docherty BN RGN RSCN Dip N
Formerly Senior Charge Nurse, Dermatology
Unit, Ninewells Hospital, Dundee, UK

Una Donaldson SRN/SCM
Ward Manager, Dermatology Department,
Queen Margaret Hospital, Dunfermline, UK

Trish Garabaldinos RN ENB 393 998 934
Sister, St John's Institute of Dermatology,
St Thomas' Hospital, London, UK

Esther Hughes BN RGN RM
Senior Staff Nurse, Dermatology Department,
Queen Margaret Hospital, Dunfermline, UK

Ray Jobling MA
Senior Tutor and Lecturer in Sociology,
St John's College, Cambridge, UK

Sandra Lawton RGN OND ENB 393
Dermatology Liaison Sister, Queen's Medical
Centre, University Hospital, Nottingham, UK

Gillian Morrison RGN
Sister, Department of Dermatology, Royal
Group of Hospitals, Belfast, Northern Ireland

Helen Perfect RGN
Sister, Outpatients and Day Care Department
of Dermatology, Amersham Hospital, Bucks,
UK

Jill Peters BSc Health Studies DipNP RGN CMS ENB 393 998 934 870
Dermatology Nurse Practitioner/Community
Liaisen Sister, Daniel Turner Dermatology
Department, Chelsea and Westminster Hospital,
London, UK

Dawn Preston RGN BSC Hons Health Care Studies ENB 998 ENB 934
Clinical Nurse Manager, Dermatology
Department, Leeds Teaching Hospitals, Leeds,
UK

Fiona Pringle RGN FETC ENB 901
Formerly Surgical Nurse Practitioner, Oxford
Department of Dermatology, Churchill Hospital,
Oxford, UK

Lynette Stone CBE BA RN RM (NSW) DMS
Dentistry and Dermatology Group, Guy's &
St Thomas' Hospital Trust, Guy's Hospital,
London, UK

Julie Van Onselen RGN RSCN DipN BA(Hons) ENB N25 998
Clinical Nurse Adviser, Leo Pharmaceuticals,
Buckinghamshire; Clinical Nurse Specialist,
Department of Dermatology, Stoke Mandeville
Hospital, Aylesbury, UK

Jane Watts RGN ENB 393
Dermatology Nurse Practitioner, Department of
Dermatology, King George Hospital, Essex, UK

Maxine Whitton BA(Hons) ALA
Patient Advocate, Member of NICE Partner's
Council and AGS (Associate Parliamentary
Group on Skin), The Vitiligo Society, London, UK

Arthur Williams OBE FRPharmS
Formerly Chief Administrative Pharmaceutical
Officer, Grampian, Orkney, Shetland and Tayside
Health Boards, UK

Helen Wilson RGN
Dermatology Specialist Nurse, Prince Charles
Hospital, Merthyr Tidfil, UK

Foreword

The development of dermatological nursing in the UK over the last decade has been considerable. Through practice development and service innovation, educational initiatives, growing involvement in research and the shaping of policy, the nursing specialty has in many respects come of age. Nurses are now at the centre of the development of dermatological services, with their fundamental role in skin care, chronic illness management and ability to establish innovative services. This book is a product of such progress. The skills and expertise of the authors of this book are among those that have contributed significantly to this evolution. The quality of text is richer for this mix of expertise.

For many years dermatology nurses have been without a substantial contemporary textbook that sufficiently covers the fundamentals of the complex range of topics and issues encountered in practice. Major changes have taken place in both the patterns of care delivery, the role of the patient and family in health care and in technological developments. The response of nursing to these changes is apparent throughout this book.

The sub-title of this book, 'A Practical Guide', highlights its value as a pointer for enhancing clinical practice. However, it also makes an important contribution as a highly readable and sound theoretical background. At this time when there is universal recognition of the necessity to develop the evidence base of health care, the authors provide an effective guide to practice that is based on evidence or theoretical principles when the research base remains unclear. There is

no shortage of reading guidance throughout the book. The science and the art of nursing are nicely integrated to give the reader an informed basis for practice.

The evolving role of the nurse in playing a more direct role in providing dermatological care is apparent throughout. Such development ranges from finding systematic ways for the nurse to help those with chronic illness self-manage and cope more effectively through planned teaching, to the nurse taking a direct role in providing new treatments such as laser therapy. The ways in which the nurse can support and empower patients and their families are also evident. Attention is given to the major psychological and social reactions to having a skin condition and the implications of these for nursing. These different features of the nurse's role reflect the expansion of the nurse's core therapeutic functions as well as its extension across the traditional professional boundaries to respond to new therapeutic opportunities.

I anticipate that in the coming years dermatology nurses will greatly step up the substantial contribution they are making to the development of dermatological care itself. This will be achieved through their innovative work on the development of roles and new services. Indeed in a recent editorial in *Archives in Dermatology* Dr Robin Marks poses the question 'Who will advise patients about matters dermatological in the new millennium?'. He concludes that dermatologists will be at the tip of the iceberg in this process, with groups such as nurses playing a central role.

There is little doubt that nurses will continue to gain prominence as a key specialist resource for both patients in the community and primary care services, where most skin care is delivered. The quality of this care will be highly dependent on the effective education of both dermatology nurses and the generalist nurses in the commu-nity or hospital, with whom they share their expertise. This book will make a very valuable contribution to this important process by helping to capture and communicate nursing expertise. It is a pleasure to recommend this book to you.

Southampton 2000   Steven Ersser

REFERENCE

Marks R 2000 Who will advise patients about matters dermatological in the new millennium? Archives in Dermatology 136: 79–80

Preface

Skin conditions are very common, accounting for 15% of all patients who attend for a consultation in primary care. Skin conditions are an underestimated source of physical suffering, psychological distress and often have far reaching social implications. Any skin condition can have a profound impact on quality of life for many people and their families.

Nurses play a major role in helping patients to cope with the physical, psychological and social effects of skin conditions. An All Party Parliamentary Group on Skin report (1997) endorsed this by stating that nurses are an essential resource for dermatology at every level from specialist nurse to the community. Nurses play a vital role in dermatology: they are the key to educating and informing patients, especially on individual and effective treatment regimens.

Every nurse in all of the healthcare settings requires knowledge and expertise in dermatology nursing skills. Nurses in primary and secondary care settings will constantly be caring for patients with skin conditions. Primary care nurses, especially nurse practitioners, practice nurses and health visitors advise and support patients with common skin conditions on a daily basis. Many primary care nurses identify dermatology as an area of need and are developing skin clinics on the same lines as other chronic disease management clinics such as asthma and diabetes.

The role of the specialist dermatology nurse within dermatology departments and some primary care has expanded in recent years. There have been many dermatology nursing innovations, including nurse-led clinics in patient education, minor surgery and phototherapy, the expansion of day care services and liaison nursing, which are all outlined in Chapter 16, 'Dermatology nursing'.

This book is written for all nurses by some of the most experienced nurses in the field of dermatology throughout the UK. All the authors are members of the British Dermatological Nursing Group (BDNG). The BDNG was established in 1989 as an independent specialty group for nurses and healthcare professionals with an interest in dermatology. The BDNG has been established within the associate membership groups of the British Association of Dermatologists (BAD), who share headquarters and the annual conference with the BDNG. The aims of the BDNG are to:

- promote the development of the highest standard of care for the patient receiving dermatological care
- promote the development and recognition of the nurse's role in dermatology, for the benefit of the patient
- promote and support the education of nurses for their role in dermatology
- promote and support research into all aspects of dermatology nursing and dermatological patient care
- provide a source of expertise for nurses facing clinical and managerial challenges in the field of dermatological nursing
- provide a forum for the dissemination of developments and knowledge in the field of dermatological nursing.

The aim of this book is to give the reader a theoretical knowledge to dermatology conditions, with research based guidelines to current treatment and practices. *Dermatology Nursing* will also highlight current issues in dermatology. The book has a practical approach, emphasizing nursing care, and should be complemented with other medical dermatological textbooks.

Dermatology Nursing covers a general introduction to dermatology from Chapters 1–8, including: Skin – its structure, function and related pathology; Assessment of the dermatology patient; Treatment issues and systemic therapy relating to dermatology; Phototherapy; Dermatological surgery and cryosurgery; Psychosocial issues in dermatology; Age-specific issues in dermatology; and Care of the acutely ill dermatology patient.

There are over 1000 skin diseases but the large majority of dermatological workload in primary and secondary care, estimated at 70%, is concerned with nine categories of skin disease (Williams, 1997). All these common dermatological conditions except leg ulcers are covered in Chapters 9–13, including treatment and nursing management of psoriasis, eczema, acne and rosacea, skin cancer, infections and infestations. Other skin conditions including epidermolysis bullosa and other bullous diseases, lichen planus and sclerosus, pruritus, urticaria, alopecia and vitiligo are addressed in Chapters 14 and 15.

The book is written as a practical nursing guide to dermatology nursing. All chapters include clear guidance on nursing and patient care. The book is illustrated throughout with clinical slides, as dermatology is such a visual specialty. A feature of the book is the emphasis on patient education, which is included in all chapters. At the end of each chapter there is a signpost box indicating any additional information on the chapter topic which is included in other chapters. This is a useful resource as there is inevitably some overlap and signposting to other chapters will help the reader to gain a comprehensive dermatological nursing knowledge. It should be noted that both propriety and generic drug names are used in the book as the text would cease to be practical (particularly with topical preparations) if only generic names were used.

The book does not include chapters on leg ulcers, pressure sores, burns management or plastic surgery, as these areas are related to dermatology but are all entire specialist areas in their own fields. There are obvious overlaps between these three specialist nursing areas and dermatological nursing and it is acknowledged that some specialist dermatological nurses may have roles and skills relating to these areas, particularly leg ulcer care. There is already an excellent range of nursing textbooks covering these areas but no up-to-date textbooks on dermatological nursing.

Finally, as the editors, we have achieved an ambition for dermatology nursing in producing a book for the specialty and for all nurses. We foresee that this book will be an essential resource and guide for every bookshelf in every ward, clinic and health centre within primary and secondary care. We believe that it is essential for every nurse to have an understanding of healthy skin care and common dermatological conditions to provide improved services and enhanced skin care for all patients.

2000   Esther Hughes and Julie Van Onselen

REFERENCES

All Party Parliamentary Group on Skin 1997 An investigation into the adequacy of service provision and treatments for patients with skin diseases in the UK. APPG, London
Williams HC 1997 Dermatology – Health care needs assessment. Radcliffe Medical Press, Oxford

Acknowledgements

We would like to thank all the contributors, who are among the key dermatology nurses and patient advocates in the UK and whose expertise has made this book possible; all our dermatologist and other colleagues, including Dr Peter Adnitt, Dr Sheena Allan, Dr Anthony Bewly, Dr Bill Cunliffe, Dr Kate Dalziel, Dr Rodney Dawber, Dr Olivia Dolan, Dr John Harper, Dr Alison Layton, Dr Ravi Ratnavel, Dr Nerys Roberts, Dr Sheena Russell, Dr Riadh Wakeel, Mark Timms, Arthur Williams and Jean Mackenzie, who have assisted authors in clinical content and provided slides for the chapters; Stuart Robertson, Medical Photographer at St John's Institute of Dermatology, and Dr Tony Burns, Consultant Dermatologist, for their generous help in providing many of the slides for illustrating this book; Dr Paul Buxton, Consultant Dermatologist, Royal Infirmary, Edinburgh and Former Consultant Dermatologist, Queen Margaret's Hospital, Fife, who provided the original inspiration for this textbook; and Dr Steven Ersser, Head of Nursing Development, School of Nursing and Midwifery, University of Southampton, for writing the foreword and all his support for the book.

1

Skin: its structure, function and related pathology

Esther Hughes

The skin is the largest organ in the body and covers an area of approximately 2 square metres. It weighs approximately 2.5 kg and contains over a million nerve endings. It has the inherent ability to regenerate itself and, to a certain degree, repair any damage that is inflicted upon it through the course of daily living. Its structure and function are vital for helping to maintain the homeostasis of the body.

Before gaining a knowledge and insight into the manifestations of skin disease, we must first have an appreciation of the structure and function of the normal skin.

THE ANATOMY OF THE SKIN

- The epidermis
- The dermis
- The skin appendages

The skin is composed of two distinct layers: the outer layer, the epidermis, and the inner layer, the dermis. The epidermis consists of cells that migrate from the basal layer to the surface. During this process, the nuclei of the cells are lost and the cells dramatically change in shape. The thickness of this layer is dependent upon the site; it is very thick on the soles of the feet and the palms of the hands. The epidermis has no direct blood supply but is nourished by the blood vessels found within the dermis.

The dermis, a thicker layer than the epidermis, contains fibrous connective tissue, smooth muscle (attached to hair follicles), blood vessels, lymphatics and nerves. It is the connective tissue support for the epithelium and allows the skin a degree of movement over the underlying organs.

Below the dermis, there is subcutaneous tissue which binds the skin to the organs below. This layer is mainly composed of loose connective tissue and adipose tissue, vitally important in the conservation of body heat. Its amount varies greatly between individuals and is also dependent on the region of the body.

The epidermis

The epidermis is composed of five distinct layers: the stratum corneum, the stratum lucidum, the stratum granulosum, the stratum spinosum and the stratum basale (Fig. 1.1).

Stratum corneum

This is often called the horny layer as it is composed of fully keratinized, dead cells. This outermost layer is shed as flakes of keratin. It can be noticeably removed by abrasive action on the skin, e.g. drying the body with a towel after bathing.

As these cells are lost from the surface of the skin they are replaced by others which migrate from the deep layers to the surface. In some hereditary conditions, e.g. ichthyosis, there is a disorder of the keratin layer. The skin cells are easily damaged and trauma to the skin can often result in infection.

Stratum lucidum

This layer is not found in most of the epidermis. It occurs within the thickened skin of the palms of the hands and the soles of the feet. It is composed of cells which are packed closely together, with characteristic flattened nuclei.

Stratum granulosum

Often called the granular layer, this layer contains flattened cells thought to be in the transitional stage between the cells of the stratum spinosum and the stratum corneum. The nuclei within these cells have a shrivelled appearance.

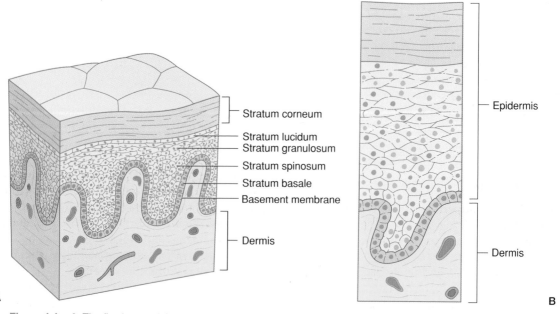

Figure 1.1   **A**: The five layers of the epidermis. **B**: The epidermis and the dermis.

Stratum spinosum

This is a relatively deep layer composed of cells which have a rounded appearance, termed prickle cells. They are loosely packed together and connected by bridges. Clefts exist between the cells, where pigment granules can be found.

Stratum basale

The basal cell layer, also called the stratum basale, is generally composed of a single row of columnar-shaped cells.

Melanocytes are to be found in this deep layer and in the underlying connective tissue of the dermis. They are responsible for the production of melanin, a pigment which determines skin colour. The pigment is usually dark brown or black. Occasionally, it may be found in the cells of the cuticle, where it is yellow and gives the appearance of freckles. The number of melanocytes present in cells is equal in all races; therefore, it is the activity and production of melanin that is increased in the darker-skinned races.

The dermis

Like the epidermis, the dermis is found in varying degrees of thickness. It is very thick on the soles of the feet and the palms of the hands but is of a delicate nature on the eyelids, scrotum and penis.

The dermis gives the skin its elasticity due to a network of elastic fibres but it is extremely tough because it is composed of dense, fibrous connective tissue. This connective tissue is found in two distinct layers: the papillary layer and the reticular layer.

The papillary layer

This is the thin, superficial layer which lies next to the epidermis. It is a highly vascular area and also has a greater water content than the more dense reticular layer.

The collagen fibres within the papillary region are arranged very loosely. The surface area of this layer is greatly increased by small, finger-like projections called papillae which project into the epidermis. Many of these papillae contain loops of capillaries; others contain receptors to pain (pacinian corpuscles) and touch (Meissner's corpuscles). On the palms of the hands and soles of the feet, the papillae rest on ridges which make loops and whorls on the epidermal surface. The patterns within these are unique and specific to each individual and are genetically determined. For this reason their indentations are used as 'fingerprints' in the process of identification.

The reticular layer

This is the deep layer which makes up about 80% of the dermis. The collagen fibres within this region are thickly arranged and interlaced which allows for strength and flexibility in all directions. The gaps which are produced as a result of this interlacing contain sweat glands, adipose tissue, hair follicles, nerves and blood vessels.

Collagen gives the skin its strength. Occasionally there is an alteration in the collagen structure, giving rise to characteristic reddened streaks known as striae. They are common in situations where the skin is stretched to the extreme, e.g. pregnancy, and, whilst initially red, will fade to silvery white with age. They are also a known side effect of overusage of topical steroids.

The skin appendages

These include the nails, the sweat glands, the sebaceous glands and the hairs. We will look at each of these in turn.

The nails

The nails are flattened epidermal structures with a horny texture found on the dorsum of the distal regions of the fingers and toes. In other animals they are found as claws or hooves. They are embedded into the skin by a root.

The area visible to the naked eye is the nail body, which has a free border at the distal extremity of the nail. It is composed of a greatly thickened stratum lucidum. Underneath most of the body there lies a thick vascular area which accounts for the pinkness of the nail. The area that extends over the nail matrix, near to the root, is of a less vascular nature. This area is whitish and is termed the lunula, because of its moon-like shape. Growth of the nail is dependent upon the proliferation of the cells at the root of the nail. The thickness of the nails is determined by the proliferation of cells which lie beneath the lunula.

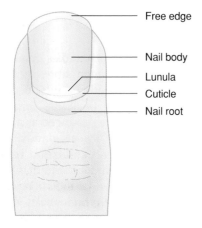

Figure 1.2 The fingernail viewed from above.

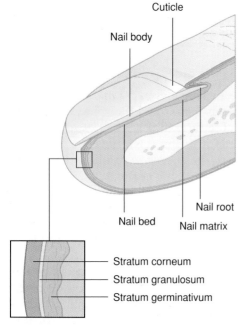

Figure 1.3 Sagittal section of fingernail.

The nail is surrounded by nail folds on three sides. The fold at the nail base, overlapping the lunula, is known as the eponychium or, more commonly, the cuticle.

Sweat glands

There are 2–3 million sweat glands contained within the skin and they can be found over the entire skin surface, excluding the lips and some areas of the genital organs. The sizes of the glands differ; large glands can be found in areas where perspiration is increased, e.g. axillae, palms, soles and forehead.

There are two different kinds of sweat gland: eccrine glands and apocrine glands.

Eccrine glands. These are the most common glands and are found in great numbers on the palms of the hands, soles of the feet and forehead. They are also found in smaller numbers on the back and neck. Each gland consists of a body (the secretory part), which lies within the dermis, and a duct which opens onto the surface of the skin in a funnel-shaped pore.

The glands become active, responding to an increase in body temperature, either through physical exercise or as a direct result of an increase in the temperature of the environment. They are also activated in periods of emotional stress, causing the familiar 'sweaty palms'.

In older people, the activity of the sweat gland is diminished and for this reason the elderly can often have difficulty in controlling body temperature.

The fluid secreted by the eccrine glands is commonly known as sweat. Sweat consists mostly of water although there are minute quantities of salts and metabolic wastes (ammonia, urea and uric acid) present. This demonstrates the excretory function of sweating. Sweat is usually of an acidic nature, with a pH of 4–6.

Apocrine glands. Apocrine glands are larger than eccrine glands and are found mainly in the axillae, the groin and around the nipples. These glands are usually associated with hair follicles, as their ducts empty into them. Inactive during childhood, they begin to function at puberty, under the influence of androgens. When the external temperature is elevated they also produce secretions, although they have a limited role in the process of thermoregulation.

They are activated under the influence of the sympathetic nervous system in times of emotional stress or pain and during sexual arousal. They are known to change in size in accordance with the stages of the menstrual cycle and are often likened to the sexual scent glands which are common in other animals.

The secretion from the glands is similar to the sweat produced by the eccrine glands, with the addition of a few proteins and fatty substances. For this reason it often has a characteristic 'milky' appearance and is odourless. There are, however, large numbers of bacteria located in these gland regions. These bacteria can act on these secretions and the decomposition of this material can cause an unpleasant body odour.

Other structures are modified apocrine glands. These include the mammary glands responsible for the secretion of milk and the ceruminous glands of the external ear canal which secrete cerumen, more commonly called earwax.

Sebaceous glands

Sebaceous glands are common all over the body excluding the palms and soles. They appear as large glands on the upper chest, face and neck but are much smaller on the trunk and limbs. Like the apocrine glands, they usually empty their secretions into the follicles of the hair. The lips, corners of the mouth, the glans penis and the labia majora do not contain hair. The sebaceous glands attached to these structures empty their secretions directly onto the surface of the skin.

Structurally, they are alveolar glands, although functionally they are holocrine glands. The central cells of the alveoli accumulate fatty lipids until they are fully engorged. The cells eventually swell and burst, releasing a secretion known as sebum. The lipid-rich, oily sebum travels along the length of the hair shaft to the skin surface.

Sebum oils the skin and hair, preventing the skin from drying out and the hair from becoming brittle. It also has a bactericidal action, as it contains substances toxic to bacteria. If sebum accumulates and blocks a sebaceous gland, it forms a whitehead. A blackhead is then formed as the blocked sebum oxidizes and dries.

The sebaceous glands are stimulated by the sex hormones, especially androgens. They are relatively inactive before adolescence but they become apparent at puberty, when acne is a troublesome complaint.

Hair

As with the other skin appendages, hair is common on most areas of the body but is absent from the soles of the feet, palms of the hands, nipples, lips and some parts of the external genitalia. Surprisingly, areas of the body that would appear hairless, e.g. the eyelids, do contain hair. These hairs are, however, too short to appear beyond the follicle.

There are millions of hairs over the whole body but in general they can be classified as either vellus or terminal. Vellus hair is pale, fine hair which constitutes the body hair of infants, children and adult females. Terminal hair is much coarser and longer. This type of hair is found on the scalp and eyebrows (and axillae and pubic regions in the adult). It also appears on the legs, arms, chest and face of the adult male under the influence of androgens, particularly testosterone.

Structure. Hairs are strands of hard, keratinized cells. Each hair consists of a shaft and a root. The shaft is the area of the hair which is visible to the eye. It extends beyond the surface of the skin and is usually made up of a medulla, cortex and cuticle. The medulla, which is not present in fine hair, is the innermost layer of large cells. Between the cells, there are pockets of air.

The cortex lies next to the medulla and forms the greatest part of the hair shaft. The cells here are very flat and are arranged in numerous layers.

The outer part of the shaft, the cuticle, comprises a single layer of overlapping cells. This prevents hairs from matting together. The shape of the hair shaft determines whether the hair is curly, wavy or straight. The root of the hair is the part which is found below the surface of the skin. It lies within the hair follicle.

The wall of the hair follicle is made up of two layers: an outer layer of connective tissue and an inner epithelial root sheath. This inner layer is further divided into an internal and external root sheath. The base of the hair follicle is enlarged, forming a hair bulb. A finger-like area of dermis protrudes into the base. This is known as the papilla and contains a network of capillaries that nourish the cells within the follicle and a plexus of sensory nerve endings.

Bundles of smooth muscle cells are associated with each hair follicle. Found below the duct of the sebaceous gland, they are known as the arrector pili and are responsible for raising the hair when the external temperature falls or when the individual experiences fear. This is achieved as a direct result of these muscles contracting, pulling the hair follicle into an upright position. The surrounding skin surface is dimpled in appearance, commonly known as 'goose bumps'. This mechanism is especially effective in some animals as air is trapped under their layer of fur, providing insulation from the cold.

Hair follicles have a cyclical nature, with periods of activity and inactivity. When the hair follicle is active, the group of cells (known as the matrix) covering the papilla divide by mitosis, causing the older cells to be pushed upwards. The hair thus increases in length. The cells furthest from the papillae, receiving no nourishment, die and become keratinized. These cells become united to the hair.

At times of inactivity (i.e. no period of mitosis) the shaft of the hair may break away from the matrix and commence its journey along the follicle. The hair may be pushed out of the follicle by the newly growing hair (when follicle activity commences again). More commonly, it is removed from the follicle by pulling, combing or brushing the hair. Loss of hair, alopecia, results from a number of conditions.

Hair colour is determined by melanin, produced by melanocytes present within the hair

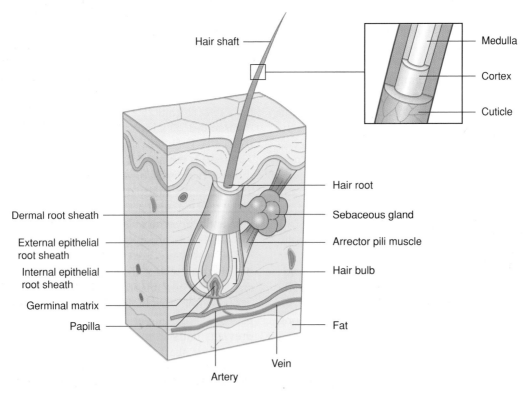

Figure 1.4   How the hair follicle relates to the epidermal and dermal layers.

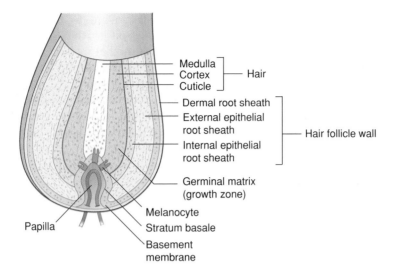

Figure 1.5 The hair follicle wall and hair bulb.

follicle. With ageing, the amount of melanin diminishes and the hair becomes grey or white.

THE FUNCTION OF THE SKIN

The skin has many important functions, which can be broadly classified as follows.

1. Protection
2. Temperature regulation
3. Sensation
4. Endocrine – vitamin D production
5. Psychosocial/sexual

Protection

This again can be divided into three groups.

1. Protection from physical damage, trauma and infection
2. Immune function
3. Inflammation and repair

Protection from physical damage, trauma and infection

The skin provides protection in the following ways.

● Its surface epithelial layer forms a protective barrier against the invasion of chemicals and microorganisms. Infection usually only occurs when this surface layer is broken.

● The subcutaneous fat layer protects the underlying tissues from trauma, providing a deep cushioning effect. It also provides protection from the cold.

● It protects the individual from dehydration; there is the prevention of internal fluids escaping, and also unwanted fluids from the external environment gaining access within the body.

● There is protection from the harmful effects of overexposure to UVB radiation by the action of the pigment, melanin.

● The lipids (fatty acids, triglycerides and waxes) and organic salts which are secreted by the sebaceous and sweat glands have a pH value of 4.5–6. This acts as an acid 'mantle' for the skin, with both antifungal and antibacterial properties.

● Evaporation of sweat, produced by the skin in extreme heat, protects the skin from overheating and regulates skin temperature.

● The normal skin pathogens (surface flora) of the skin help to prevent the overactivity of endogenous pathogens, which are potentially more harmful.

The normal skin flora. The large expanse of the skin as a covering provides great potential for the colonization of bacteria.

Bacteria have a greater chance of survival in a moist, damp environment; consequently, the numbers of bacteria in the skin are dependent on the body site. Areas of dry skin may contain a few hundred bacteria per square centimetre whilst moist folds can be colonized by several million bacteria per square centimetre.

One of the most common groups of bacteria resident on the surface of the skin is the staphylococcal species. This group of bacteria occur in large numbers due to their salt tolerance. They include *Staphylococcus aureus, Staphylococcus epidermis, Staphylococcus haemolyticus* and *Staphylococcus hominis* (arms and legs).

Some other bacteria found on the skin are listed below.

1. Micrococcus groups, e.g. *Micrococcus luteus*
2. *Propionibacterium acnes* (greasy areas)
3. *Propionibacterium avidum* (armpit)
4. *Propionibacterium granulosum* (side of nose)
5. Gram-negative bacilli

Yeasts. Yeasts can be found in the region of the trunk and ear, whilst moulds are common between the toes.

Immune function of the skin

Humans have a well-developed, complex immune system. This system has the potential to recognize harmful substances which may enter the body and then eliminate them. Despite this, our immune system does not only work in a beneficial manner. Damage which results from the immune system acting against the body is known as hypersensitivity. There are four different types of hypersensitivity reaction.

Type I   Anaphylaxis/Immediate hypersensitivity. This is the basis of all atopic allergic reactions. Atopy can be found in 10% of the population and includes eczema, hay fever, asthma and food allergies. Within all, there is an initial exposure to an extrinsic allergen (antigen), e.g. pollen, seafood. This antigen stimulates the production of IgE antibodies which adhere to the surface of mast cells in particular areas (nose, conjunctiva, gut). The individual is now primed for the development of an anaphylactic reaction (Fig. 1.6).

On reexposure to the allergen, the antigen attaches itself to the IgE antibodies. Powerful chemical mediators are released from the cell. These often act locally, causing streaming eyes and a runny nose in hay fever, wheeze (caused by constriction of smooth muscle in the bronchi) in asthma and diarrhoea in food allergies. In extreme cases, the results can be severe and life-threatening.

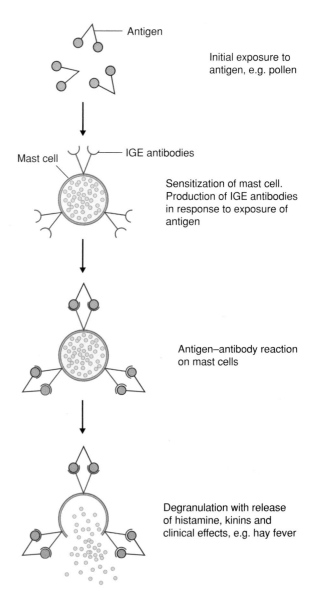

Antigen

Initial exposure to antigen, e.g. pollen

Mast cell

IGE antibodies

Sensitization of mast cell. Production of IGE antibodies in response to exposure of antigen

Antigen–antibody reaction on mast cells

Degranulation with release of histamine, kinins and clinical effects, e.g. hay fever

Figure 1.6   Type I anaphylactic hypersensitivity reaction.

Type II   Cytotoxic hypersensitivity. With this type of reaction, the cells are attacked by antibodies which enter the system and are either damaged or destroyed by phagocytosis. An example of this is Rhesus incompatibility. During pregnancy, trauma involving the placenta may result in Rhesus-negative cells from the fetus crossing the placental barrier to the Rhesus-positive mother. Rhesus-negative antibodies are produced by the mother and maintained within her circulation. In subsequent pregnancies, these antibodies may cross the placental barrier and cause haemolysis of fetal erythrocytes and, in extreme cases, death of the fetus (Fig. 1.7).

Type III   Immune complex-mediated hypersensitivity. This type of reaction occurs when antibodies within the circulation combine with antigens to form immune complexes. This type of hypersensitivity is the major cause of glomerulonephritis. An inflammatory reaction occurs, due to the activation of complement. There is often cellular damage.

These immune complexes can be of two types.

1. *Soluble* – when there is an antigen excess, soluble immune complexes form which can circulate within the blood and lead to serum sickness.
2. *Insoluble* – with an excess of antibody, precipitates can form between antibody and antigen known as the Arthus reaction precipitates. These are normally deposited at specific sites, often in organs, giving rise to vasculitis. Following inhalation of an exogenous antigen, e.g. wood dust, an Arthus reaction can take place in the lung. The damage caused here can produce restrictive airways disease, e.g. woodworker's lung (Fig. 1.8).

Type IV   Delayed-type hypersensitivity. Delayed-type hypersensitivity is distinct from the first three types as T-lymphocytes and no antibodies are involved in the process.

The Mantoux reaction (tuberculin test) is included in this group. Upon initial exposure to the antigen (tubercle bacilli), the T-lymphocytes become specially sensitized to this antigen. These specialized cells can remain dormant within the circulatory system for many years. On reexposure to the antigen (i.e. the injection of tubercle protein onto the skin) these specialized T-cells react with the antigen at the skin surface.

Macrophages and inflammatory exudate accumulate at the site, under the direct influence of agents known as lymphokines. These lymphokines each have unique properties to enhance this process. The degree of tissue damage is directly proportional to the severity of the reaction; in extreme cases there may be necrosis and ulceration of the skin (Fig. 1.9).

Inflammation and repair

Inflammation is the response of living tissue to cellular injury. Repair is the process by which lost or destroyed cells are replaced. We will look briefly at the process of inflammation, before describing the process of repair within the skin.

Inflammation. Inflammation can be produced by:

- physical agents, e.g. extreme heat, radiation
- chemical agents, e.g. acid, poisons
- microbial infections
- tissue necrosis: a loss of blood supply leading to cell death
- hypersensitivity reactions: the body's immune system damaging the body.

Inflammation demonstrates the following signs and symptoms:

- heat – caused by vasodilatation
- redness – caused by vasodilatation
- swelling – result of increased interstitial fluid from exudation
- pain – thought to be due to pressure from exudation on the nerve endings
- loss of function – results from a combination of the above factors.

Inflammation may be either acute or chronic.

Acute inflammation. Lasting from a few minutes to a few weeks, acute inflammation has the following main features.

1. *Vasodilatation* – there is an opening of previously inactive capillary beds and an increase in

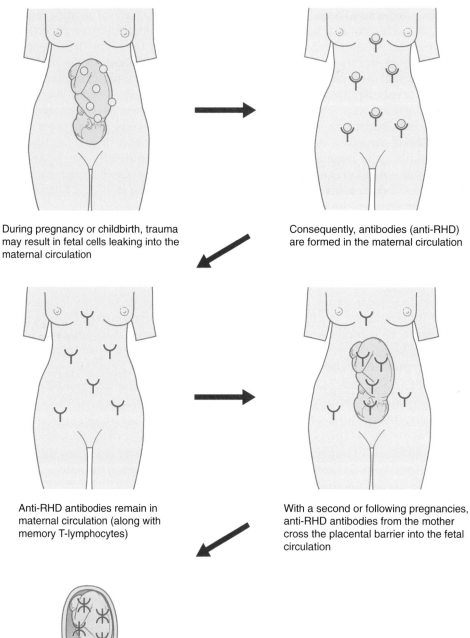

During pregnancy or childbirth, trauma may result in fetal cells leaking into the maternal circulation

Consequently, antibodies (anti-RHD) are formed in the maternal circulation

Anti-RHD antibodies remain in maternal circulation (along with memory T-lymphocytes)

With a second or following pregnancies, anti-RHD antibodies from the mother cross the placental barrier into the fetal circulation

Fetal red blood cells become haemolysed. In severe cases, the fetus dies ('Hydrops fetalis')

Figure 1.7 Cytotoxic hypersensitivity, e.g. Rhesus incompatibility.

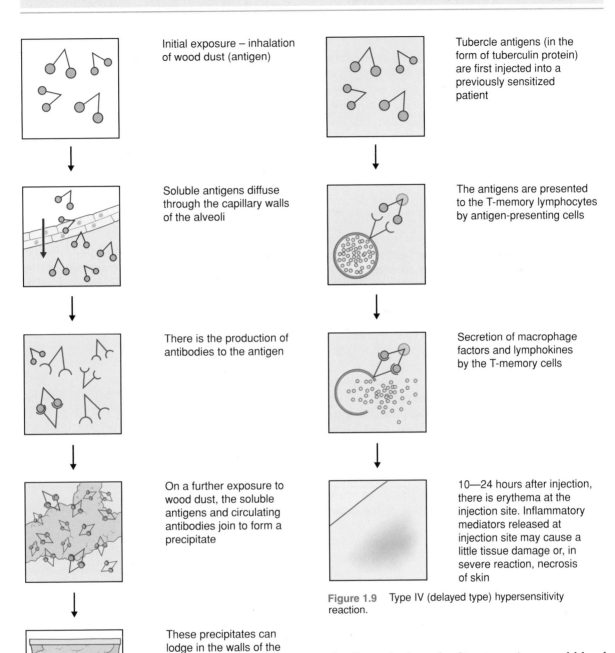

Initial exposure – inhalation of wood dust (antigen)

Soluble antigens diffuse through the capillary walls of the alveoli

There is the production of antibodies to the antigen

On a further exposure to wood dust, the soluble antigens and circulating antibodies join to form a precipitate

These precipitates can lodge in the walls of the alveolar capillaries causing local damage (fibrosis and restrictive airways disease). There is also the release of inflammatory mediators causing tissue damage

Figure 1.8   Type III immune complex-mediated hypersensitivity reaction.

Tubercle antigens (in the form of tuberculin protein) are first injected into a previously sensitized patient

The antigens are presented to the T-memory lymphocytes by antigen-presenting cells

Secretion of macrophage factors and lymphokines by the T-memory cells

10—24 hours after injection, there is erythema at the injection site. Inflammatory mediators released at injection site may cause a little tissue damage or, in severe reaction, necrosis of skin

Figure 1.9   Type IV (delayed type) hypersensitivity reaction.

the flow of others, leading to an increased blood flow to the site.

2. *Increased vascular permeability* – the blood vessels are weaker than normal and thereby allow plasma proteins and leucocytes to escape from the circulatory system.

3. *Emigration of leucocytes and plasma proteins* – on leaving the circulatory system, the plasma

proteins and leucocytes congregate at the site of the injury. This constitutes an inflammatory exudate. This process is effected by the production and release of a number of substances known collectively as chemical mediators. Examples of these include complement and kinin (plasma derived) and histamine, prostaglandins and leukotrienes (cell derived).

Chronic inflammation. Unlike acute inflammation, chronic inflammation is a direct result of prolonged, sustained injury of many weeks' or months' duration.

1. *Involvement of the immune system* – cells within the immune system react to certain antigens, e.g. microorganisms, and become precommitted to produce an immunological reaction to them. In autoimmune disease, the body produces an immunological reaction to its own tissues.

2. *Involvement of mononucleur phagocytes* – commonly known as scavengers because of their role in phagocytosis, macrophages are also vitally important in the process of inflammation. They become activated, increasing in size and allowing the secretion of a number of products involved in the inflammatory process. Examples of these include comprehensive proteins, tissue factor, factors V, VII, IX and X (coagulation), interferon and interleukin-1. Again, these products can cause considerable harm when activated in the autoimmune diseases.

3. *Connective tissue synthesis and parenchymal regeneration (repair)* – this involves the proliferation of fibroblasts, the budding of new capillaries and phagocytosis by macrophages. The repair of the skin is described in detail below.

Repair. As we have already noted, the skin has the ability to repair itself. This can take place by two different methods: primary union (first intention) or secondary union (second intention).

Primary union. This type of healing occurs within cleanly excised wounds, e.g. surgical incisions. The edges must be closely situated together, with minimal trauma or damage to the tissues around the wound.

Within the first 24 hours, the wound line will fill up with blood clots, as there will have been some small blood vessels damaged at the time of the incision. The scab which forms on the surface of the wound is a direct result of the coagulation of blood. It is an important feature as it helps to keep the wound clean.

The fibrin network within the blood clot acts as a frame for building the new epithelial surface. The capillary buds, fibroblasts and epithelial cells migrate to various sites along this framework. Over the next few days, the new epithelial layer grows from one single column of cells to the many layers found within the normal epidermis.

The epidermis should be strong enough to allow the sutures to be removed from 7–10 days after the incision, depending on the site of the incision. Sweat glands, hair follicles and sebaceous glands which may have been destroyed have the ability to regenerate themselves.

Unfortunately, the elastic structure of the dermis cannot reconstruct itself and its tensile strength and elasticity will not be regained, even if the wound heals well.

Secondary union. Secondary intention healing results when dead tissue, necrosis or infection is present within the wound. This must be removed before the wound can heal and therefore healing takes place over a much longer period of time.

The margins of the wound are usually significantly apart and, as a result, a very large amount of granulation tissue is needed to cover the site. The degree of scarring will be determined to some extent by the amount of tissue which has been lost. Debris and exudate are first removed from the wound by phagocytosis. Granulation tissue is then allowed to grow to 'fill in' the lesion. Contraction often takes place within large areas; the fibroblasts within the granulation tissue contract and help to shrink the wound. The epithelium regenerates to cover the surface. There is often a greater loss of function within these larger wounds and an increased likelihood of significant scar tissue.

Complications. If there are excessive amounts of wound granulation tissue (overgranulation) at the base and edges of the wound, the growth of the new epithelium may be hindered. The resulting overgranulation sits 'proud' above the level of the normal skin and hence is often given the term 'proud flesh'.

The excess formation of collagen fibres within the wound can often produce a raised, tumour-like keloid scar. Keloid scars are more common amongst negro populations and their formation still remains misunderstood.

Finally, if the collagen bundles thicken and shorten as they are laid down within the wound, a contracture develops. They often develop when extensive burns heal and the resulting disfigurement can cause great distress. There can often be an associated loss of function, especially if the joints are affected.

Temperature regulation

Body temperature depends on heat lost or heat gained. Heat can be lost or gained by four different mechanisms:

- radiation
- conduction
- convection
- evaporation.

The skin is an important feature within each of these processes.

Radiation

Heat is emitted from the surface of all objects in the form of electromagnetic waves. Usually the skin surface is warmer than the surrounding surfaces and therefore heat is lost from the skin. The converse is true, however, when on a warm day the skin receives heat as a direct result of radiation from the sun.

Conduction

The transfer of thermal energy when objects are in contact with each other is known as conduction. Our skin therefore transfers thermal energy when it comes into contact with another surface, e.g. a chair. As most of the time the skin is in contact with the air, heat is lost to the air, as air temperature is usually lower than the skin temperature.

Convection

Dependent upon the temperature and movement of air (or water) next to the body, heat may be gained or lost by convection. Hot air around the surface of the body rises and is replaced by cooler air, which in turn heats up; this is a constant process. Heat loss is made more difficult because the individual is usually wearing clothes and a layer of air can then become trapped. Heat loss is made easier by the introduction of external agents, e.g. extractor fans or wind.

Evaporation

The skin can lose water by the process of evaporation in two different ways: sweating and insensible loss. Sweating, as we have already noted, occurs when the sweat glands produce a secretion called sweat. This covers the body surface area and evaporates, absorbing heat in the process (the heat of vaporization).

Insensible loss is water loss which occurs daily unnoticed by the individual. It is lost through the slightly permeable barrier of the skin, the lungs and the buccal mucosa.

Thermoregulation is the process whereby the body maintains a homeostatic body temperature. It is controlled by the hypothalamus, which is activated when triggered by a decrease or an increase in body temperature. There are temperature receptors within the skin (peripheral receptors) which aid this process. Receptors within the hypothalamus, spinal cord and abdominal organs (central receptors) help to regulate the core temperature.

The core temperature of the body is kept at a relative constant of 37°C. Skin temperature is largely dependent upon the temperature of the environment. To reduce heat loss, skin temperature must be reduced and conversely, to gain heat, skin temperature must be increased. This is controlled by the dilatation or constriction of blood vessels to the surface of the skin, under the direct influence of the sympathetic nervous system. As the volume of blood flowing to the skin from the core increases, there is a direct rise in the temperature of the skin to approach that of the core.

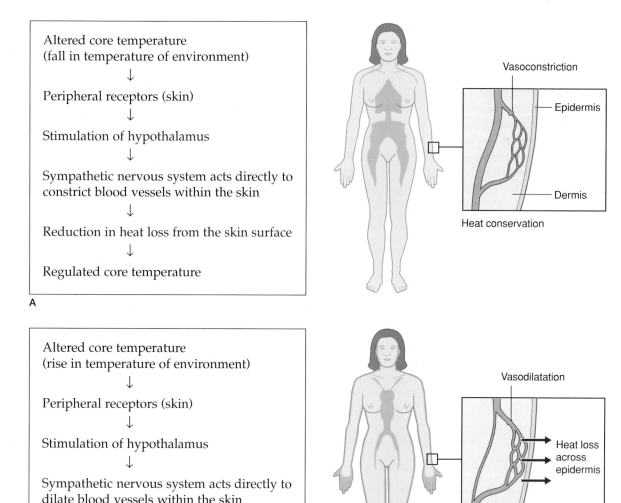

Altered core temperature
(fall in temperature of environment)
↓
Peripheral receptors (skin)
↓
Stimulation of hypothalamus
↓
Sympathetic nervous system acts directly to
constrict blood vessels within the skin
↓
Reduction in heat loss from the skin surface
↓
Regulated core temperature

A

Vasoconstriction
Epidermis
Dermis
Heat conservation

Altered core temperature
(rise in temperature of environment)
↓
Peripheral receptors (skin)
↓
Stimulation of hypothalamus
↓
Sympathetic nervous system acts directly to
dilate blood vessels within the skin
↓
Increase in heat loss to the skin surface
↓
Regulated core temperature

B

C

Vasodilatation
Heat loss
across
epidermis
Increased heat loss

Figure 1.10   A: Mechanism of heat gain. **B:** Mechanism of heat loss. **C:** Heat conservation and heat loss in the skin.

Sensation

The skin is the largest sensory organ within the body, containing a number of receptors (afferent nerve fibres) important in sensation. Some of these fibres have a protective function, as in pain or itch, whilst others are important in touch and pressure.

As we have already seen, there are also receptors important in maintaining body temperature.

Pain

Pain can be classified as either visceral (relating to the organs within the thoracic or abdominal cavity) or somatic (relating to the bodily framework or outer surfaces). It is the latter which is associated with the skin. Somatic pain may be superficial (acute) or deep (chronic). The somatic receptors are free nerve endings, known as Meissner's corpuscles.

Superficial (acute) pain. The pain fibres responsible for this type of pain are known as A-delta fibres. They are relatively finely myelinated fibres, responsible for the transmission of very rapid nerve impulses. Usually restricted to a local area (the epidermis or mucosa), this pain tends to be sharp but usually disappears after the stimulus for the production of pain is removed.

Deep (chronic) pain.   The pain fibres responsible for this type of pain are small, myelinated C fibres. They are thinly myelinated and transmit impulses very slowly. The pain produced is more diffuse and continues for longer periods, even after the stimulus has been removed.

The pain receptors responsible for this type of pain are found within the deep layers of the skin (Fig. 1.11).

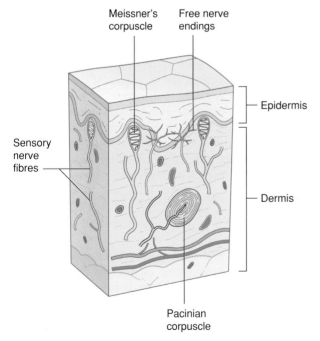

Figure 1.11   Touch and pressure receptors in the skin.

Itch

Itch spots can be found in recognized areas of the body. Within these areas, there are many unmyelinated fibres with naked endings. Mild stimulation of these areas, e.g. movement across the skin, can produce an itch. Itching is not only produced by mechanical stimulation but also by a variety of chemical factors. Injury to the skin can produce large volumes of histamine which can be responsible for a severe itch within the area. The kinins produced in inflammation can be responsible for itching. Elevated levels of bile salts can also produce an itch.

Scratching the area of skin responsible for the itch can give relief. It is thought that scratching activates nerve impulses that block the impulses created by the itch. This mechanism is thought to be similar to that of the inhibition of pain. Scratching the area should, however, be discouraged as there is an increased likelihood of the skin surface being broken and hence the possibility of infection. Rubbing the area can often produce the same result without the complication of the skin surface being broken.

Touch and pressure

Touch and pressure are two closely connected sensations. Both rely on a degree of physical force from the tissues to generate a nerve impulse. Within regions of the body there are specific touch spots; the areas most sensitive to touch contain the greatest number of nerve endings. The density of these structures is high in some areas, e.g. lips, nipples, fingertips, but lower in other areas, e.g. the back. Tactile corpuscles can be found around the base of the hair follicles. In hairless areas, they are known as Meissner's corpuscles.

Within areas of sensitive skin, there are clusters of Meissner's corpuscles making up the aforementioned touch spots. Shaving an area of skin markedly reduces the tactile sensibility of that area; a single hair can contain over a dozen nerve terminal endings.

Where there is firm pressure, the corpuscles activated are known as pacinian corpuscles.

They are found in large amounts in the tissues of the feet and hands and also in the tendons and joints.

Whilst humans' most sensitive touch organs are their fingertips, some animals, e.g. the cat, rely on highly developed tactile hairs (whiskers) to touch objects within the environment. We also have the inherent ability to touch an object without seeing it and identify it correctly. This is known as stereognosis.

Endocrine – vitamin D production

Vitamin D is an essential requirement for the normal development of the skeletal system. The skin plays an important part in the regulation of vitamin D within the body.

On exposure to sunlight, particularly ultra-violet B (UVB) radiation, a substance found within skin cells, 7-dehydrocholesterol, is converted into cholecalciferol. This is the precursor to vitamin D.

Cholecalciferol is then transported to the liver and kidneys via the bloodstream. On reaching these organs it is activated and converted into vitamin D. Vitamin D regulates calcium and phosphorus levels, controlling the absorption of these substances from the small intestine. In this way the amount of minerals needed for the healthy development of bone tissue is maintained.

During the first half of the 20th century, within the inner cities there was a rise in levels of industrial pollution which often led to a blanket of smog covering the city. This dense layer of fumes prevented individuals residing in these areas receiving sufficient sunlight to synthesize vitamin D.

As a direct result, a disease characterized by softening of the bones, called rickets, became prevalent amongst children of the inner-city population. It was easily cured by provision of vitamin D supplements and ensuring an adequate intake of calcium and there was a notable decrease of the disease in the postwar period. It is rarely seen today in Britain, although it may develop in the preterm infant.

Psychosocial/sexual

Psychosocial function

From our earliest moments our skin is important to the way in which we relate to others. As soon as possible after delivery, a mother is encouraged to have intimate contact with her newborn. This skin-to-skin contact is known to help the bonding process; indeed, sometimes when contact is lost, e.g. the baby is nursed within an incubator, the bonding process is thought to be hindered. A small child enjoys the security that touch can bring and feels safe when holding hands with his parents or siblings.

Affection is denoted by touch: the stroking of a child's cheek or the close, intimate cheek-to-cheek contact between adults. The simple act of touch at the bedside of a terminally ill patient can often mean more than any words.

Skin helps us to fairly accurately determine the sex, race and age of our fellow beings and can also denote, to a degree, physical health and well-being. Over the centuries, the skin has displayed the influences fashioned through culture and society. As the skin is important in mating signals amongst animals, so too visual signals between the sexes are displayed on the skin.

Egyptian paintings from many centuries ago have shown that females reddened their lips to enhance their signal. The painters of the 17th century highlighted the sexuality of their female studies by reddening their cheeks.

Hundreds of years later, the upper-class ladies of society spent hours whitening their faces to indicate their aristocracy. It was only the lower-class peasants, who spent hours toiling outdoors, who developed weatherbeaten brown faces. Before social functions, however, these upper-class ladies would pinch their cheeks, encouraging blood flow to the area and so gaining a high-coloured 'flush'.

With the development of cosmetics, enhanced visual signals became easier for women to achieve. Blemishes could easily be covered up, or 'beauty spots' created with the use of the make-up pencil.

Moving into the 20th century, it is interesting to note that the bronzed look, so despised in earlier years, was now seen as an attractive feature. With the increase in foreign travel and the development of the use of sunbeds, a tanned skin is easier to achieve and maintain. Only in more recent years, as the dangers of exposure to the sun became recognized, has there been a tendency amongst some to revert back to a pale skin.

Hair, too, has been important throughout the ages. From earliest times, many would pledge their love by giving their partner a lock of hair.

Baldness amongst the male species meets with different reactions. Some see it as a sign of ageing, with a loss of sex appeal, and will therefore go to great lengths to try to inhibit the process. Others believe that baldness happens to only the most virile of men, as they have a higher level of androgens. This would seem a small price to pay for a partner with increased sex drive!

Society and fashion place great demands upon hair and its style. Current trends will denote colour and length. Some religious groups believe that men should completely shave the head whilst in biblical times, the apostle Paul noted that it was shameful for a man to have long hair; rather this was the glory of the woman.

Sexual function

During puberty, important changes take place between the sexes to further differentiate them and help them achieve their full sexual roles.

The female develops pubic and axillary hair and increased breast tissue. This acts as a visual stimulus to the male but also plays an important part during periods of sexual activity. As the female becomes aroused, her breasts enlarge due to vasocongestion. The nipples, too, become erect and can increase by up to a centimetre in length. This swelling makes their surface more responsive to the skin-to-skin contact between both parties. Additionally, the majority of women show a 'sex flush', a rash similar to measles, due to increased blood flow through the skin. Tactile stimulation of the clitoris and perineal area also serves as a sexual stimulus. This stimulus triggers off parasympathetically controlled reflexes which produce an inflow of blood to the area. This causes the labia to swell and the clitoris to become erect.

In the male counterpart, pubic and axillary hair also develops. Hair often develops to a greater or lesser degree on the arms, legs and chest of the male.

The male penis consists of a glans, shaft and root. In the relaxed state, the glans is covered entirely by a loose sheath of skin known as the prepuce or, more commonly, the foreskin. This maintains the sensitivity of the tip of the penis during sexual activity when, in an erect state, it comes into contact with the female genitals. It also acts as a protective layer at all times. During arousal, there is an increased blood flow to the penis, with a reduced output. This causes the penis to become erect, enabling penetration of the vagina. During pelvic thrusting, the penis causes powerful contact sensations, as it rhythmically massages the highly sensitive folds of skin, the labia, at the female orifice.

Signpost Box

page 3	Ichthyosis	→ Chapter 7
page 3	The skin in pregnancy	→ Chapter 7
page 3	Overuse of topical steroids	→ Chapter 3
page 5	Acne	→ Chapter 11
page 6	Hair growth	→ Chapter 15
page 7	Alopecia	→ Chapter 15
pages 7, 16	Skin cancer	→ Chapter 12
page 8	Atopic eczema	→ Chapter 10
page 13	Keloid scars	→ Chapter 5
page 15	Infection in broken skin	→ Chapter 10

FURTHER READING

Marieb E N 1998 Human anatomy and physiology, 4th edn. Benjamin Cummings, California, pp 142–147

Robbins S L, Kumar V 1987 Basic pathology, 4th edn. W B Saunders, Philadelphia, pp 50–54, 137–144

Shier D, Butler J, Lewis R 1996 Human anatomy and physiology, 7th edn. William C Brown, Dubuque, Iowa, pp 162–176

Tannock G W 1995 Normal microflora. Chapman & Hall, London, pp 4–8

Van de Graaff K, Fox S 1995 Concepts of human anatomy and physiology, 4th edn. William C Brown, Dubuque, Iowa, pp 138–148

Williams P L 1996 Gray's anatomy, 38th edn. Churchill Livingstone, New York

2

Assessment of the dermatology patient

Jill Peters

INTRODUCTION – HOW TO CARRY OUT A CONSULTATION

This chapter will take you through the different stages of carrying out a consultation. This will include the initial opening, through the history taking and then the physical examination with particular consideration given to describing the presenting condition. How to make a diagnosis will also include relevant investigations. The plan of nursing care is also based on the psychological assessment of the impact of the disease on the patient/client (for ease, the term 'patient' will be used) and how much intervention will be required. A glossary of dermatological terminology will assist you in the description of the presenting skin condition or enable you to interpret a dermatological consultation report from a dermatology nurse practitioner/clinical nurse specialist or dermatologist.

The previous chapter will have given you insight into the structure and different functions of the skin, drawing together the physical and psychological aspects.

The ability to carry out a comprehensive examination is essential to all nurses. Early assessment enhances patient care, before the patient seeks help.

Environment

A warm and private room with good natural lighting or artificial lighting that will not change the natural colour of the skin is essential (Lawton

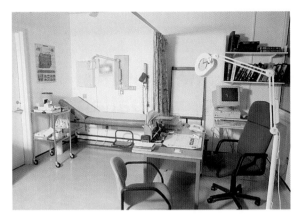

Figure 2.1 Dermatology treatment room.

1998) (Fig. 2.1). A good magnifying lamp is useful when assessing lesions and also allows the use of perpendicular lighting when looking for subtle skin changes. A pump-up couch ensures the patient can lie down so that the skin can be assessed in a relaxed manner. The couch should be sited so that you stand to the patient's right or can walk around it. It is easier to palpate the liver and spleen when examining a patient from the right. The use of a blanket to ensure modesty should be offered. If assessing patients in their own homes try to use natural light; you could always return with a portable lamp.

It is dangerous practice to look at a patient's lesion/rash in isolation without comparing it with the rest of their skin (Epstein 1985, Peters 1998). The chance of detecting a melanoma is 6.4

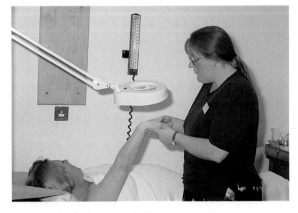

Figure 2.2 Patient examination.

times greater with a complete skin examination than with a partial examination of just exposed skin (Rigel et al 1986).

Make patients feel welcome and reassured by your manner, indicating that you are willing to listen to their story and acknowledge the value of what they have to say. A well and robust patient may feel embarrassed or angry about their skin condition, whilst a systemically ill patient will be relieved to receive nursing care. Some patients perceive the nurse as someone who cares and is interested in them. Patients often think that the doctor is too busy to have time for them and they are often willing and happy to see the nurse instead (Poulton 1995).

The assessment should start at the onset of the meeting between patient and nurse. Consider their physical bearing and posture, which can indicate unhappiness, loss of self-esteem or confidence, anger or embarrassment. The skin is the window into the patient's inner feelings, which are also often reflected through their facial expression (Mairis 1992) before they first speak.

Consultation with a dependant as the patient

If the patient is a child or there is a carer or translator present, note who is giving the history. Give priority to information from the patient but ask for evidence from the carer to consolidate this. Assess whose needs you will have to meet to achieve a successful consultation.

These consultations can take longer but should not be rushed in case anything is missed. Play is often useful to put children at their ease. If children undress in their mother's lap they will probably be safer and happier than if they are forced to lie on the couch. Toys in the consultation room are a must so that the child can play happily, thus giving time for the parent/carer to listen and ask questions about the care required (Campbell & Glasper 1995).

Written information

Written information regarding diagnosis, how to carry out the treatment and practical advice for environment changes can be read by the patient at a later date. A contact number to ring for advice often gives confidence and reassurance. Patients are often interested in the patient support groups for practical and psychological advice.

If the patient is already receiving care from the district nurses or health visitors then ensure that their community care communication book is updated with the necessary information to allow for seamless care and good communication.

HISTORY TAKING

The history taking is an important starting point as its purpose is to elicit information from patients as to why they are there and to evaluate what they say in the context of their general health and their beliefs. Record the patient's own words in the notes whenever possible as this may indicate the patient's level of understanding and ensure the language used by the nurse can be understood. It is usual to ask open questions initially and then more closed, directed questions when seeking specific information, for example about symptoms.

Documentation of information

- Date and time of consultation (UKCC 1998)
- Identification information: *age, date of birth, marital status, occupation and religion*
- Source of referral: *self, accident and emergency, general practitioner, district nurse, health visitor or other*
- Source of history: *patient, carer, relative, friends or letter*
- Reliability: *patient vague on details, gets lost in the story or differs from information in referral letter*
- Chief complaints: *use patient's own or identify their goals, e.g. came for a check-up*
- Presenting illness: *it is helpful to use a structured model to ensure everything is recorded correctly. It is essential that nothing is overlooked. Listening to the patient shows that the therapeutic relationship has begun. Note significant negatives (absence of certain symptoms that will aid in differential diagnosis) (Bates 1995)*

Ask the patient to tell you about their skin complaint and record it in their own words.

- What is their main problem? *Every patient is different so do not assume that what you perceive is right*
- When and where did it first start? *Site and timing are important*
- What did it look like and is it different now? *There will have been a time lapse and you may therefore miss diagnostic signs*
- What time lapse has occurred since the onset of the rash – hours, days or months?
- How long was the lesion present on the skin?
- Site of initial lesion? Has the rash spread over the body and in what kind of distribution? *Pattern of the rash aids diagnosis*
- Has this ever occurred previously and what was the outcome? *Previous diagnosis and treatment*
- Had anything occurred prior to the occurrence? *Any symptoms like tingling, pruritus, tenderness, localized temperature or any systemic symptoms like a fever or joint soreness*
- Does the rash improve at weekends or when on holiday? For instance, *irritant contact dermatitis*
- Travelled abroad recently or in forested areas? For example, *Lyme disease*

Establish the baseline severity of a symptom, which can be reused in subsequent consultations to indicate a remission. For example, using a scoring system of 0–10 where 0 equals the best their skin has been and 10 the worst their skin can be, a patient might give a figure of 7. This can be used on subsequent visits to achieve an understanding of the patient's perception of their skin condition. This also works for intensity of itch, scaling or erythema.

- Any new activity, hobby or job? *DIY, model making, catering*
- Any activities that they can no longer do? *Swimming, socializing*
- Any new medication or anything taken that was purchased over the counter or any recreational drugs? *Ibuprofen*

- Sun exposure. Have they lived abroad, what sun protection factor is used and does it influence the skin condition in any way? *Lived in Australia, SPF 15, hat and clothing, etc.*
- Sexuality may also influence some diseases, causing them to worsen or change their presentation. For example, *psoriasis with HIV infection*
- Any family history of 'atopy', 'psoriasis', 'skin cancer', depending on the presenting condition?
- Have they had to take time off work or could it be work related? *Indication of severity and possible diagnosis*
- What do they think is wrong with them? What are their health beliefs? *Insight into the patient's expectation of the consultation*
- Ask what initiated their enquiry. Any fears or anxieties?
- Past history
- General state of health and their beliefs – 'fit and healthy'
- Adult illness
- Psychiatric illness
- Accidents and injuries
- Operations
- Hospitalizations not already described
- Current medications: what *medication are they taking orally or topically, from the general practitioner or as over-the-counter products? With any topical medication, ask how often they have used it and what effect it had.*
- Allergies: *any – explore their interpretation of these*
- Smoking: *an area to explore is the impact of smoking on the skin. Palmar/plantar pustular psoriasis is strongly linked to smoking (Williams 1994)*
- Alcohol: *an area to explore is the impact of alcohol on the skin (Higgins et al 1992). For patients with chronic psoriasis, alcohol damage to the liver may prevent systemic medication being given in the long term. Patients with eczema often mention their skin is drier the day after alcohol has been drunk*
- Dietary intake: *patients often relate how their skin gets worse after certain foods. Food intolerance is more likely in people who have other hypersensitivities but this is different from allergy*

- Immunizations: *such as tetanus, diphtheria, polio, measles, rubella, mumps, influenza, hepatitis B*
- Sleep patterns: *what are the usual hours of bedtime and awakening? Has this altered? Daytime naps, difficulties in falling asleep or staying asleep? This may indicate that they spend most of the night scratching and are thus tired in the day*
- Exercise and leisure activities: *hobbies or sports? Have they stopped these activities?*
- Home situation and significant others: *who can help you? Anyone at home with you?*
- Daily life: *what is a typical day?*

Psychosocial history

Throughout the history taking, note the posture, tone of voice, eye contact (or lack of it) and the words used. Gauge the psychosocial impact of the condition. Build up a picture of lifestyle and how much intervention the patient is asking for. Anxiety, fear, feelings of loss of control and confusion as to why they are suffering can lead a patient to be angry (Bates 1995). It is important to recognize and acknowledge this and carefully explain every procedure. Allow the patient to respond to reduce their anxiety.

Scores to evaluate the effectiveness of therapy and nursing intervention can be remeasured on subsequent consultation but reliability may depend on the skills of the scorer. It is easier to establish a therapeutic relationship if the same practitioner sees the patient and carries out the scoring at every consultation.

The original evaluation scoring models were developed as measuring tools used in clinical trials in the 1970s and thus were based on physical presentation. The later models developed in the 1990s take psychological, social and economic impact into account.

The psychological impact of skin disease can leave invisible scars and in some cases it may be helpful to use a general questionnaire to measure the impact, e.g. the Dermatology Life Quality Index (Finlay & Khan 1994), or one that is disease specific such as the Assessment of the Psychological and Social Effects of Acne (Fig. 11.11) (Cunliffe 1994).

The Psoriasis Area and Severity Index (PASI)

Four main anatomic sites are assessed.

1. the head (h)
2. the upper extremities (u)
3. the trunk (t)
4. the lower extremities (l)

Roughly corresponding to 10%, 20%, 30% and 40% of the body surface area (BSA) respectively.

Each BSA is then assessed using a four-point scale where:

```
0 = no symptoms
1 = slight
2 = moderate
3 = marked
4 = very marked
```

for the following:

```
E = erythema
I = induration
D = desquamation
A = area.
```

The score varies in steps of units from 0.0 to 72.0. The highest score represents complete erythroderma.

Dermatology life quality index (DLQI)

The aim of creating the DLQI was to meet the need for a short, simple and validated questionnaire to measure the impact of skin disease on patients' quality of life (Finlay & Khan 1994).

Each question was designed to refer to the experience of the previous week. The scoring is based on each question having four alternative responses scored from 0 to 3. The maximum score is 30, representing maximum handicap.

DLQI question topics

1. Symptoms, including itchiness, soreness, pain
2. Feelings of embarrassment or self-consciousness
3. Interference with shopping or looking after home or garden
4. Clothes
5. Social or leisure activities
6. Sport
7. Effect on working or studying
8. Problems with partner or close friends or relatives
9. Sexual difficulties
10. Treatment effects

NB: Finlay & Khan have copyright of the DLQI and it must not be copied without permission from the authors.

For use with children, there is the Children's Dermatology Life Quality Index (CDLQI) (Lewis-Jones & Finlay 1995). The authors of this are now working on a cartoon version. The scoring is the same as for the DLQI.

Holistic review

Although the patient has presented with a skin condition, you may need to consider a complete systems review (see Box 2.1). A skin condition may be the presenting symptom of a systemic disease, e.g. tiredness and dry skin could be due

Box 2.1	Review of systems
General	Usual weight, any loss or gains noticed by clothing tightening or loosening. Weakness, fatigue or fever
Head	Headaches, head injury
Eyes	Vision and recent changes, glasses, contact lens, blurred vision, pain, specks, flashing lights, glaucoma, cataracts, crusting or dryness
Ears	Hearing, tinnitus, vertigo, earaches, scaling, infection, discharges, itching or lumps
Nose and sinuses	Frequent colds, nasal stuffiness, discharge, itching, hay fever, nosebleeds, sinus trouble
Mouth and throat	Condition of teeth and gums, ulcers, blisters, discharge, tongue sore or changed appearance, sore throats, hoarseness
Neck	Lumps, swollen glands, goitre, pain or stiffness
Breasts	Lumps, increase in size, pain or discomfort, nipple discharge, self-examination

Box 2.1	Review of systems *(continued)*
Respiration	Cough, sputum (colour and quantity), shortness of breath, date of last chest X-ray
Cardiac	Discomfort or palpitations, swelling of extremities, date of last ECG or echo
Gastrointestinal	Trouble swallowing, heartburn, appetite, nausea, vomiting, regurgitation, vomiting of blood, indigestion. Bowel habits: frequency, colour, texture, size, haemorrhoids, constipation, diarrhoea, bleeding. Abdominal pain, excessive belching or passing wind
Urinary	Frequency of micturition, burning or pain on micturition, urgency, hesitancy, dribbling, incontinence, blood seen or loss of pressure
Genital	Discharge from or sores on penis, loss of tissue structures, testicular pain, swelling of glans, loss of hair. History of sexually transmitted diseases and treatment. Sign of circumcision, sexual preference, interest, activity and satisfaction. Any problems
Female	Age at menarche, regularity, amount, frequency and duration of periods, breakthrough bleeding or after intercourse, last menstrual period, dysmenorrhoea, premenstrual tension. Age at menopause, symptoms or postmenopausal bleeding. Discharge, itching, loss of tissue structure, pain on intercourse, lumps or sores. History of sexually transmitted diseases and treatment. Number of pregnancies, delivery or spontaneous and induced abortions. Sexual preference, interest, activity and satisfaction. Any problems

Box 2.1	Review of systems *(continued)*
Peripheral vascular	Leg cramps, local heat, varicose veins, past clots in veins, pigmentation changes, loss of sensation, skin dryness or irritation
Musculoskeletal	Muscle or joint pain or swelling, stiffness, backache. If present, describe location, frequency and intensity, swelling, redness or limitation of movement
Neurological	Fainting, blackouts, seizures, weakness, paralysis, numbness or loss of sensation, tingling or 'pins and needles', tremors or other involuntary movements
Haematological	Tiredness, easily bruises or bleeds, past transfusions and any reactions to them
Endocrine	Heat or cold intolerance, excessive sweating, tiredness or hyperactivity, excessive thirst or hunger
Psychiatric	Nervousness, tension, mood swings.

to hypothyroidism. The patient may be too embarrassed to mention certain symptoms unless specific questions are asked, e.g. vulval itching in lichen sclerosus.

Specific considerations when taking a history of a child

Taking a history for a child is very different, as you have to rely on the observations of the parent/carer. Also, if there is a language deficit, you may not be talking to the child's main carer. Relationships within the family may be complex, with different agendas being followed which have nothing to do with the presenting condition.

Bates (1995) suggests that the following points could be included in the general history taking. As you become more experienced, you will learn to follow your intuition and focus on certain areas.

- Identifying data: *nickname, identification of parents or carer, contact numbers, their occupation and work hours*
- Chief complaint: *have the concerns been raised by the patient, a parent(s) or someone else, e.g. school-teacher?*
- Present illness: *include how all members of the family respond to the patient's symptoms. What do they think? Is there any secondary gain for the patient?*
- Birth history: *first 2 years of life, important for identifying lack of bonding and reaching of milestones*
- Prenatal history: *maternal illness before and during pregnancy, exacerbation or remission of skin condition. Parental attitude concerning pregnancy, parenthood or this particular child. Any difficulties in bonding due to guilt feelings (the parent feels they have given the child the condition, affecting their ability to cope) (Peters 1997)*
- Feeding history: *breast feeding frequency and duration of feeds, use of complementary or supplementary artificial feeds. Any difficulties encountered (regurgitation, colic, diarrhoea). Timing and method of weaning*
- Artificial formula feeds: *type, concentration, amount and frequency. Timing and method of weaning. Any problems encountered. Did the child's skin become red and the child irritated following each feed?*
- Vitamin or iron supplements given: *type, amount, frequency and duration*
- Solid foods: *types and amounts of baby food given, when introduced, infant response, introduction to table foods, self-feeding. Parent and infant response*
- Childhood eating habits: *likes and dislikes, specific types and amounts of food eaten. Parental attitude to eating in general and towards the child*
- Parental response to eating problems: *use of a diary over a 7–14-day period for accurate assessment of food intake or to record how the child or its skin reacts to certain foods. What have they removed from the diet and is there any supervision from a dietician? Exclusion diets must be supervised because nutritional deficiencies can cause long-term problems in growth (Atherton 1994)*
- Growth and developmental history: *particularly important during infancy and childhood.*
Dealing with problems of delayed physical growth, psychomotor and intellectual retardation and behaviour disturbances.
- Physical growth: *actual weight and height at birth, at regular intervals and 10 years. History of any rapid gains or losses, tooth eruption and loss pattern*
- Developmental milestones: *record of milestones and when they were achieved*
- Social development
- Sleep: *amount and pattern during the day and night, any alterations. Do they sleep with their parents?*
- Schooling: *experience with socialization by teachers and peers, any bullying, name calling*
- Personality: *loss of confidence, isolation or frustration. No special friends*
- Allergies: *medication, asthma, hay fever and urticaria, allergic rhinitis, food intolerance and insect hypersensitivity*
- Immunizations: *specific dates of administration of each vaccination so a record can be maintained for ongoing boosters. Some parents worry if the skin is bad and may avoid the immunizations. Explore their fears*

CLINICAL EXAMINATION

It is important to explain to the patient why you require them to undress down to the underwear for a full examination of their skin. A gown or blanket should be available to ensure modesty and warmth. Be aware of cultural and religious differences, as well as embarrassment, especially if the patient perceives their problem to be localized, e.g. a wart on the finger (Epstein 1985). An information leaflet explaining the importance of a full skin examination, sent with the appointment letter, may help to pave the way. A female chaperone may be reassuring for the female patient, enabling her to relax, particularly if the practitioner is male and especially if the genital area needs to be examined.

Try to put the patient at ease. They might make embarrassed comments about their hygiene, e.g. 'my feet smell', indicating nervousness. Remember, the skin can be painful so be gentle but sure in your movements.

Anything seen should be recorded on a body map, including length and diameter.

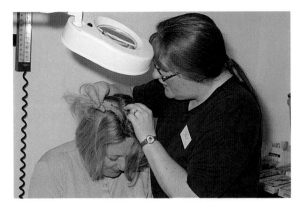

Figure 2.3 Examination of the hair and scalp.

Closer examination of the lesions takes place after the general survey (see Box 2.2). This gives a picture of the patient's skin, extent of the condition and any particular landmarks, scars, tattoos and any sign of Köebnerization or atrophy. Questions can be asked during this time and patients often volunteer information that they had not thought essential.

Remember that the skin does not lie but it can mimic different rashes. The patient often denies scratching but excoriations are evidence that cannot be dismissed. Do they scratch more at night? Is anyone around them also scratching (scabies)? Making a diagnosis is a process of elimination through history taking and clinical presentation.

The glossary on page 37 contains words commonly used when describing the skin and lesions found on its surface and Fig. 2.6 shows common presentation of skin lesions. Otherwise, write what you see literally and what you feel on palpation.

Focus on the presenting condition and identify the primary lesion and its anatomical position. Is it a generalized or localized rash (see Box 2.3). Endogenous rashes are usually symmetrical, e.g. psoriasis. Exogenous rashes may affect only one side, e.g. tinea. Herpes zoster is restricted to a dermatome (Ashton 1998). Does it affect the skin and the mucosa in the mouth? Remember to check for pemphigoid, pemphigus and lichen planus.

Distribution

What is the distribution of the presenting condition? Does this give a clue to the diagnosis, e.g.

Box 2.2 Clinical examination

Examination procedure	Action
Carry out the examination from the right side of the couch, using the skill of touch.	This light surface palpation allows you to assess the texture and extent of the lesions.
Start from the nails. Move from the fingertips to the finger webs, then palms and dorsum, moving up both arms.	Are the cuticles intact? Any pitting, onycholysis, extra lines? Check for signs of lesions or damage on both flexural and extensor sides, into the axilla.
Check the scalp.	Parting the hair to examine the hair shaft, feel the texture of the hair. Note the pattern of thinning around the hairline and behind the ears. Any bald patches?
Examine the face.	Note not only any obvious lesions but also pay attention to the eyes, including lash and eyebrow. Check around the nasolabial folds and also the oral mucosa and tongue. It is important not to miss the primary lesion or an initial symptom.
Work your way down the trunk.	Start from under the chin, into both axillae, down the chest wall, across the abdomen to the pelvic area. This ensures no area is missed.
Start again at the nails on the feet and work your way up the front of the legs.	Check in between the toes and on the soles of the feet for moles. Raise the patient's awareness for monitoring.
Ask the patient to turn over or stand so you can examine from the nape of the neck to the feet.	Be methodological, ensuring that no skin is left unexamined.
When examining the genital area, be respectful and gentle.	Ask the patient to point to the areas of concern. For close examination, gloves should be worn if the skin is ulcerated or broken (universal precautions).

Box 2.3 Labelling of lesions by configuration and distribution (adapted from Hill 1998)

Configuration	The arrangement or pattern of lesions in relation to other lesions
Distribution	The arrangement of lesions over an area of skin
Annular	Ring-shaped
Gyrate	Ring spiral shape
Linear	In a line
Nummular, discoid	Coin-like
Polymorphous	Occurring in several forms
Punctate	Marked by points or dots
Serpiginous	Snake-like
Solitary	Single lesion
Satellite	A single lesion in close proximity to a larger group
Grouped	Cluster of lesions
Confluent	Joined up
Diffuse	Widely distributed, spreading
Discrete	Separate from other lesions
Generalized	Total body area
Localized	Limited areas of involvement which are clearly defined
Symmetrical or asymmetrical	Distributed bilaterally or unilaterally
Zosteriform	Band-like distribution along a dermatome

---

sun-exposed areas such as face, nape of neck, dorsum of the hands and V of the neck with sparing under the chin and other shaded areas. Is there a marked line perhaps indicating contact allergy, e.g. just above the wrists from the wearing of rubber gloves.

Making a contact dermatitis diagnosis is like good detective work. The history and initial presentation are essential and affect the decision to order patch testing. The interpretation depends on the relevance to that patient. Someone with atopic eczema is not exempt from developing contact dermatitis.

Arrangement

How are the lesions then arranged? As an individual discrete lesion, e.g. psoriasis or lichen planus, or in a coalescent form with small papules, e.g. eczema?

Shape

Is the lesion annular or linear (Köebnerized psoriasis) or grouped (herpes virus simplex)? Is Köebner's phenomenon present (lesions on sites of previous trauma such as surgical scars or tattoos, i.e. psoriasis or viral warts)? Are there signs of burrows in the skin webs or along the side of a finger or in a linear pattern under the axilla (scabies)?

What does the skin look and feel like?

What is age related, and thus normal, and what is abnormal? Learn to recognize what is normal across the spectrum of pigmented skin and then what is abnormal will stand out. Sun-damaged skin shows earlier signs of ageing.

Box 2.4 Skin phototypes based on a person's own estimate of sunburning and tanning

Skin type I	Always burns
Skin type II	Sometimes burns, sometimes tans
Skin type III	Always tans, never burns
Skin type IV	Never burns, always tans
Skin type V	Moderately and heavily pigmented
Skin type VI	Black African skin

Pigmentation

It is important to be aware of the range of skin colour (differences in pigmentation) in the human race. Depigmentation may follow inflammatory changes and is often seen after herpes zoster and eczema in people with darker pigments. An understanding of the normal pigmentation allows detection of change; palpation is often useful in darker pigmented skins (Baxter 1993) (Box 2.5).

The skin tells its own story but often takes its time to reveal itself; patients may make several visits before a diagnosis is made. The skin has the ability to mimic different skin diseases. If misdiagnosed and treated, it can then change clinical

Box 2.5   Changes in pigmented skin

Condition	Colouration
Pallor	Ashen grey in black skin, yellow-brown in brown skin. They are both dull looking.
Inflammation	Hyperpigmentation in black or brown skin but lighter on tips of nose, in front of and behind ears. Use of palpation to detect increased warmth.
Erythema	Purplish tinge, difficult to see dark area, macular, local or generalized. Palpate for increased warmth with inflammation, for taut skin and hardening of deep tissue.
Purpura	Jet-black in lighter negroid skin
Oedema	Lightens the skin, weals appear pale. Slick tight skin. Palpate for warmth of oedema.
Jaundice	Yellowing of the sclera of the eyes, junction of hard and soft palate and also in palms.

presentation. The presenting skin disorder can be a symptom of systemic disease and thus the assessment process should be more than skin deep, e.g. acquired ichthyosis = lymphoma.

Describing the lesion/rash

- Is the skin smooth, uneven or rough to the touch?
- Has the skin lost turgor or elasticity? Lift a fold of skin, release it and note its reaction.
- Are the skin lines accentuated? Has the skin become lichenified (check the nails – are they shiny or dirty, often the signs of a scratcher?) or is it very dry and looks like crazy paving (eczema craquele)?
- What colour pigmentation is seen? Assess what is normal for that patient and what is abnormal – erythema, jaundice, blanching, pallor. If the skin is hyperpigmented you need to identify the normal skin colour of the patient, e.g. pityriasis versicolor.
- Any sensitivity to touch, tingling or pain?
- Is the skin moist or dry, sweaty or oily?

- Is the skin hot or cold to the touch (touch the lesions and compare with other areas of the skin not involved and note the difference)?
- Is there excessive scaling in between the skin creases – possible fungal infection?
- Have the lesions been changed through trauma from scratching or previous topical therapy?
- Inspect one that has not been altered – what does it look like, feel like?
- What is the surrounding skin like? Is the margin of the lesion smudged or excoriated?
- Are there signs of picking or rubbing?
- Is there anything on the surface of the lesion or contained within it and could it be swabbed for further investigation?
- Is there any scale, crusting or weeping?
- Colour of the lesion, e.g. yellow = xanthomas (lipid deposits) or sebaceous gland. Pigmented lesions, e.g. blue-black for cellular blue naevus or red in strawberry naevus (see Chapter 12 for suspicious symptoms or signs in a naevus).
- Is the edge pearly, i.e. basal cell carcinoma (see Chapter 12)?
- Does the skin smell? Is it distinguishable from the smell of old skin or is it indicative of infection?

Excoriations/lichenified skin

Pruritus or itch is a very common complaint and it is important to differentiate between generalized or localized itch. Identify excoriations on the skin to ascertain if there is any local inflammation surrounding the excoriated skin. The history should enable you to establish the differential diagnosis: physiological change due to ageing; scabies; eczema; lichen simplex; lichen sclerosus; urticaria or scratching from habit which changes acute disease to chronic; pruritus due to metabolic disorders (blood tests would support this finding).

It is important to explore the itch cycle and identify with the patient a pattern of behaviour. Insight gained by the patient into the problem itself will lead to change. A combined approach including education about the disease, the role and application of topical emollients (to prevent rubbing in) and topical steroids with behaviour modification

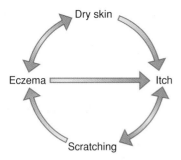

Figure 2.4   The itch–scratch cycle in eczema.

(habit reversal) will help to change damaging behaviour caused by scratching to healing through non-damaging behaviour (Bridgett et al 1996).

If the patient can identify with the itch–scratch cycle (Fig. 2.4) and understand the damage done to the skin by scratching or rubbing, they will understand that to allow the skin to heal they have to change their behaviour. Any patient with an acute inflammatory disease should be taught about the itch–scratch cycle as part of their therapy programme. A better understanding will reduce the occurrence of lichenification and allow them to deal with acute flares of their symptoms rather than a chronic condition.

Feel the lesion

- Use deep palpation by compressing the lesion between finger and thumb. How thick is it and how deep?
- A soft lesion can be compressed easily and feels like your lips. A normal lesion is just like squeezing your own cheek.
- A firm lesion can only just be compressed and it has a certain degree of infiltrate, like urticaria weals.
- A hard lesion cannot be compressed as it contains fibrous tissue like a histocytoma.
- Induration of the lesion is a palpable thickening in the lesion itself, like squamous cell carcinoma.

Infection

The role of infection as a cause of inflammation needs careful consideration. First, the patient has to understand how infection acts as a trigger for their inflammatory disease; for example, *Staphylococcus aureus* has been identified as a super-antigen for patients with atopic eczema, and pharyngitis group A beta-haemolytic streptococcus can trigger guttate psoriasis. Secondary infection introduced by scratching allows the skin to be infected by *Staphylococcus aureus*. The use of antimicrobial emollients can reduce colonization and the role of staphylococcus as a super-antigen (Whitefield 1998) but sensitization can occur more easily in an atopic person.

Secondary crossinfection can occur in people with an acute flare of eczema. The dryness and breaks in the skin from scratching allow bacteria colonization. Herpes is a viral infection triggered by contact with others with the active virus (cold sores), giving rise to eczema herpeticum.

Some infections can interfere with the healing process and thus do require antibiotic therapy, based on sensitivities and swabs to check if the course needs to be lengthened. Avoid using shorter, more frequent courses as this could lead to resistance.

Patients who have frequent admissions to hospital or who have broken skin and increased exfoliation are at risk of developing methicillin-resistant *Staphylococcus aureus* (MRSA). This is a human pathogen resistant to a number of antibiotics, including methicillin. It can either cause a serious infection or can be carried by a patient who remains asymptomatic. The use of an antimicrobial emollient can decrease the episodes of antibiotic therapy and decrease the probability of MRSA within dermatological patients.

Characteristics affecting the nails

Observation of the nails starts with the colour and shape. To check the capillary return, apply pressure to the nail, blanching the nail bed underneath.

Look for pigment changes such as a longitudinal band of pigmentation. This is normal in people with skin types III–V (brown nails). For abnormal lesions of pigmentation in the nail bed where the pigment extends into the surrounding tissue, the differential diagnosis could be acral lentiginous melanoma. HIV-positive patients who develop skin lesions could have Kaposi's sarcoma.

Smaller streaks of brown or red could be splinter haemorrhages, which result from trauma or are a sign of infection, e.g. bacterial endocarditis.

Any changes to the surface of the nail (Fig. 2.5) can give clues about skin diseases. Psoriasis causes pitting of the nails and onycholysis. Tinea can also cause hyperkeratosis of the nail plate and onycholysis (Table 2.1). Onycholysis can also be caused by repeated pressure trauma, e.g. jogging.

White spots within the nails usually follow trauma to the nail and grow out slowly with the nail. They also can be caused by overvigorous repeated manicuring.

Paronychia is inflammation of the proximal and lateral nail folds. The cuticles may have disappeared and the folds are swollen and sore. People who regularly immerse their hands in hot water are susceptible to developing this, particularly diabetics. Candida infections can cause painful paronychia; it is also associated with HIV disease and mucosal candidiasis.

In Terry's nails, otherwise known as 'half-and-half' nails, the proximal two-thirds of the nail plate is white, whereas the distal third shows the red colour of the nail bed. This is fairly rare but may be a manifestation of congestive heart disease. In the classic half-and-half presentation the distal half is pink or brown and is sharply demarcated from the proximal half, which is dull and white and obliterates the lanula. Ten percent of patients found with this have uraemia of chronic renal failure. The differences between the two condition presentations are not clear and are still debated (Fitzpatrick et al 1997).

Beau's lines are transverse depressions in the nails associated with acute severe illness. The lines emerge from the proximal nail folds weeks later and grow out with the nail.

Mees' lines are transverse white lines associated with acute or severe illness, also seen in arsenic poisoning. The lines emerge from the proximal nail folds and grow out with the nails.

Periungual telangiectasia occurs when the capillary loops of the proximal nail folds become tortuous and dilated. There are degrees of severity and it can be caused by repeated injury from infection but also is a characteristic of dermatomyositis/lupus erythematosus.

Characteristics affecting hair

Androgenic alopecia is the normal progressive balding that occurs through the combined effect of a genetic predisposition and the action of androgen on the hair follicles in the scalp. Observe for normal presentation of hair and then look for any abnormalities.

The increase of hair in abnormal places, e.g. on a woman across both breasts and down the umbilicus to the groin, could indicate hirsutism. Loss of hair from normal areas may occur either in the form of bald patches in alopecia or a general thinning across the scalp. The progressive balding in males has been classified into grades I–VII (Staughton 1988). Women who present with androgenic alopecia accompanied by acne, hirsuties and menstrual irregularity would need to be investigated for a hormonal disorder, e.g. ovarian tumour (Staughton 1988).

When examining the scalp and other body hair, you need to consider its pattern. Is the texture

Table 2.1 Classifications of onychomycosis (adapted from Baran et al 1998)

Classification	Major clinical features
Distal and lateral subungual onychomycosis (DLSO)	1. Subungual hyperkeratosis 2. Onycholysis 3. Paronychia
Superficial white onychomycosis (SWO)	May differ in colour depending on the dermatophyte
Proximal subungual onychomycosis (PSO)	Subclassified as: 1. without paronychia 2. with candida paronychia 3. with non-dermatophyte mould paronychia
Endonyx onychomycosis (EO)	Lamellar splitting of the plate
Total dystrophic onychomycosis (TDO)	1. Secondary total dystrophic onychomycosis 2. Primary total dystrophic onychomycosis

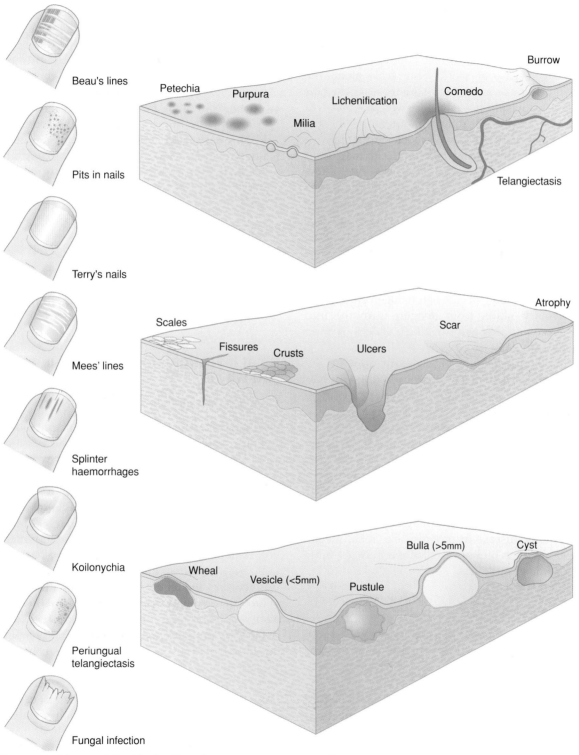

Figure 2.5 Characteristics affecting the nails.

Figure 2.6 Common presentations of skin lesions.

correct for the position of hair on the body? Does the hair shaft break easily? Has the colour greyed prematurely? Are there signs of scarring from hair loss or erythema, which could mean inflammatory disease at work? Skin scale along the shaft (pityriasis amiantacea) often breaks the hair due to its weight but once removed, the hair will regrow and underlying inflammatory disease may be identified, e.g. seborrhoeic dermatitis.

Patients often bring hair that has been shed prior to their visit to support their story. If infection were present, then the debris would need to be sent to the laboratories. Changes might be linked to other ongoing medical conditions or medication so the history should always be thorough. Hair shaft deficits can be psychological, as in trichotillomania.

Stress or an acute illness or pregnancy can cause an acute shedding of club hair (telogen effluvium). Secondary shifts from anagen (growth) into catagen and telogen (resting) phases see an increase in daily loss of hair and, if severe, generalized thinning. Following chemotherapy, anagen effluvium can occur with generalized loss of hair involving the whole scalp. There are many drugs that can induce an alopecia of this type, e.g. ACE inhibitors, heavy metal poisoning.

The scalp and hairline should always be examined as many skin disorders affect either the scalp or the hair, e.g. lichen planus or discoid lupus erythematosus. Lesions may be hidden by the hair, so part the hair and move around the scalp. Lesions of the scalp may be a symptom of a systemic disease in progress, e.g. renal metastases are often highly vascular and may resemble pyogenic granulomas.

Examination tips

- The blanching test is a test for erythema. Apply firm pressure and then release; if redness turns white (blanches), it indicates erythema, especially in those with skin types IV–V.
- If a lesion is covered by a crust then it should be removed to examine what is underneath.
- If the skin does not look scaly initially, stretch the skin between thumb and index finger and release 2–3 times and then observe closely. If

scaling occurs, then consider pityriasis versicolor.
- When trying to make a differential diagnosis on a scaly rash, pick the scale off. If profuse scale detaches or bleeding occurs, then it is likely to be psoriasis.
- When examining bullae, try dislodging the epidermis by finger pressure in the area of a lesion, leading to erosion of the bulla. This is known as the Nikolsky sign which is positive for pemphigus and erythema multiforme but negative for pemphigoid.

INVESTIGATIONS

Investigations can assist with the process of elimination or act as supporting evidence for a working diagnosis. Interpreting the results is important, identifying the relevance to the current clinical picture and the patient.

What investigations should you order and why?

Bacterial investigation

Primary bacterial infection such as staphylococcus may be the trigger factor in atopic eczema or scalded skin infection. Streptococcus may be the trigger factor in guttate psoriasis.

Think carefully in secondary infection such as staphylococcus imposed on eczema as in some conditions the pus is sterile, i.e. pustular psoriasis.

Distinguishing between colonization and infection is important. Wounds colonized by bacteria will heal without antibiotics (Collier 1994). Infected skin will require antibiotics. Identification of growth sensitivity is just as important as known allergies when making the treatment choice. Although remember that natural skin flora contains bacteria.

When taking a bacterial swab from skin, ensure that the swab tip is moist, either with normal saline (Rudensky et al 1992) or transport medium. To collect the bacteria, roll the swab in a zig-zag motion across the skin, rotating it between the fingers (Cooper & Lawrence 1996), covering all the skin.

Viral investigation

Primary viral infection includes herpes zoster (shingles). Secondary infection is exemplified by herpes simplex on top of eczema, which results in eczema herpeticum. Look for the characteristic disseminated punched-out vesicles. Pierce a vesicle and swab the fluid inside.

Mycology investigation for fungus or yeast

Mycology investigation supports clinical findings in some cases. In others, it ensures the correct systemic or topical therapy. The most common reason for treatment failure is misdiagnosis (Goodfield 1998) so skin scrapings, nail clippings or hair debris should be sent.

- Skin scrapings – use a blunt blade at a 45° angle to remove skin cells without cutting. Place onto black filter paper.
- Nail clippings – use nail clippers. Place specimen of nail on black filter paper.
- Hair debris – use a stiff toothbrush to collect skin, exudate and hair.

Mycology culture takes 4–5 weeks; dermatophytes grow more slowly than bacteria. However, microscopic investigation takes 2 weeks and can identify yeast infections and indicate a possible positive culture.

Woods light examination

This is often carried out to identify bacterial, fungal or yeast infections (Table 2.2). In order to

Table 2.2 Woods light examination

Disease	Flourescent colour	Aetiology
Erythrasma	Coral red	Bacterial infection *Corynebacterium minutissimum*
Pityriasis versicolor	Scales are blue-green	*Pityrosporum ovale* yeast
Tinea capitis	Greenish	Microsporum
Porphyria	Orange-red in urine	Elevated porphyrins

carry out the test, you need a Woods light (UVL handset) and a darkened room. Ensure the patient is lying comfortably whilst you fluoresce the skin with the UVL light.

The Woods light can also be used to measure the depth of melanin in the skin, since variations in the epidermal pigmentation are more apparent under Woods light than under visible light (as in vitiligo) (Rook et al 1992).

Common blood tests performed in dermatology

The list shown in Table 2.3 is not exhaustive but indicates the most relevant tests to be carried out when considering a dermatological diagnosis or related systemic disease.

Diagnostic biopsy

The decision to carry out a biopsy is dependent on the differential diagnosis. A biopsy may allow you to confirm your diagnosis so that you can make an informed decision on treatment required.

Table 2.3 Common diseases and blood tests

Test	Pruritus	Atopic eczema	Alopecia	Urticaria	Erythroderma
FBC	*	*	*	*	*
Albumin					*
U & E	*			*	*
ESR	*			*	*
IgE		*			
LFT	*			*	*
Thyroxine TSH	*		*	*	
Ferritin	*		*		*
Antinuclear factor			*	*	

Lawrence (1996) states that the correct interpretation of histological changes in the skin is dependent on the operator choosing the right biopsy site and obtaining an adequate specimen (see Chapter 5).

Skin samples can sent for:

- histological interpretation
- culture for bacterial infections
- immunofluorescence (detecting the presence and positioning of substances, e.g. antigens, antibodies, cell components for diagnosis of blistering conditions).

Porphyrin studies

Patients who present with fragile skin on sun-exposed sites (vesicles and bullae with pain) require diagnostic investigations to check for the levels of excreted porphyrins in the faeces and urine (Table 2.4). The results should indicate what type of porphyria the patient has.

It is important to ensure that the samples are protected from the light as ultraviolet light can destroy the porphyrin in the specimens. Cover the specimen pot completely with tin foil. The same applies to blood samples.

Dermographism

Although only 4.2% of the general population have positive dermographism (Fitzpatrick et al 1997), symptomatic dermographism is a nuisance. Stroke the skin firmly with a wooden stick; after 5 minutes linear urticaria signs will appear. The weal should be pink and raised, lasting about 30 minutes. This is a positive diagnostic test, helpful in urticaria.

Table 2.4 Diagnosis based on elevated levels of porphyrins

Type of porphyria	Sample	Levels
Congenital erythropoietic or cutanea tarda	Urine and plasma	Increase of uroporphyrin
Variegate or erythropoietic protoporphyria	Faeces	Moderate increase of protoporphyrin
Variegate or intermittent acute	Urine	Increase in porphobilinogen

Diascopy

Using a glass microscopic slide, press firmly over a skin lesion. This will enable you to determine whether the redness in a macule or papule is due to erythema (capillary dilatation) or to purpura (extravasation of blood). It is also helpful for detection of the glassy yellow-brown appearance of papules in sarcoidosis, tuberculosis of the skin, lymphoma and granuloma annulare.

Acarus hunt

Patients with persistent itch should be closely examined for burrows. The search for mites in burrows is difficult because they live in the stratum corneum. Once you have found a likely burrow, add a few drops of 5% potassium hydroxide which will dissolve the keratin. Then scrape the cells onto a microscopic slide and examine under a microscope for positive identification. You can clearly see the mite or its larvae on the slide.

Köebner or isomorphic phenomenon

This is the occurrence of an inflammatory skin condition at the site of previous trauma, i.e. a surgical scar. This is particularly characteristic in psoriasis, lichen planus and sarcoid.

Patch testing

Allergy patch testing is one of the investigations carried out to detect contact allergy of the delayed sensitivity type. This is a type IV delayed type of hypersensitivity. The investigation is quite time consuming for the patient as it takes several appointments. Patch tests are usually read at 48 and 72 hours and up to a week later. Contact urticarial reactions can be read at 30 minutes. Patients are often convinced that they have an allergy as they want to blame 'something' for the condition of their skin.

The procedure of patch testing is explained in greater detail in Chapter 10.

IgE antibodies

IgE is the classic anaphylactic antibody of humans and mediates most anaphylactic (immediate) actions. IgE is present in normal serum in very small quantities (10–70 μg/100 ml). IgE is the antibody formed by atopic persons to a wide number of common allergens. Non-atopic persons also form IgE antibody as a result of vaccinations, e.g. tetanus.

Radioallergosorbent test (RAST)

Some amounts of IgE are too small to be detected by conventional techniques but by using antibody reagents with radioisotopes, amounts of IgE proportional to the amount of radioactivity of the total IgE can be measured. This gives a definite confirmation for those allergic to cat and dog dander, house dust mite, peanuts, milk, egg white, etc. A positive result can mean that changes to lifestyle may be required to avoid these allergens. A negative result should reassure the patient that they need not restrict their life.

Prick testing

This procedure is used to detect immediate hypersensitivity type I reactions. The substitute antigens used in this procedure can cause a potentially fatal anaphylactic reaction. The relevance of a positive result to the cause of the condition under investigation is debatable (atopic eczema or urticaria).

Erythrocyte sedimentation rate (ESR)

The mechanism of this blood test is not fully understood but it is useful as a non-specific indicator of systemic disease. In dermatology, it is helpful when considering whether more extensive investigation is required in a patient with pruritus of unknown cause. An ESR above 50 mm/h is nearly always associated with some significant illness, i.e. vasculitis, systemic lupus erythematosus or malignant neoplasm.

Ovacysts and parasites Sellotape test

This is a simple but sometimes awkward investigation. The aim is to try to capture the worm on a piece of Sellotape for identification in the laboratories. A piece of Sellotape is stuck across the anal orifice overnight in the hope that the worm will poke its head out and stick to the Sellotape.

CONCLUSION

At the end of the consultation, you will have taken a complete and detailed history, carried out an examination and filled in a body diagram or free drawing to illustrate location, size, severity and clinical signs (e.g. Fig. 2.7). As you go through this process, you are categorizing the clinical signs and symptoms in a process of elimination to create a list of possible differential diagnoses.

You may need to carry out investigations to support the differential diagnosis list and make a final decision based on the findings. You may have to review the patient at a later date as some investigations take time.

Treatment of the final condition may start immediately, before all the evidence is collated, because of the clinical picture and your intuition.

Decisions about the intervention required should be discussed with the patient. Some insight will have been gained as to the patient's wishes from their description of the disease, its symptoms and how it affects their daily life. The personal distress that a condition causes may be more important in some cases than the clinical severity. People have different coping mechanisms and thus all react differently to their condition. Discuss the different treatment options (Box 2.6) with the patient. Explain about the disease process, how the treatment will work, its application and expected duration. This approach will enable the patient to make an informed choice and participate in their own care. If the patient understands not only how a medication will work but also how to apply it, they are likely to carry out the treatment in a more effective way.

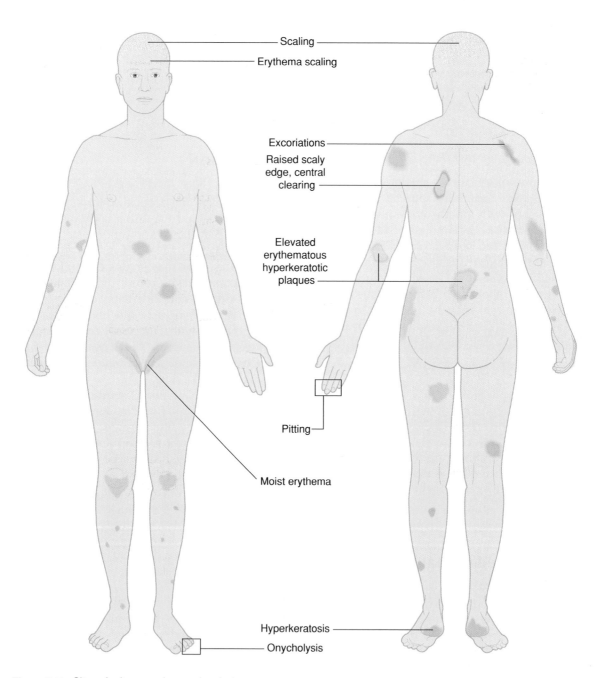

Scaling

Erythema scaling

Excoriations

Raised scaly
edge, central
clearing

Elevated
erythematous
hyperkeratotic
plaques

Pitting

Moist erythema

Hyperkeratosis

Onycholysis

Figure 2.7   Sites of primary and secondary lesions.

Box 2.6   Dermatology treatment options

- Topical therapies
- Local dermatological surgery
- Phototherapy
- Systemic therapies
- Teaching and demonstration sessions
- Dermatological day care
- Inpatient care
- Community liaison supervision
- Shared care with community nurses
- Referral to plastic surgeons
- Referral to other medical teams

Building a good therapeutic relationship between the patient and practitioner will enhance the advice and treatment the patient is given. Follow-up visits help to reinforce the treatment programme chosen and enable the patient to seek alterations to the programme if their expectations are not met.

Signpost Box

page 23	Psoriasis	→ Chapter 9
page 24	Lichen sclerosus	→ Chapter 15
pages 27, 34	Contact dermatitis and patch testing	→ Chapter 10
page 27	Skin types and sunburn	→ Chapter 12
page 28	Strawberry naevus	→ Chapter 7
page 28	Basal cell carcinoma	→ Chapter 12
page 28	Ageing skin	→ Chapter 7
pages 29, 32	Infection	→ Chapter 13
page 29	Squamous cell carcinoma	→ Chapter 12
page 29	Guttate psoriasis	→ Chapter 9
page 29	Eczema Herpeticum	→ Chapter 10
page 30	Hair	→ Chapter 15
page 34	Type IV hypersensitivity	→ Chapter 1
page 32	Pemphigoid, Pemphigus	→ Chapter 14

Written information about diagnosis or the different elements which make up a treatment programme will support the information given in the consultation and act as a reminder for the patient at home.

Lifestyle is important to everyone and health education about how diseases are caused enables the patient to make an informed decision about the value of their health.

GLOSSARY

Primary lesions		Examples
Abscess (>1 cm)	Pus-filled lesion (pseudocyst)	
Blister (>1 cm)	Fluid-filled lesion	Pompholyx
Bulla (<1 cm)	Fluid-filled lesion, circumscribed elevation, over 0.5 cm in diameter containing a liquid	Herpes zoster Pemphigoid Pemphigus Bullous impetigo
Macule	Stain (<1 cm), change in colour only, surface is flat and does not blanch	Brown lentigo *Cafe-au-lait* Drug rash Secondary syphilis Hypopigmented (vitiligo) Purpura
Nodule (>1 cm)	Rounded elevated solid lesion, thickness = diameter	Erythema nodosum Rheumatoid nodules Kaposi's Lipoma Cancer
Papule (<1 cm)	Any raised lesion or scaly, crusted, keratinized or macerated surface.	Skin colour white, pink, yellow Skin tags or warts Brown colour – melanoma, naevus, seborrhoea
Patch (>1 cm)	A large macule, change in colour only, surface is always normal	Mycosis fungoides (stage 1)
Plaque (>1 cm)	Raised, flat-topped lesion, diameter = thickness	
Pustule (<1 cm)	Pus-filled lesion	
Vesicle (<1 cm)	Contains clear fluid	

Secondary lesions

Atrophy   A diminution of tissue

Erosion   Superficial or total loss of epidermis or mucous membrane; heals without scarring

Fissuring   Slits through the whole thickness of skin due to excessive dryness or inflammation

Ulcer   Full-thickness loss of epidermis and upper dermis; heals with scarring

General

Acantholysis   The separation of keratinocytes in the epidermis by loss of intercellular connections, permitting the cells to become round and hyaline

Allergen   An external substance which stimulates an immunological response

Alopecia   'Fox mange' – a fall of hair

Annular   Round or ring shaped

Asymmetrical   One side more involved than the other

Atopy   'No (without) place'. An inheritable clinical state associated with eczema, asthma and hay fever

Burrow   Linear lesion caused by parasites 3–5 mm long

Callus   Hyperplasia of the stratum corneum due to physical pressure (keratoderma)

Carbuncle   A necrotizing infection of the skin and subcutaneous tissue composed of a group of furuncles (boils)

Cellulitis An inflammation of cellular tissue

Coalescing   Lesions merging into one another

Comedone   Papule plugging sebaceous follicle, containing sebum and cellular debris. Closed comedone = whitehead. Open comedone = blackhead

Crust   Outer layer consisting of dead cells and serum

Cutaneous   Appertaining to the skin

Cyst   A closed cavity or sac lined with epithelium containing fluid, pus or keratin

Dermatome   Cutaneous nerve distribution on one side of the body

Discoid   Disc shaped

Discrete   Separate lesions

Disseminated   Discrete lesions scattered over a wide area

Emollient   Moisturizer which stays on the skin, reducing scaling and water loss

Erosion   Loss of epidermis, which heals without scarring

Erythema   Redness of the skin caused by vascular congestion or perfusion

Erythroderma   A generalized redness of the skin, associated with desquamation

Excoriation   Any loss of skin substance produced by scratching

Exfoliation   The splitting off or separation of keratin and epidermal skin surface in scales or sheets

Fibrosis   The formation of excessive fibrous collagen

Fissure   Any linear gap or slit in the skin surface

Fistula   An abnormal passage from a deep structure to the skin surface

Flexure   Area of skin against skin, e.g. axilla, groin

Furuncle   A localized pyogenic infection originating in a hair follicle

Gangrene   Death of tissue, associated with the loss of blood

Gel   Semi-solid colloidal solution

Generalized   Widespread eruption covering at least 50% of body surface

Granuloma   Chronic inflammatory tissue composed of macrophages, fibroblasts and granulation tissue

Guttate   Drop-like

Haematoma   Localized tumour-like collection of blood

Horn   A keratosis which is taller than it is broad

Infarct   An area of coagulation necrosis due to localized ischaemia

Keloid   Elevated progressive scar formation without regression

Keratoderma   Hyperplasia of the stratum corneum

Kerion   A nodular inflammatory, pustular lesion due to a fungal infection

Lesion   Any area of skin with changed colour, elevation or texture that is surrounded by normal skin

Lichenification   A chronic thickening of the epidermis with exaggeration of its normal markings, often as a result of rubbing or scratching

Milium   A tiny white cyst containing lamellated keratin

Necrobiosis   Partial degeneration of tissue, such as swelling and degeneration of collagen

Necrosis   Death of tissue or cells

Ointment   Oil-based preparation – emollient

Onycholysis   Nail separation from nail bed

Papilloma   Nipple-like projection from the surface of the skin

Petechia   A punctate haemorrhagic spot 1–2 mm in diameter

Poikiloderma   Dermatosis characterized by variegated cutaneous pigmentation, atrophy and telangiectasia

Pruritus   An irritating skin sensation which elicits the scratch response

Purpura   Discolouration of the skin or mucosa due to extravasation

Pus   Yellowish viscid fluid formed by the liquefaction of dead tissue

Pyoderma   Any purulent skin disease, either bacterial or non-bacterial in origin

Rash   A collection of many lesions, some of which are coalescing

Regionalized   Local to any one area of the body, e.g. face

Scale   A flat plate or flake of stratum corneum

Scar   Fibrous tissue replacing normal tissue destroyed by injury or disease

Sclerosis   Induration or hardening of the skin

Sinus   A cavity or channel that permits the escape of fluid

Stria   A linear, atrophic, pink, purple or white streak or band on the skin due to changes in the connective tissue

Symmetrical   Both sides involved to a similar extent

Telangiectasia   A visible vascular lesion formed by dilatation of small cutaneous blood vessels

Tumour   An enlargement of the tissues by normal or pathogenic material or cells that form a mass

Turgor   Rigidity due to the uptake of water into living cells or tissues

Ulcer   A defect or loss of dermis and epidermis producing sloughing of necrotic tissue

Vegetation   A growth of pathological tissue consisting of multiple, closely set papillary masses

Verruca   An epidermal tumour caused by a papilloma virus

Vibex   A narrow linear mark, usually haemorrhage from scratching

Weal   An elevated, white, compressible, evanescent area produced by dermal oedema

---

REFERENCES

Ashton R 1998 The art of describing skin lesions. Dermatology in Practice 6(2): 11–14

Atherton D 1994 Eczema in childhood: the facts. Oxford University Press, Oxford

Baran R, Hay R J, Tosti A, Haneke E 1998 A new classification of onychomycosis. British Journal of Dermatology 139(4): 567–571

Bates B 1995 A guide to physical examination and history taking, 6th edn. Lippincott, Philadelphia

Baxter C 1993 Observing the skin. Community Outlook 3(1): 19–20

Bridgett C, Noren P, Staughton R 1996 Atopic skin disease: a manual for practitioners. Wrightson Biomedical, Petersfield, Hampshire

Campbell S, Glasper E A 1995 Nursing assessment and communication. In: Campbell C S, Glasper E A (eds) Whaley and Wong's children's nursing. Mosby, St Louis

Collier M 1994 Assessing a wound. Nursing Standard 8(49): 3–8

Cooper R, Lawrence J 1996 The isolation of bacteria from wounds. Journal of Wound Care 5(7): 335–340

Cunliffe W J 1994 New approaches to acne treatment. Martin Dunitz, London

Epstein E 1985 Crucial importance of the complete skin examination. Journal of the American Academy of Dermatology 13(1): 150–153

Finlay A Y, Khan G K 1994 Dermatology quality of life index (DLQI) – a simple practical measure for routine clinical use. Clinical and Experimental Dermatology, 19: 210–216

Fitzpatrick T B, Johnson R A, Wolff K, Polano M K, Suurmond D 1997 Colour atlas and synopsis of clinical dermatology, 3rd edn. McGraw-Hill, New York

Goodfield M 1998 Superficial infections. Prescriber Journal 38: 183–189

Higgins E M, Du Vivier A W P, Peters T J 1992 Skin disease and alcohol abuse. Alcohol and Alcoholism 27 (suppl): 95

Hill M J (ed) 1998 Dermatology nursing essentials: a core curriculum. Jannetti, New Jersey

Lawrence C M 1996 An introduction to dermatology surgery. Blackwell Science, Oxford

Lawton S 1998 Assessing the skin. Professional Nurse 13(4) (suppl): S5–S7

Lewis-Jones M S, Finlay A Y 1995 The children's dermatological life quality index (CDLQI): initial validation and practical use. British Journal of Dermatology 123: 942–949

Mairis E 1992 Four senses for a full skin assessment: observation and assessment of the skin. Professional Nurse 7(6): 376–380

Peters J 1997 Treatment strategies. Community Nurse 3(8): 38–40

Peters J 1998 Assessment of patients with a skin condition. Practice Nurse 15(9): 525–530

Poulton B 1995 Keeping the customer satisfied. Primary Health Care 4(5): 16–19

Rigel D S, Freidman R J, Kopf A W et al 1986 Importance of complete cutaneous examination for the detection of malignant melanoma. Journal of the American Academy of Dermatology 144(5): 857–860

Rook A, Wilkinson D S, Ebling F J G 1992 Diagnosis of skin disease. In: Champion R H, Burton J L, Ebling F J G (eds) Textbook of dermatology, 5th edn. Blackwell Science, Oxford

Rudensky B, Lipschitts M, Isaacsohn M, Sonnenblick M 1992 Infected pressure sores: comparison of methods for bacterial identification. Southern Medical Journal 85(9): 901–903

Staughton R C D 1988 The colour atlas of hair and scalp disorders. Wolfe, London

UKCC 1998 Guidelines for records and record keeping. United Kingdom Central Council, London

Whitefield M 1998 Effectiveness of a new antimicrobial emollient in the management of eczema/dermatitis. Journal of Dermatological Treatment 9: 103–109

Williams H C 1994 Smoking and psoriasis. British Medical Journal 308: 428–429

3.1

Treatment issues relating to dermatology

Rebecca Davis

INTRODUCTION

The nursing role in educating patients in the management of skin disorders is of immense importance. 'In dermatology, nurses are possibly the most important persons in the medical team' (Seville & Martin 1981).

It is essential to ensure that the social, economic and psychological needs of patients are balanced with the medical management. Patients must feel that they are able to influence the treatment plans, not least taking account of their lifestyle. The majority of topical medications have to be used in a specific manner, often at regulated times and usually in conjunction with other preparations. Without sufficient information the patient can be left feeling isolated and unable to cope, at which point many people stop their treatment. Likewise, the patient may use the treatment but if they do not see immediate results they may become unmotivated and stop medication.

The nurse who is well informed will be able to provide the patient with advice, written and verbal, and ensure that the patient has contact with the clinic/surgery if they are unable to manage both physically and emotionally. Prescribed systemic medication especially must be complemented with time spent explaining the medication to the patient, including for example what side effects the patient may expect to experience and stressing the importance of attending for regular monitoring if necessary.

Compliance is a term used to describe whether a patient uses their medication as prescribed.

Many factors that affect the likelihood of compliance are outside the control of the patient or the dermatology team: social and marital status, language difficulties, previous experiences of medicine. Patients with chronic conditions in particular are less likely to comply with their treatment, perhaps due to disillusionment after years of therapy or the complicated regimens that are required. In addition, dermatology patients often have numerous treatments to use which lead to confusion and poor compliance. The clinic nurse is well placed to assess patients who are less likely to comply and provide them with better support and information, ensuring that they are able to contact the clinic/surgery should they have difficulty with their treatment. Written information for all patients who attend is an extremely important reinforcement for the information given in clinic.

BASES FOR TOPICAL TREATMENTS

The vehicle used to deliver the topical treatment to the skin will affect the efficacy of the treatment, drug stability and the patient compliance. Topical medications are available in a variety of vehicles (bases) (Box 3.1). Griffith & Wilkinson (1998) stated that an ideal vehicle should be:

- easy to apply and remove
- non-toxic
- non-irritant
- non-allergenic
- chemically stable
- homogeneous
- bacteriostatic
- cosmetically acceptable
- pharmacologically inert.

EMOLLIENT THERAPY

Emollients are one of the most important tools in controlling and managing dry skin conditions as they are effective rehydrating agents. There are three main emollient types:

1. soap substitutes (Box 3.2)
2. bath additives (Box 3.3)
3. skin moisturizers (Boxes 3.4, 3.5).

Box 3.1 Bases for topical treatments (adapted from Stone et al 1989, Pariser 1991)

- OINTMENTS – greasy base ideal for dry skin. Occlusive properties increase hydration of the skin. Unsuitable for infected, intertriginous and hairy areas.
- CREAMS – contain oil, water, emulsifier (prevents the oil and water separating) and preservative (prevents bacterial growth). Ideal for wet or infected skin.
- LOTIONS – an oil and water preparation with more water than oil. The liquid consistency means that application with cotton wool is often necessary. Suitable for hairy areas.
- SOLUTIONS – alcohol or water. For hairy areas. The alcohol content can cause stinging to cracked or raw skin.
- GELS – liquify when applied to the skin. Often used on hairy areas and the face.
- PASTES – mix of powder in a greasy base.
- Also mousses, tape, bandages.

Box 3.2 The use of soap substitutes

- Washing and bathing are opportunities for moisturizing.
- Soap is alkaline which has a drying effect on the skin. A soap substitute should be used instead.
- Covering the affected areas with the soap substitute prior to contact with water can help to prevent stinging.
- Moisturizing bars will cleanse like soap but have a neutral pH and contain a moisturizer so can be used once the condition is controlled.

Box 3.3 Bath oils

- Bath oil should be used each time the patient bathes.
- The patient should soak in the warm water for 10 minutes.
- Bath oils can make the bath slippery so patients should be warned.
- Some bath oils contain additives: antipruritic and antistaphylococcal. They should be used for the limited prescribed time only.
- Many bath oils contain fragrance which is a known sensitizer.
- Once the skin condition is controlled the bath oil should be continued.

Box 3.4   Moisturizing ointments

- Greasy, insoluble in water.
- Do not contain preservatives.
- Provide a barrier over the skin so rehydrating the skin by reducing evaporation.
- Not easily washed off.

Box 3.5   Moisturizing creams

- Oil in water or water in oil preparations.
- Contain preservatives to maintain their stability.
- Easily washed off once applied and so require reapplying after handwashing.
- Feel cool and soothing when applied.

Box 3.6   Application of emollients

- Applied direct to the skin.
- Apply 'Thinly, quickly and frequently' (Bridgett et al 1996).
- Always apply in a downward motion in the direction of the hair growth.
- Avoid vigorous rubbing which may cause plugging of the hair follicles and then infection (folliculitis).
- Always apply after a bath.
- Do not stop once the condition is controlled. Emollients will help to prevent future exacerbations.

Patients require frequent education and reminders of the importance and effectiveness of these products (Box 3.6). If used in combination (the bath oil, soap substitute and moisturizer), they will aid the rehydration of the skin and have a beneficial antiinflammatory effect which can also help to reduce the need for topical steroids.

The skin acts as a barrier between the internal milieu and the outside world, preventing the invasion of foreign particles and loss of body fluids. A dry skin (asteatosis) has a damaged barrier function, allowing water loss, cracking and reduction in elasticity. As water is lost through the skin surface, the corneocytes (keratinocytes that are in the upper layer of the epidermis and no longer have their nuclei) shrink, causing cracks to appear on the skin surface (Cork 1997). The cracking of the stratum corneum allows a greater surface area for microbial organisms and infection becomes more likely (Figs 3.1, 3.2, 3.3). A layer of emollient over the skin surface will trap water, preventing evaporation, and so restore the skin's natural barrier surface.

Dry skin is often itchy. The response to this is to scratch, sometimes until pain is felt. Scratching may cause injury to the skin surface which in turn can allow the development of skin infection

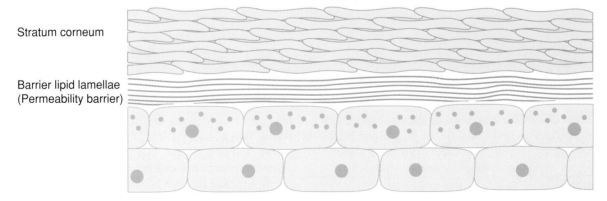

Stratum corneum

Barrier lipid lamellae (Permeability barrier)

Figure 3.1   The stratum corneum provides the barrier to water loss and is composed of extracellular lipids and corneocytes. It can therefore be visualized rather like a brick wall with corneocytes forming the bricks and the lipids forming the mortar. The lipid is extruded from the lamellar bodies into the intercorneocyte space to form highly organized multilamellar bilayer structures. These lipids layers are the most important component of the epidermal barrier (reproduced with permission from Cork 1997).

Loss of water from corneocytes

Changes in epidermal lipids

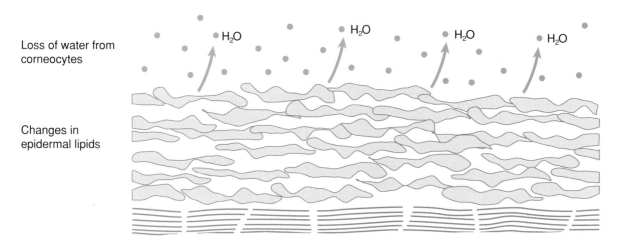

Figure 3.2 There are changes in the epidermal lipids in atopic eczema which result in a defective epidermal barrier and an increase in loss of water from the stratum corneum. As a result the corneocytes shrink and cracks open in between them which permit the penetration of irritants or allergens. These substances then gain access to antigen-presenting cells and trigger the development of eczematous lesions (reproduced with permission from Cork 1997).

Occlusive emollient

Water trapped under emollient passes into corneocytes

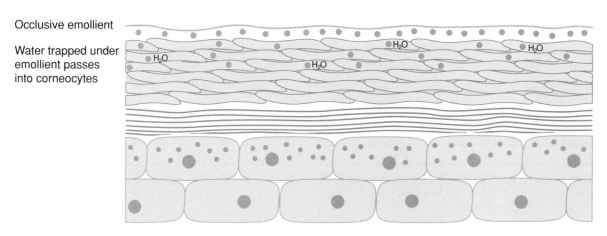

Figure 3.3 Emollients provide an oily layer over the surface of the stratum corneum which traps water underneath it. The water passes back into corneocytes and as a result they swell up, closing the cracks in between them. This results in restoration of the epidermal barrier and therefore prevents penetration of irritants and allergens which would have triggered the development of eczematous lesions (reproduced with permission from Cork 1997).

which also in turn may make the skin more irritated. Patients may be said to be caught in the 'itch–scratch' cycle. Emollients can have a soothing, cooling and occlusive effect that helps to reduce the irritation of dry skin and restore the barrier function.

With the vast array of emollients on the market (Box 3.7), it can be difficult to choose the one which would be most appropriate. Ointments are most effective for very dry, flaky skin; creams are useful when the patient finds ointments too greasy. Patient choice is extremely important. Creams contain preservatives to maintain their stability; patients may become sensitized to the preservatives, causing a contact eczema.

Emollients must be acceptable to the patient cosmetically and be effective. Often patients are offered a sample selection of emollients to try

Box 3.7 Emollients commonly used in dermatology for dry skin conditions

Bath additives	Oil	Add oil to bath water	Used in bath water	Alpha Keri Bath Aveeno Balneum Diprobath E45 bath Emulsiderm Emulsifying ointment Hydromol emollient Oilatum
Soap substitutes	Usually oil and water preparations but may be grease based	Moisturize skin when washing rather than experiencing the drying effect of soap	Used whenever washing hands or body	Aqueous cream Dermol Shower E45 wash Emulsifying ointment Epaderm Oilatum shower gel
Moisturizing creams	Oil and water preparations	Cool and soothing on application Contain preservatives Cosmetically acceptable	Use whenever skin feels dry particularly when the condition is 'weeping'	Aveeno Cetomacrogol cream Dermatological cream Dermol 500 Diprobase cream E45 cream Hydromol cream Neutrogena Unguentum Merck
Moisturizing ointments	Grease based	Hydrate the skin effectively Cannot be washed off easily	Used on very dry and/or inflamed skin	50:50 White soft paraffin: liquid paraffin Dermamist (spray) spray Diprobase ointment Epaderm

prior to being issued with a prescription. This allows them to decide which moisturizer is the most acceptable and provides them with some control over the management of their condition. Many patients find that whilst a greasy ointment is the most effective, it may not be cosmetically acceptable to use at school or work. These patients could be advised to use the ointment at night and a lighter cream during the day. It is important to stress to patients that the use of moisturizers should never be a once-a-day treatment; every time their skin feels dry they should reapply the moisturizer. This necessitates carrying around a supply of emollient, small tubes or pots that fit into a pocket or bag.

Emollients within a container can become a source of infection if the patient dips their hand repeatedly into the container. Skin scales and bacteria, in a moist environment, provide an arena for further bacterial growth. The patient is thus using a contaminated emollient which could lead to the skin becoming infected. Some manufacturers have addressed this problem by providing the emollient in a pump dispenser or aerosol. However, for those in a conventional container, the patient must be educated about decanting the emollient into a smaller pot, using a clean utensil which can be cleansed.

The use of emollients is best discussed early on in the treatment. Patients who improve rapidly may not attend further clinics and the patient should be advised to continue with their emollients even when their condition is controlled (Box 3.8).

TOPICAL STEROIDS

Topical steroids are glucocorticoids which have been used for over 40 years. They can be fluorinated or non-fluorinated. Generally, the fluorinated steroids may have an increased probability of side effects in comparison to the non-fluorinated

---

Box 3.8 Emollient routine

- Bathe in warm water with an added emollient (oil).
- Use a soap substitute for washing.
- Pat dry with a soft towel.
- Apply the emollient liberally to the skin.
- Wait for at least 20 minutes before applying other treatments. Using them together will dilute their effect.
- Reapply emollients at regular intervals throughout the day to protect the skin from irritants and to rehydrate the skin.

---

steroid of the same potency though fluorinated steroids may be more effective as glucosteroids. Half of all prescriptions written by dermatologists are for topical steroids (Pariser 1991).

Topical steroids are important for their anti-inflammatory, immunosuppressive, vasoconstrictive and antimitotic effects and are useful in the treatment of eczema and some inflammatory dermatoses (Box 3.9). However, there is widespread concern about their use due to their perceived potential side effects (Box 3.10). Many people are aware that 'steroids will thin the skin' and as a result are often reluctant to use the treatment. In reality, this should only be a problem if a potent topical steroid is used in the same area for an extended period of time. Patients should have the opportunity to discuss the use of topical steroids and their side effects. In that way any fears the patient may have can be addressed and the treatment used appropriately.

Once applied to the skin, the steroid is partially absorbed through the epidermis by percutaneous absorption, which has many stages. The penetration may be through the follicles or the epidermis or by passive diffusion (Morris 1998). Areas with increased numbers of hair follicles and a thin epidermis, e.g. the scalp and axillae, have a more rapid absorption. Palms and soles with a thick epidermis and no hair follicles are unable to absorb topical steroids. Hydration of the skin also affects the speed of percutaneous absorption. Plastic occlusion may occasionally be used as a therapeutic service to increase absorption.

The process of steroid action is not completely understood but the three stages currently

---

Box 3.9 Considerations when prescribing/using topical corticosteroids

Age	• Stronger preparations should not be prescribed for infants in primary care • Children not responding to mild/moderate steroids should be referred to a specialist • Mild/moderate steroids should be adequate for adults • Potent/very potent steroids should be used with caution and for limited periods only
Site	• Absorption is increased in certain sites such as the face and flexures • On the face 1% hydrocortisone should be used in all age groups (specialists only should use stronger preparations) • Care should be taken when using potent preparations in adolescents who are at risk of developing striae atrophicae • Long-term use around the eyes should be avoided due to the risk of glaucoma • Palms/soles – potent preparations may be used for a longer period
Extent	• The potential for systemic absorption increases with extent and severity • Monitor the number, strength and size of tubes used (excessive/ underuse of treatment)
Type	• Ointments are preferable to creams (better penetration and fewer problems with sensitization)
Method of application	• Treatment should be no more than twice daily. Some preparations are once daily • Using the fingertip method regulates the amount used (Fig. 3.4) • Used with wet wrap bandaging (see p. 159) • Under film occlusion in certain areas, e.g. palms/soles (widespread occlusion is not recommended)

Box 3.10 Potential side effects from using topical steroids

Spreading and worsening of untreated infection
Thinning of the skin
Irreversible striae atrophicae and telangiectasia
Contact dermatitis
Perioral dermatitis
Acne at the site of application
Mild depigmentation

accepted are explained by Griffith & Wilkinson (1998) as follows: receptor binding, synthesis of specific mRNA and synthesis of protein. Whilst there are antiinflammatory properties of steroids that have a beneficial therapeutic effect, the process is still being studied.

Patients require to know how much topical steroid to use, to which areas and how frequently. When dispensed, the preparation may have instructions stating 'apply sparingly'; whilst this is helpful in preventing the patient from using it as liberally as a moisturizer, it does not provide the information required. Many manufacturers now include diagrams of the 'finger tip unit', illustrating how much steroid to use, and this information can be reinforced by the nurses.

The finger tip unit (Fig. 3.4), devised by Long & Finlay (1991), offers a method for measuring out an amount of topical steroid per section of the body. The finger tip unit is equivalent to a gram of topical steroid and is measured from the end of the adult index finger to the first joint. The measurement is based upon the use of a 5 mm nozzle. Each part of the body is then allotted a number of finger tip units. This has proved an effective and easy-to-explain method to allow patients to use their medication confidently.

Topical steroids are grouped into different strengths (Table 3.1). The strength of the steroid should be reduced as the condition improves until it can be stopped. In an acute flare the most effective treatment will be a potent or very potent topical steroid, which will be stepped down to moderate and mild steroids plus emollients as the condition improves. Emollients should, of course, be used throughout. It is more effective to use a more potent steroid for a shorter duration than mild steroids over a prolonged time. If the steroid is stopped abruptly the patient may experience a rebound reaction where the condition flares again very rapidly. In extreme cases patients may experience an Addisonian crisis, due to the body's natural production of steroids being suppressed as the patient uses the topical steroids.

Potent and very potent topical steroids should not be applied to the face, genitals or flexures

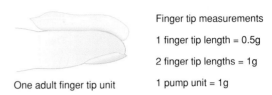

Use the adult finger tip unit (FTU) as your guide

One adult finger tip unit

Finger tip measurements

1 finger tip length = 0.5g

2 finger tip lengths = 1g

1 pump unit = 1g

The diagrams of the child (below) show how many adult finger tip units of cream or ointment are required to cover each area of the child's body

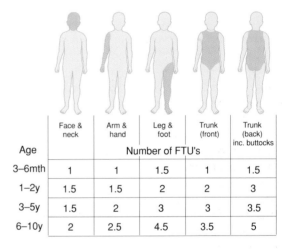

Age	Face & neck	Arm & hand	Leg & foot	Trunk (front)	Trunk (back) inc. buttocks
			Number of FTU's		
3–6mth	1	1	1.5	1	1.5
1–2y	1.5	1.5	2	2	3
3–5y	1.5	2	3	3	3.5
6–10y	2	2.5	4.5	3.5	5

Topical steroids: single application requirements

Child aged 4

Adult

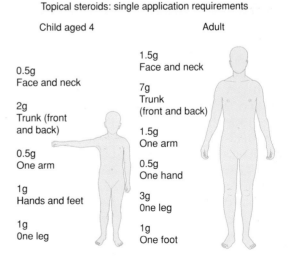

0.5g
Face and neck

2g
Trunk (front and back)

0.5g
One arm

1g
Hands and feet

1g
One leg

1.5g
Face and neck

7g
Trunk
(front and back)

1.5g
One arm

0.5g
One hand

3g
One leg

1g
One foot

Figure 3.4 The finger tip unit (reproduced with permission from Long & Finlay 1991).

Table 3.1 Potencies of topical steroids

Potency (strength)	Steroid preparation	Combination preparations
Very potent	Dermovate Nerisone Forte	Dermovate NN
Potent	Betacap Betnovate Bettamousse Cutivate Elocon Locoid Nerisone Proaderm Steidex Synalar	Aureocort Betnovate C Diprosalic Fucibet Locoid C Lotriderm Nystradermal
Moderate	Betnovate RD Eumovate Modrasone Synalar 1:4	Trimovate
Mild	Hydrocortisone Synalar 1:10	Daktacort Fucidin H

due to the potential side effects as the skin in these areas is already thinner than that of the trunk and limbs and the lower strengths are usually effective. Flexural areas may also have an occlusive effect which increases the absorption of the steroid. Children will usually require only mild and moderate topical steroids; occasionally a stronger one is prescribed by their dermatologist or paediatrician.

The vehicle base for the topical steroid is very important as it influences the delivery of the steroid to the skin. Topical steroids should be applied approximately half an hour after moisturizing, as this ensures that the steroid is applied across the skin surface evenly but is not diluted by excessive emollients. Controversy remains about mixing steroids with emollients prior to application. Whilst this is common practice, there is concern that the steroids become unstable with this procedure so application of the steroid after the emollient is recommended. The majority of steroids are contained within creams or ointments and the general rule is that ointments are best. Some steroids are delivered via a special topical tape. Gel and lotion preparations allow application to hairy areas but some lotions are alcohol based and may cause stinging on open or cracked skin.

Topical steroids can be manufactured as combination preparations – steroid/antibiotic or steroid/antifungal. These can be extremely effective in treating a localized infection without the need for systemic treatment. Long-term use of topical antibiotics may cause bacterial resistance so should only be used for a short course when infection is present.

OTHER TOPICAL TREATMENTS
Coal tar

Synonyms: crude coal tar, liquor picis carbonis, oil of Cade

Tar is used for the treatment of psoriasis and chronic eczema. It is obtained by the distillation of coal, wood or shale. Tar has an antiinflammatory and antipruritic effect. It also helps to reduce scaling due to its antimitotic effect on keratinocytes, thus preventing rapid cell turnover (psoriasis sufferers have a cell turnover of 4 days compared with a normal adult of 28 days). Crude coal tar does need to be applied accurately (Seville & Martin 1981) as applications can cause skin irritation and photosensitivity. If the patient is intolerant to tar the skin will become erythematous. It should be avoided if the skin is excoriated or if the condition becomes unstable, erythrodermic, pustular or infected.

Tar can be used in the form of solutions, ointments, bath additives, impregnated bandages and shampoos. It forms an important part of both the Ingram's Regimen (tar bath, UVB therapy followed by dithranol application) and Goeckerman's Regimen (tar bath, UVB therapy followed by application of crude coal tar), which incorporate the photosensitive aspect of tar.

Although coal tar preparations have been used for many years, concerns have been raised recently about possible long-term carcinogenicity. The long-term toxic effects must be considered when using tar products (Arnold 1997). Whilst the treatment can be effective many people find their use unacceptable as a result of odour and staining of clothes. Inpatient and day-care facilities are able to employ more tar than patients at home would be willing to use. When used as an outpatient treatment, clearance may take months as the tar strengths are weaker (Penzer 1996).

Dithranol products

Synonyms: Anthralin, Dithrocream, Micanol

Dithranol is a preparation used for the treatment of large, chronic, thick plaques of psoriasis. It is a synthetic derivative of tar and may be prepared in a number of bases, the most common being Lassar's paste (a combination of zinc and salicylic acid). The dithranol should only be applied to the affected areas. The area surrounding the plaque may be covered with ichthammol 1% in zinc oxide to prevent the spread of dithranol to unaffected skin. Dithranol must not be applied to psoriasis on sensitive areas such as the face, genitals, axillae, etc. It is not suitable for use in unstable psoriasis, e.g. Erythrodermic, Pustular.

Once applied, the dithranol can stay on the skin from 30 minutes (known as short-contact treatment) to overnight. The advantage of short-contact treatment is that on its removal the patient is able to continue for the day without further treatment. If the dithranol is left on for longer contact then talc should be applied over the dithranol and then covered with a stockinette or tubinette body suit to prevent spread of the treatment onto unaffected skin and reduce the staining of clothing. Dithranol staining of the skin will remain for 10–14 days after treatment is finished before fading.

Dithranol in Lassar's paste should be removed using oil but other cream preparations can be washed off with warm water.

Vitamin D analogues

Synonyms: calcipotriol, tacalcitol

These can be used for psoriasis plaques. These are the newer preparations and are more acceptable to patients due to their absorption on the skin surface and low odour. They can be used successfully by the patient in their own home with minimal disruption to their lifestyle.

Tacalcitol is limited to 10 g per day and should be applied once a day.

Topical retinoids (vitamin A analogues)

Topical retinoids are used for treating acne and psoriasis. The preparations may cause redness, scaling and irritation of the skin. If the gel is applied at night and the skin washed in the morning, the unsightly scaling and peeling that occurs as the drug acts will happen when the patient is asleep and so will not be a cosmetic problem. Overuse of these substances increases the irritation; only a fine layer should be applied to the affected area. If more is used, the surrounding skin can become irritated and reddened. These treatments will also increase the photosensitivity of the skin so sun avoidance advice should be provided and sunscreens used on exposed skin.

Retinoids are contraindicated in women who are pregnant or are likely to conceive as they are teratogenic. Women of childbearing potential who use retinoids must receive contraception advice prior to commencing treatment.

Keratolytic agents (salicylic acid, benzoyl peroxide)

Salicylic acid is used for hyperkeratotic skin conditions. It helps to control scaling but can cause irritation. Hyperkeratosis most commonly occurs on the scalp, soles and palms and salicylic acid is most often used in these areas. It can be used as a combination product, e.g. with tar, or steroids.

Benzoyl peroxide can be an effective acne treatment as it combines the keratolytic effect which unblocks the pilosebaceous follicles with an antibiotic effect. Patients should be warned of the possibility of bleaching that can occur occasionally (Layton 1996). The skin can become dry with the use of this preparation so patients should use a non-greasy emollient.

Topical antibiotics

These are used for treating localized bacterial infections (Table 3.2). If the infection does not

Table 3.2 The use of topical antibiotics (adapted from Killen et al 1998)

Antibacterial agent (some brand examples)	Usage
Bacitracin (Polyfax)	Gram-positive infections
Neomycin sulphate (Naseptin)	Aerobic Gram-positive and some aerobic Gram-negative infections
Silver sulphadiazine (Flamazine)	Gram-negative and -positive infections
Erythromycin (Benzamicin)	Acne vulgaris
Chloramphenicol (Actinac)	Superficial bacterial infections and acne
Tetracycline hydrochloride (Aureomycin)	Superficial bacterial infections
Mupirocin (Bactroban)	Antistreptococcal and antistaphylococcal
Fusidic acid (Fucidin)	Superficial skin infections
Aminoglycosides (Cicatrin)	Broad spectrum. May cause nephrotoxicity and ototoxicity if used on large areas

improve or becomes widespread then systemic antibiotics may be required. The widespread use of topical antibiotics is not encouraged due to the risk of bacterial resistance to the antibiotics. The treatment should be for a short course and not continued by the patient indefinitely. Patients can become sensitized to certain antibiotics.

Many topical antibiotics are available as combination therapies with topical steroids which can be an effective treatment for infected eczema.

Topical antifungals

These are used to treat tinea (fungal) infections of the skin, hair and nails. A combination antifungal and topical steroid can be an effective treatment as the infection is treated at the same time as the irritation and inflammation are relieved. Skin scrapings, nail clippings or scalp brushings are required to determine a suitable antifungal treatment. If the infection is widespread or does not respond to the topical treatment, systemic treatment will be required.

Topical antivirals

Aciclovir is the antiviral commonly used for the treatment and prevention of the herpes simplex (cold sore) virus. For widespread herpes simplex infections, for example eczema herpeticum, systemic aciclovir is always required.

OVER-THE-COUNTER (OTC) PRODUCTS

The cost of topical treatments (Table 3.3) whether bought over the counter or on prescription, can be so high that many patients will use sparse quantities so the treatments become virtually ineffective. Other patients may use only selected items from their prescription to help reduce the cost but this again will make their treatment less effective. If a patient has to pay prescription charges, they should be advised to obtain a pre-

Table 3.3 The cost of emollients (as at April 2000)

Emollient	Quantity	Retail price (£)	Price per 100 g or ml
Alpha Keri	480 ml	11.33	2.36
Aveeno Bath	250 ml	7.19	2.88
Aveeno Cream	100 ml	6.35	6.35
Balneum Bath	500 ml	10.68	2.13
Dermamist	250 ml	16.92	6.77
Dermol	500 ml	11.97	2.39
Dermol Shower	200 ml	7.04	3.52
Diprobase Cream	500 g	12.20	2.44
Diprobase Ointment	50 g	2.78	5.56
Diprobath	500 ml	13.22	2.64
E45 Bath	500 ml	7.15	1.43
E45 Wash	250 ml	4.49	1.79
E45 Cream	500 g	8.79	1.76
Emulsiderm	1 l	13.95	1.39
Epaderm	500 g	11.45	2.29
Hydromol Bath	1 l	15.65	1.56
Hydromol Cream	500 g	22.21	4.44
Lipobase	50 g	3.61	7.22
Oilatum Bath	500 ml	8.06	1.61
Oilatum Cream	80 g	4.90	6.12
Oilatum Gel	125 g	8.53	6.82
Unguentum Merck	500 g	18.70	3.74

payment certificate (currently form FP95 available from the Post Office or pharmacy). After an initial payment, they can have all their prescriptions free within an agreed time limit up to a year.

Many patients prefer to buy their treatments as OTC medications. It is possible to buy emollients, mild topical steroids, some acne and psoriasis treatments over the counter. This can be cheaper than the prescription charge and it reduces time spent waiting at the surgery and pharmacy. Nurses should be aware of the dermatology products that are available as OTC preparations so that they are able to provide accurate advice and information. Pharmacists are able to advise patients on the most suitable products available and how to use them.

Signpost Box		
page 43	Barrier function of skin	→ Chapter 1
page 44	Eczematous lesions	→ Chapter 10
page 44	Itch–scratch cycle	→ Chapter 2
page 45	Wet wrap bandages	→ Chapter 10
page 45	Topical steroids	→ Chapter 3.2
page 48	The skin in psoriasis	→ Chapter 9
page 49	Skin awareness	→ Chapter 12
page 49	Bacterial, fungal and viral infections	→ Chapter 13

REFERENCES

Arnold W P 1997 Tar. Clinics in Dermatology 15: 739–744

Bridgett C, Noren P, Staughton R 1996 Atopic skin disease: a manual for practitioners. Wrightson Biomedical, Petersfield, Hampshire

Cork M J 1997 The importance of skin barrier function. Journal of Dermatological Treatment 8: S7–S13

Griffith W A D, Wilkinson J D 1998 Topical agents. In: Champion R H, Burton J L, Burns D A, Breathnach S M, (eds) Textbook of dermatology, vol 4, 6th edn. Blackwell Science, Oxford

Killen G, Christensen I, Vargo N 1998 Treatment modalities. In: Hill M J (ed) Dermatological nursing essentials: a care curriculum. Dermatology Nurses Association, USA

Layton A 1996 Acne: assessment and treatment. Community Nurse 1(7): 36

Long C C, Finlay A Y 1991 The finger tip unit – a new practical measure. Clinical and Experimental Dermatology 16(6): 444–447

Morris A 1998 Effects of long term topical corticosteroids. Dermatology in Practice 6(3): 5–8

Pariser D M 1991 Topical steroids: a guide for use in the elderly patient. Geriatrics 46(10): 51–63

Penzer R 1996 Psoriasis. Nursing Standard 10(29): 49–53

Seville R, Martin E 1981 Dermatological nursing and therapy. Blackwell Science, Oxford, Chs 1, 3, 22

Stone L A, Lindfield E M, Robertson S 1989 A colour atlas of nursing procedures in skin disorders. Wolfe Medical, London

Drugs used systemically in dermatology

Lynette Boardman   Arthur Williams

INTRODUCTION

Many patients with skin complaints will be managed with topical therapies and will not require systemic drug therapy. However, some suffer conditions which are too widespread or severe to respond to topical therapy and may need oral or parenteral therapy.

The reasons for prescribing any medication should always be explained carefully to a patient in order to maximize adherence to the regimen; it is vital to listen to any concerns that the patient may express of history of allergic reactions.

A number of agents used to treat dermatological conditions also require careful monitoring of the patient for adverse reactions and interactions with other drugs. It is not possible or appropriate to list every adverse reaction to the agents discussed but important parameters to be monitored in each case will be identified.

Since patients are often receiving treatments over long periods, it is important that all healthcare professionals involved with the patient understand their responsibilities. Local arrangements will obviously vary but use of 'shared care protocols' may help to ensure that the necessary monitoring is performed.

The text will also include key facts for patients boxes containing information to be conveyed to patients to ensure safe usage of their therapy. Coordination between medical, nursing and pharmacy staff helps to ensure the patient receives consistent and correct verbal and written information.

From 1999 all medication in the UK must legally be supplied with patient information leaflets. Some agents used to treat dermatological conditions are not actually licensed for these purposes; the patient may find such package inserts confusing and will require specific information directly from the health-care professionals.

Systemic medication should be prescribed at dosages which take account of the patient's age, weight and ability to eliminate the drug via the hepatic and renal routes. Specialist advice should always be sought when prescribing for children, pregnant and breastfeeding women and those with specific susceptibility to adverse reactions or drug interactions.

ANTIHISTAMINES

Antihistamines provide symptomatic relief of pruritus and hypersensitivity reactions such as urticaria and angiooedema. Antihistamines are also used for treatment of itch in atopic dermatitis, especially in children. Although the underlying disease state may be unaltered, antihistamine use may reduce the self-inflicted damage of scratching and allow sleep for both the patient and other family members.

Antihistamines block the H_1-type receptors for histamine in the skin. Some antihistamines also affect receptors in the brain to cause sedation which also contributes to the relief of symptoms. Sedative antihistamines such as hydroxyzine create difficulties if daytime activities involve coordination or concentration, e.g. driving. Paradoxically, stimulant actions may occur in some patients, especially children, rather than the sedative effects expected (Parfitt 1993).

Antihistamines which do not have significant central nervous system activity include terfenadine, cetirizine, loratadine, acrivastine, mizolastine and fexofenadine.

Trials of various antihistamines may be necessary to find the most effective for any particular patient; some antihistamines act at receptors for chemicals other than histamine which may increase efficacy, e.g. cyproheptadine. Ranitidine, which blocks H_2 receptors for histamine, is occasionally used for patients with urticaria in combination with an antihistamine (Kobza Black 1997).

Adverse reactions and interactions need careful consideration; some antihistamines show anticholinergic actions leading to blurred vision and urinary retention. Photosensitivity may occur with some antihistamines such as trimeprazine (alimemazine) and promethazine (Parfitt 1993).

Terfenadine has been associated on rare occasions with cardiac arrhythmias; this drug should therefore be avoided in patients with preexisting cardiac problems. For this reason terfenadine is now only available on prescription. It should only be used in doses recommended by the manufacturer and never if metabolism is impaired by hepatic problems or by drugs which are metabolized by the same liver enzyme systems. This includes drugs such as erythromycin and itraconazole. Grapefruit juice increases plasma concentrations of terfenadine, which may cause cardiac reactions (Shenfield & Gross 1999).

Fexofenadine is a metabolite of terfenadine which has been developed to retain the antihistamine activity but apparently avoids the cardiac effects.

Topical application of antihistamines is best avoided because of the incidence of hypersensitivity problems.

Key facts

- Some cold and hay fever remedies contain antihistamines. Check with the pharmacist before using these as well as the prescribed antihistamine.
- For non-sedating antihistamines (see above) – although drowsiness is rare take care when driving and avoid alcohol intake.
- For sedative antihistamines – if drowsiness occurs do not drive or operate machinery. Avoid alcohol intake.
- For terfenadine – do not take more than 120 mg terfenadine daily.
- Remind the doctor and pharmacist about antihistamine use when any other medicines are prescribed or bought.

TRICYCLIC ANTIDEPRESSANTS

Some tricyclic antidepressant drugs such as amitriptyline, doxepin and nortriptyline have antihistamine-type actions and have therefore been used in relief of conditions such as urticaria (Kobza Black 1997). Doses are low compared with those needed for depression but sedation, confusion and anticholinergic effects do pose problems for older patients (Spigset & Martensson 1999).

SYSTEMIC CORTICOSTEROIDS

Systemic corticosteroids are used less frequently than topical corticosteroid preparations in dermatology. Severe, acute or unresponsive conditions may necessitate systemic corticosteroids. Dosage should be kept to the minimum needed to control the disease state; in some conditions use of other immunosuppressants such as azathioprine with the corticosteroid enables lower doses to be used.

Hydrocortisone is the 'natural' corticosteroid produced by the adrenal cortex. It is administered intravenously in anaphylaxis and angiooedema. Hydrocortisone has mineralocorticoid side effects which preclude its use for disease suppression. It may be required short term when a patient on oral steroids cannot receive treatment by mouth.

Prednisolone is the most commonly used oral steroid in the UK. Patients who suffer gastrointestinal side effects may prefer the enteric-coated preparation although this does not guarantee protection from peptic ulceration.

Methylprednisolone may be administered intravenously when very high doses of corticosteroid are needed. Slow administration is necessary to avoid cardiovascular collapse.

The mechanisms by which corticosteroids achieve their effects are complex (Haynes 1990). Antiinflammatory activity involves inhibition of 'chemotactic' substances which attract leucocytes to the site of inflammation as well as those with more direct actions. Immunosuppressive effects probably involve disruption of the 'lymphokine' chemical messengers between leucocytes.

Adverse effects of corticosteroids are well characterized, particularly effects on the endocrine system. Long-term therapy may result in cushingoid features and suppression of the normal adrenal response. Other serious consequences of corticosteroid use include increased susceptibility to infections; chickenpox poses a particular problem for those mixing with children. Latent tuberculosis may be reactivated.

Corticosteroids should not be commenced without careful consideration of the patient's medical history; bone loss, muscle weakness, impairment of glucose tolerance, gastrointestinal irritancy, growth suppression and mood changes are some of the important issues to consider.

Stopping corticosteroid therapy also requires care; not only may the disease relapse but adrenal response may be impaired. Gradual withdrawal is recommended for patients taking steroids for more than 3 weeks or on high doses (e.g. more than 40 mg prednisolone daily).

Key facts for patients

- If you have been taking the medication for more than three weeks, you will need to reduce the dose gradually, unless your doctor has advised you otherwise.

- Always read the patient information leaflet that is given with your medication. Always ensure that you carry the steroid card that is given with your medication.

- You must always mention to medical staff that you have had a course of steroids, for one year after you have stopped taking the treatment.

- If you come into contact with anyone with an infectious disease, or if you suddenly become ill, whilst on the treatment, you must contact your doctor immediately.

- If you have never had chicken pox you should avoid contact near people with either chicken pox or shingles. If contact is made with these people, you must see your doctor urgently.

- Always make sure that the information on the steroids card that you carry is up-to-date.

(Based on British National Formulary guidelines for all patients treated with systemic steroids, especially for more than 7 days.)

Topical corticosteroids

Oral mucosal lesions may require topical corticosteroid therapy but ointment and cream preparations are not suitable for this purpose. The steroid triamcinolone is marketed in an adhesive paste Orabase; other more potent steroids have also been formulated extemporaneously with Orabase.

If lesions are widespread, soluble tablets of betamethasone or prednisolone have been used as oral rinses. Patients should avoid swallowing the products as far as possible to avoid systemic effects.

Corticosteroid inhaler preparations have also been sprayed directly at mucosal lesions. The use of any corticosteroid preparation in the mouth could, however, mask any underlying infection.

Sometimes a high concentration of corticosteroids is required within a specific lesion, e.g. a keloid scar. Triamcinolone is formulated as a depot injection to facilitate retention of the medicament at the injection site.

METHOTREXATE

Methotrexate is a cytotoxic agent which inhibits folic acid synthesis during the S phase of mitosis, thereby influencing DNA production and cell replication. Low-dose methotrexate has become well established as a treatment providing an effective means of controlling psoriasis. Methotrexate has particular benefit for patients who also suffer from arthritis as joint problems may respond along with skin lesions. It has also proved useful for patients with pustular psoriasis, erythrodermic psoriasis or widespread plaque psoriasis unresponsive to topical therapy. Methotrexate has also been used in the treatment of scleroderma.

Methotrexate may prove hazardous to rapidly proliferating cells, such as those in bone marrow (Gawkrodger 1997). The dose is therefore kept to the minimum achieving adequate control and should be given once a week, on the same day each week.

Since methotrexate is eliminated renally, care should be taken if renal function is impaired, particularly in elderly patients. Toxicity becomes an even greater risk if the patient is dehydrated due to fever or vomiting (Gawkrodger 1997).

Blood levels of methotrexate do not indicate toxicity except in an overdosage situation but neutrophil and platelet counts indicate toxicity to the bone marrow. Mouth ulceration may also indicate adverse reactions.

Many patients experience nausea when taking methotrexate; this is not necessarily an indicator of toxicity and can sometimes be reduced by altering the fluid intake or using antiemetic agents. Some dermatologists advocate use of folic acid to reduce gastrointestinal upset.

Methotrexate presents problems for both men and women with regard to their reproductive health. Sperm may be damaged and case reports document teratogenicity.

Methotrexate may cause fibrosis and eventually cirrhosis of the liver; patients who have a high alcohol intake are at greater risk (Gawkrodger 1997). The risk also increases with the cumulative dose of methotrexate. Standard liver function tests identify patients with preexisting damage to the liver and any inflammatory changes but are poor indicators of fibrosis. Use of liver biopsy is controversial as this procedure itself does carry risks for the patient. Pulmonary toxicity may occur in some patients and drug interactions may occur, especially with NSAIDs.

The weekly dose of methotrexate is usually started low at 2.5 mg or 5 mg and gradually increased to a maximum dose of 20–25 mg according to results of blood tests and response. Dosage may require adjustment if the patient takes non-steroidal antiinflammatory agents or other drugs which reduce the renal elimination of methotrexate.

Methotrexate is usually taken orally but is occasionally administered intramuscularly when absorption from the gut is poor or gastrointestinal side effects are intolerable. Handling of parenteral methotrexate preparations requires operators to protect both patients and themselves when drawing up the drug and disposing of unused solution.

Monitoring guidelines

- Renal function ⎫ Weekly until patient is stabilized
- Hepatic function ⎬ and then every 2–3 months
- Full blood count ⎪ providing no other parameters
  ⎭ change
- Pregnancy testing – advisable before starting treatment in women of childbearing age

---

Key facts for patients

- Take the dose once weekly on the same day.
- Ask the pharmacist to give the dose as 2.5 mg tablets; confusion arises if 10 mg tablets are also used.
- Blood tests are important to identify any early signs of toxicity.
- Keep alcohol intake to a minimum.
- Remind the doctor or pharmacist that you are taking methotrexate when obtaining any other medicines. Do not take aspirin or ibuprofen.
- Report any abnormal bruising or bleeding to the doctor and also seek attention promptly if any coughing or infection occurs.
- Women should use adequate contraception during treatment and for 6 months after treatment has finished.
- Men should avoid unprotected sex during treatment and for 6 months after treatment has finished.

AZATHIOPRINE

Azathioprine is a cytotoxic drug used to achieve immunosuppression, either alone or often in combination with corticosteroids. This enables lower doses of steroids to be used. Dermatologists employ azathioprine in the control of bullous disorders and various other conditions such as Behçet's disease, dermatomyositis, severe atopic dermatitis and occasionally in psoriasis (Parfitt 1993).

Azathioprine is metabolized in the liver to cytotoxic compound mercaptopurine (Parfitt 1993); both these agents affect the production of RNA and DNA and thus replication of cells. Azathioprine may therefore cause bone marrow toxicity (Gawkrodger 1997) and gastrointestinal irritation. Rarely, patients lack a particular enzyme needed for metabolism and are therefore at particular risk of toxicity.

Azathioprine sometimes causes hepatic damage and may occasionally initiate a hypersensitivity reaction involving major organ systems.

Azathioprine is given by mouth in doses calculated according to body weight. Dosage should be adjusted if the patient has significant renal impairment. Azathioprine should be avoided in pregnancy where possible because of the theoretical risk to developing cells

NB: As with all prescribing, unofficial abbreviations should not be used.

Monitoring guidelines

- Full blood count – weekly for first 8 weeks of treatment and then at least every 3 months
- Renal function – to ensure dose is not excessive
- Liver function

Key facts for patients

- Blood tests are important to identify early signs of toxicity.
- Report any abnormal bruising or bleeding to the doctor and also seek attention promptly if any infection occurs.
- Report any other unusual side effects, e.g. severe aches and pains or infectious, to the doctor.

CICLOSPORIN

Ciclosporin is a potent immunosuppressant which is licensed for use in severe psoriasis and atopic dermatitis where no other treatment is appropriate. The mechanism of action in skin disease is not fully established but it is known to affect T-lymphocytes and lymphokine production (Creamer & Barker 1997). Ciclosporin has less risk of toxicity to bone marrow than cytotoxic immunosuppressants such as azathioprine.

Ciclosporin has been reformulated into the Neoral product which was designed to provide more steady blood concentrations. Treatment with Neoral should commence with a dose not exceeding 2.5 mg ciclosporin per kg per day in two divided doses. The dose may gradually be increased to 5 mg per kg per day if necessary.

Short courses are used by some dermatologists to minimize toxicity. At present, ciclosporin is only licensed for use for an 8-week period in treatment of atopic dermatitis; there is no time limitation for psoriasis use.

Measurement of blood levels of ciclosporin is required if conversion between different brands of ciclosporin is undertaken (bioavailability differences). Predose levels are occasionally measured if serious toxicity is suspected. Ciclosporin is extensively metabolized in the liver. Drug interactions occur between ciclosporin and many other drugs which use the same enzyme systems for metabolism, thereby altering the ciclosporin levels.

Ciclosporin may cause nephrotoxicity and renal function should be monitored carefully before starting treatment and at regular intervals; if the glomerular filtration rate falls, dosage adjustment must be made whilst damage is reversible (Gawkrodger 1997). Additional care is needed if other drugs are in use which also have nephrotoxic effects, such as non-steroidal antiinflammatory agents. Actions within the kidney may also lead to hypertension and hyperkalaemia (Gawkrodger 1997).

Ciclosporin has been associated with various other adverse effects including nausea, headaches, tremor, gum hypertrophy and raised blood levels of urate, lipids and glucose. Doses of ciclosporin used in transplant recipients may predispose patients to malignancy; this is less likely in doses used in dermatology but exposure to ultraviolet light (including sunlight) should be minimized. Ciclosporin is contraindicated if infection is present.

Monitoring guidelines

- Renal function (every 2 weeks for first 3 months then at least every 2 months)
- Blood pressure (regularly for all patients, frequently if any other risk factors)
- Serum potassium (frequency depends on renal function)
- Baseline hepatic function, lipid levels, blood glucose and urate

---

Key facts for patients

- Blood tests are important to identify any early signs of damage to the kidneys.
- Blood pressure may be raised and needs to be checked regularly.
- Remind the doctor or pharmacist that you take ciclosporin when obtaining any other medicines.
- Protect the skin from exposure to the sun. Do not use sunbeds.

ISOTRETINOIN (ROACCUTANE) AND ACITRETIN (NEOTIGASON)

Isotretinoin and acitretin are retinoids (chemicals related to vitamin A) licensed for use in the UK under the supervision of dermatologists. Treatment cannot be initiated in the community. In the UK, isotretinoin is used orally in treatment of severe acne and occasionally for disorders of keratinization; acitretin is used in treatment of psoriasis and disorders of keratinization. Acitretin has also been investigated for various unlicensed conditions including treatment of warts. Etretinate was used in the UK until the mid-1990s but has now been replaced by acitretin which is the active metabolite of etretinate.

Retinoids used topically for moderately severe acne include isotretinoin, tretinoin and the retinoid-related compound adapalene whilst tazarotene may be used for both acne and psoriasis (Marks 1999). Topical tretinoin has also been used in cosmetic dermatology to reduce pigmentation and sun damage.

Retinoids have complex actions involving alteration of keratinization and epidermal differentiation; thus both isotretinoin and acitretin may cause drying of the nasal mucosa, the lips and the conjunctiva. Photosensitivity may be increased whilst hair loss may affect some patients. This is usually reversible on discontinuation or even dose reduction (Smith 1995).

The drugs undergo metabolic changes in the liver but also have the potential to cause hepatic damage. Raised serum lipids may occur and the drugs should be discontinued if triglycerides are significantly increased since pancreatitis could occur.

Muscle and bone pain pose problems for those participating in sports.

The main group of patients for which these drugs require care are young women as significant teratogenic effects may occur. Small amounts of acitretin can undergo metabolism to etretinate. This concentrates in adipose tissue and therefore undergoes slow elimination from the body; the risk of teratogenic damage may continue for months after use. Patients on isotretinoin may become more susceptible to depression.

An unusual but serious problem of retinoids is benign intracranial hypertension; this risk may be increased by concomitant use of tetracyclines.

Monitoring guidelines

- Hepatic function (pretreatment 1 month after starting treatment and then 3-monthly)
- Lipid levels (cholesterol and triglycerides)
- Pregnancy testing in women of childbearing potential

Key facts for patients

- Women must use adequate contraception during treatment and for the stated period afterwards (1 month for isotretinoin and 2 years for acitretin).
- Keep alcohol intake to a minimum.
- Soreness of the lips and nostrils can be alleviated with lipsalve and soft paraffin (Vaseline).
- Soreness of the eyes can be alleviated with moisturizing eyedrops.
- Protect the skin from exposure to the sun. Do not use sunbeds.
- Wax depilation should be avoided during treatment and for 2 months afterwards.
- Do not take large doses of vitamin A (more than 5000 units daily).
- Do not give blood whilst taking the medication (risk of drug present causing teratogenic effects if given to pregnant woman)
- Inform the doctor or pharmacist of retinoid use if other medication is prescribed or bought.

OTHER DRUGS USED TO MODIFY DERMATOLOGICAL DISEASE

Dapsone is an antiinfective agent but finds use in dermatology to suppress bullous disorders (Chren & Bickers 1990). It should be avoided in

patients lacking the glucose-6-phosphate dehydrogenase enzyme; this can trigger haemolytic anaemia. Haematological monitoring is also necessary to check for methaemoglobinaemia. Sulfapyridine and sulfametopyridazine (both unlicensed drugs) are also used to treat dermatitis herpetiformis (Parfitt 1993).

Studies have shown that sulfasalazine, also from the sulphonamide group, is of benefit to some psoriasis patients (Parfitt 1993).

Hydroxyurea, a cytotoxic agent, is occasionally used as a second-line treatment for psoriasis. Careful monitoring of blood count is needed; dosing needs to take account of renal impairment as the drug is eliminated via the kidneys (Gawkrodger 1997).

Cyclophosphamide, also a cytotoxic agent, has been used as an intermittent or 'pulse' therapy for bullous disorders, dermatomyositis and lupus. Cyclophosphamide is administered intravenously, accompanied by mesna treatment if the patient has any susceptibility to urinary or renal problems. Haemorrhagic cystitis due to urothelial toxicity may develop due to a cyclophosphamide metabolite. Mesna reacts with this metabolite, preventing local toxicity.

Intravenous human normal immunoglobulin administered in high doses (such as 0.4 g per kg per day) also has the ability to suppress bullous disorders and other severe conditions. This highly expensive treatment is used in specialist centres as short-course treatment over a few days and repeated after a few months. The patient requires significant fluid intake with the immunoglobulin and must also be monitored carefully for hypersensitivity reactions (Leighton & Jolles 1998) or raised blood pressure.

Thalidomide has significant teratogenic risk. It is not licensed for use in the UK but has been used for the treatment of various conditions such as Behçet's disease and certain cases of leprosy. Careful monitoring for neurological damage using electromyelograms is necessary. Patients need to be aware of sedative and neurological effects and the drug must be avoided in women of childbearing potential.

Hydroxychloroquine and *mepacrine* are antimalarial agents used in treatment of lupus (Chren

& Bickers 1990). Baseline eye examination and reporting of any visual changes should ensure early detection of the rare retinal damage which can occur with hydroxychloroquine (Jones 1999). Patients on mepacrine should minimize alcohol intake as alcohol metabolism may be impaired.

ANTIMICROBIAL AGENTS

Treatment of specific infections is discussed in Chapter 13. Details of systemic antimicrobials are discussed in the following section.

Antimicrobial agents are used to enable the immune system to control infections of the skin but care must always be taken to minimize development of resistance. Local antibiotic policies are designed to reduce the development of resistant organisms.

Appropriate agents should be used in adequate doses and courses; this principle applies to bacterial, viral or fungal infections. Wherever possible samples should be taken for sensitivity testing.

Antibacterial agents

Treatment of some dermatological infections demands agents with specific activity. Penicillin is required for treating the streptococcal infection of erysipelas, flucloxacillin is the first-line therapy for staphylococcal infections and metronidazole for anaerobic infections.

Other conditions may benefit from a broad-spectrum antibacterial such as amoxicillin or erythromycin. Local sensitivity patterns of organisms should be considered; for example, if resistance occurs with amoxicillin the preparation co-amoxiclav, which contains the beta-lactamase inhibitor clavulanic acid, may be useful. Hypersensitivity problems of the patient may rule out some antibacterials such as penicillins whilst adverse effects of others may require alteration of treatment; the gastrointestinal effects of some erythromycin products may be troublesome.

Occasionally, media publicity occurs over serious adverse events, eg. minocycline has been associated with autoimmune hepatitis and systemic lupus erythematosus, but such events are very rare compared with use of the drug (Gottlieb 1997). Intravenous antibacterials are only required in a few circumstances such as acute cellulitis but should always be administered at the appropriate dilution and rate. Interactions arising from the use of antibacterials should not be forgotten. Short courses of broad-spectrum antibiotics reduce the efficacy of oral contraceptives whilst the enzyme-inhibiting actions of erythromycin and ciprofloxacin cause concerns when combined with drugs where the margin between a therapeutic and toxic dose is narrow.

Longer term treatment with oral antimicrobials for acne (see Chapter 11) raises issues of continuing compliance. Patients sometimes find the dosing schedule of oxytetracycline and tetracycline difficult as no milk product or other agent containing calcium ions should be taken within an hour because absorption of the antimicrobial may be impaired. The milk restriction does not apply to minocycline (Livingstone 1997) but patients should be aware of the possibility of skin pigmentation with this drug (Archer 1998). Other longer term issues such as the need for effective contraception and minimizing sun exposure should also be discussed with patients on tetracyclines.

Topical agents

Use of topical antimicrobial agents is only appropriate if the agent is likely to penetrate to the site of infection; problems from use of topical agents vary from sensitization to systemic effects through absorption and resistance development.

Two antibacterial agents which are not available in systemic form merit special mention because of their use in dermatology. Silver sulfadiazine has proved its efficacy in treating burns patients and also those with severe exfoliative conditions. Absorption of both the sulphonamide component and silver is possible after extensive or prolonged use, leading to argyria and/or leucopenia. Silver sulfadiazine is not suitable for treating reactions such as Stevens–Johnson syndrome if caused by sulphonamides. Mupirocin has proved useful to control Gram-positive infections, particularly MRSA.

Use of other topical antibacterial products reduces the likelihood of adverse reactions and interactions. Metronidazole is effective against anaerobic organisms and is used in gel formulation for rosacea. It may also be used for treating malodorous tumours.

Clindamycin, tetracycline and erythromycin are used effectively for mild to moderate acne. Fusidic acid is useful against staphylococci and helps to control acute infective 'flares' in conditions such as atopic dermatitis. It is possible that the benefits of these agents may be limited by resistance problems in the future.

Antiviral agents

The availability of aciclovir has enabled dermatologists to control herpes infection effectively. Aciclovir is manufactured as topical formulations; it is effective for cold sore treatment if started in the 'prodromal' phase. Patients with a dermatological condition with superimposed herpes simplex or zoster infection require systemic aciclovir, especially those with zoster who need high doses.

Aciclovir is poorly absorbed from the gastrointestinal tract so oral administration necessitates a five times daily dosing schedule to achieve adequate levels. Acute conditions such as eczema herpeticum may require intravenous aciclovir. Intravenous aciclovir requires dilution with saline and administration as an infusion over 1 hour to ensure renal complications are avoided.

Valaciclovir and famciclovir are 'prodrugs' which release the active agents aciclovir and penciclovir once in the body. There is less experience with these agents but the regimen for oral use requires less frequent dosing. These agents are not available in the form of an injection.

Antifungal agents

Before using antifungal agents it is useful to identify the organisms (agents active against candida do not necessarily kill dermatophytes) and to remove any animal source of infection.

Two antifungals are made in specific 'nail applications' for use in distal nail infections (Denning et al 1995) and systemic treatment is not suitable. Amorolfine is applied as a lacquer once a week but is an expensive treatment. Tioconazole nail solution needs to be applied twice daily for months; results from studies show a low cure rate (Denning et al 1995).

Systemic therapy with antifungal agents is required in some conditions.

Terbinafine is used to treat dermatophyte infections of nails and scalp and severe or extensive infection of the body. It has a simple dosage regimen of 250 mg once daily. The course of treatment depends on the nature of the infection but courses are shorter than those required for griseofulvin. Terbinafine has less potential for drug interactions than griseofulvin. Terbinafine can cause headaches, gastrointestinal problems (including taste disturbance) and very occasional serious skin reactions such as Stevens–Johnson syndrome.

Before the availability of terbinafine, griseofulvin was used for many years to treat the same types of dermatophyte infections. Months of treatment were required for nail infections, particularly in elderly patients. Griseofulvin has other disadvantages and contraindications. Griseofulvin is still used for children since terbinafine is not licensed to treat children yet and is not available in liquid formulation (Denning et al 1995).

Ketoconazole is used frequently in topical shampoos for seborrhoeic dermatitis but the oral form is not considered suitable for treating skin infections as there are risks of fatal hepatic impairment, especially if treatment is given for more than 14 days.

Itraconazole may be used for various fungal conditions caused by candida or dermatophytes. Nail infections can be treated with continuous therapy or intermittent 'pulses' of 200 mg twice daily for 1 week followed by 3 weeks without therapy. Itraconazole may cause headaches and gastrointestinal upset; if continuous therapy is used for more than 1 month, liver function should be monitored.

Fluconazole is a fungicidal drug which is useful in a number of dermatological infections caused by dermatophyte fungi and yeast. Dosage level (adults) are of the order of 50 mg per day fo 2–6 weeks (maximum). Both itraconazole and fluconazole have the potential to cause liver damage and othe serious side effects and drug interactions (see product literature for details). Immunocompromised patients often suffer from fungal infections (AIDS patients) and may require treatment with fluconazole. An initial dose of 400 mg followed by 200 mg daily is a typical regimen.

Evening primrose oil (Epogam, Efamast)

The evening primrose plant is related to the willow family and is found at roadsides, on waste ground and sand dunes. Gamolenic acid is a constituent of evening primrose oil and is reported to help improve atopic eczema. Gamolenic acid is a part of the linoleic acid group. People with atopic eczema are less able to convert linoleic acid to gammalinoleic acid, an essential fatty acid required for a healthy skin. Many patients with atopic eczema do gain benefit from taking evening primrose oil (Say 1991). The course should be taken for approximately 3 months before its success can be evaluated.

Evening primrose oil is available on NHS prescription for the treatment of atopic eczema. The dose is 160—240mg per day in adults and 80—160mg for children. Side effects can include nausea, indigestion and headache and it should be avoided where there is a history of epilepsy or during pregnancy. Fiocchi et al (1994), in their evaluation of evening primrose oil, found a gradual improvement in the erythema, excoriations, irritation and lichenification of their patients.

ADVERSE DRUG REACTIONS INVOLVING THE SKIN

This chapter has emphasized the role of the nurse in providing information to the patient about the medication for their dermatological disorder so that adverse effects to other organs and body systems may be avoided. Nursing care is also required for patients suffering from adverse reactions which involve the skin and to prevent such reactions occurring or recurring.

Even though adverse drug reactions seem an unpredictable phenomenon, patient suffering may be minimized if prevention, early diagnosis, appropriate treatment, adequate documentation and careful reporting occur.

Prevention

Careful history taking is important with regard to previous hypersensitivities and reactions.

Patients sometimes refer to proprietary names or even descriptions of tablets and capsules. If reactions have been severe in the past, it is best to try to identify problem drugs before a new prescription is given. Cross-sensitivities between drugs may also occur; for example, penicillin and cephalosporin antibiotics contain a similar structure within their molecules and some patients may be hypersensitive to both groups of drugs.

The role of the nurse in preventing adverse reactions from topical agents by ensuring that patients use correct application techniques and suitable quantities of topical preparations has already been emphasized at the beginning of this chapter. This is especially important for patients with increased likelihood of reactions because of skin type or fragility. Many photosensitivity reactions may be avoided simply by informing people to take extra care to minimize sun exposure. The effects of photosensitizing drugs should also be taken into account for patients undergoing therapeutic ultraviolet treatment (see Chapter 4). The BNF contains excellent general guidance or the prevention of adverse drug reactions.

Diagnosis of adverse reaction affecting the skin

Adverse drug reactions vary in severity from mild irritation to life-threatening exfoliation (Smith 1994). There is a considerable range in the types of reaction that occur. Many drugs cause different reactions in patients; some have a distinct drug eruption appearance (Smith 1989) whilst others may be difficult to distinguish from naturally occurring skin disorders (Magee & Beeley 1994). Some reactions, such as oral hyperpigmentation with minocycline, occur only rarely (Eisen 1997). Careful history taking of all medication including vaccinations, over-the-counter medicines, contraceptives, herbal products and lay remedies is needed.

The likelihood of a particular type of reaction occurring from the agents used can be checked in specialized texts and with drug information centres. The CSM's Adverse Drug Reactions On-line Information Tracking System (ADROIT) facilitates the monitoring of adverse drug reactions. Some reactions occur months after starting treatment whilst other reactions may persist after medication is discontinued.

Confirmation of diagnosis could be obtained by drug 'rechallenge', i.e. giving a further dose. This is usually considered unacceptable to the patient, particularly for severe reactions (Smith 1989). Patch and prick testing are not always reliable and also pose a risk of severe reactions (Magee & Beeley 1994). Urticarial reactions due to azo dyes like tartrazine (which may be present in some pharmaceuticals) may be investigated using specially prepared oral capsules.

Treatment

If possible, the drug which may be responsible should be discontinued. This obviously depends on whether the patient can be adequately treated with alternative medication. Sometimes drugs from the same group may cause the same reactions, e.g. several phenothiazine antipsychotics may cause photosensitivity. Alternatives should therefore be selected carefully.

Treatment of severe skin damage should follow the principles set out in Chapters 8 and 14. Systemic corticosteroids may be necessary for control of severe reactions. Flamazine (silver sulfadiazine) cream should be avoided in patients with sulphonamide-induced skin problems.

In other cases symptomatic relief with antihistamines and moisturizers may be sufficient, depending on the nature of the reaction. Menthol cream (between 0.5% and 2%) relieves intense itching and mild or moderate topical corticosteroid preparations reduce the severity of inflammatory reactions.

On rare occasions, a procedure of desensitization has been undertaken when it has been imperative to continue using a drug which has caused reactions. Desensitization involves giving minute doses of drug and very gradually increasing the dose, whilst the patient is being monitored extremely carefully.

Documentation

Reactions should be recorded clearly and information passed between the health-care professionals involved with the patient. This can easily be overlooked whilst concentrating on treatment aspects. The patient or parent should be informed of the drug likely to be responsible. Some patients like to obtain 'Medicalert' jewellery to record such information; others may ask their local pharmacist to record this on their patient medication records.

All drug therapy for hospital inpatients should be prescribed and the administration recorded on the approved forms or within the computer system. All adverse reactions should be recorded within such systems.

Reporting

Within the UK, information on adverse reactions is coordinated by the Committee on Safety of Medicines who gain details of reactions via reports sent by doctors and pharmacists. Any reaction to recently marketed drugs should be reported. Serious reactions to more established therapies also require reporting. The system is voluntary. Details of the reporting system are given in the BNF which incorporates reporting forms (yellow cards).

Overall, a patient suffering an adverse drug reaction requires coordinated care by health-care staff who communicate effectively. This principle underlies the use of all the treatment described in this chapter.

It is vital that the reporting system is actively used to ensure that sufficient data is collected.

This monitoring system is designed to assist in recognizing emerging problems.

REFERENCES

Archer C B 1998 Minocycline-induced skin and tissue pigmentation. Prescribers Journal 38: 47–49

Chren M M, Bickers D R 1990 Dermatological pharmacology. In: Goodman Gilman A, Rall T W, Nies A S, Taylor P (eds) The pharmacological basis of therapeutics. Pergamon, New York, Ch 65

Creamer D, Barker J 1997 GP guide to effective psoriasis management. Prescriber 8(17): 63–68

Denning D W, Evans E G V, Kibbler C C et al 1995 Fungal nail disease: a guide to good practice (report of a working group of the British Society for Medical Mycology). British Medical Journal 311: 1277–1281

Eisen D 1997 Minocycline-induced oral hyperpigmentation. Lancet 349: 400

Fiocchi A, Sala M, Signoroni P 1994 The efficacy and safety of GLA in the treatment of infantile atopic dermatitis. Journal of International Medical Research 22(1): 24–32

Gawkrodger D J 1997 Current management of psoriasis. Journal of Dermatological Treatment 8: 27–55

Gottlieb A 1997 Safety of minocycline for acne. Lancet 349: 374

Haynes R C 1990 Adrenocorticotrophic hormone; adrenocortical steroids and their synthetic analogs; inhibitors of the synthesis and actions of adrenocortical hormones. In: Goodman Gilman A, Rall T W, Nies A S, Taylor P (eds) The pharmacological basis of therapeutics. Pergamon, New York, Ch 60

Jones S K 1999 Ocular toxicity and hydroxychloroquine: guidelines for screening. British Journal of Dermatology 140: 3–7

Kobza Black A 1997 Guide to recognition and management of urticaria. Prescriber 8(13): 25–35

Leighton C, Jolles S 1998 A review of IV immunoglobulins. Hospital Pharmacist 5: 251–255

Livingstone C 1997 Acne. Pharmaceutical Journal 259: 725–727

Magee P, Beeley L 1994 Drug-induced skin disorders. In: Walker R, Edwards C (eds) Clinical pharmacy and therapeutics. Churchill Livingstone, New York, Ch 54

Marks R 1999 The role of tazarotene in treatment of psoriasis. British Journal of Dermatology 140 (suppl 54): 24–28

Parfitt K (ed) 1993 Martindale – the extra pharmacopoeia. Pharmaceutical Press, London

Say B 1991 A panacea for all ills. Nursing Times 87(15): 58–60

Shenfield G, Gross A 1999 The cytochrome p450 system and adverse drug reactions. Adverse Drug Reaction Bulletin 194: 639–642

Smith A G 1989 Cutaneous adverse drug reactions to systemic drug therapy. Adverse Drug Reaction Bulletin 134: 500–503

Smith A G 1994 Important cutaneous adverse drug reactions. Adverse Drug Reaction Bulletin 167: 631–634

Smith A G 1995 Drug-induced disorders of hair and nails. Adverse Drug Reaction Bulletin 173: 655–658

Spigset O, Martensson B 1999 Drug treatment of depression. British Medical Journal 318: 1188–1191

FURTHER READING

Breathnach S M, Hintner H 1992 Types of clinical reaction. In: Adverse drug reactions and the skin. Blackwell, Oxford, Ch 3

4

Phototherapy

*Helen Perfect   Helen Wilson
Trish Garabaldinos*

INTRODUCTION

Phototherapy and photochemotherapy (PUVA) are widely used treatments for skin disease. Both forms of treatment can be dramatically effective and may transform a patient's life by clearing their skin disease. However, acute and chronic adverse reactions are not infrequent and expertise is required for the safe and effective delivery of these treatments. The recognition of potentially serious adverse effects, in particular skin malignancy, has led to the more controlled use of phototherapy and PUVA.

For the patient, phototherapy remains one of the most user-friendly and socially acceptable treatments, despite two or three journeys a week to hospital for up to 10 weeks. The end result is usually clearance of disease and a 'tan'. The success of treatment is reflected by the ever-expanding number of phototherapy units in the United Kingdom.

PRINCIPLES OF PHOTOBIOLOGY

Phototherapy is the treatment of skin disease by means of non-ionizing electromagnetic radiation with or without the addition of photoactive drugs. It includes photochemotherapy (PUVA), photodynamic therapy (PDT) and UVB therapy.

Photochemotherapy is the combination of a photoactive chemical and light therapy. Psoralen, a phototoxic drug, is activated by long-wave ultraviolet radiation UVA, hence the term PUVA.

Photodynamic therapy (PDT) involves exposing localized lesions or disease to certain wavelengths within the visible light spectrum in combination with a photosensitizing agent to cause energy-dependent cytotoxicity.

Phototherapy is more commonly referred to as UVB therapy. It involves exposing the skin to a midwave ultraviolet radiation.

The ultraviolet spectrum

The UV spectrum is arbitrarily divided into three subregions: UVA 320–400 nm, UVB 280–320 nm and UVC 200–280 nm. However, the visible light spectrum is becoming more important as research is developing uses and procedures for various conditions in the medical field.

The UVC region represents the part of solar radiation which is filtered by the atmosphere before it reaches the earth's surface. The UVB region is separated from UVA because of the effect these wavelengths have on human skin. The amount of UVB radiation needed to cause reddening of skin is about 100–1000 times less than the amount of UVA needed to produce the same effect (Fig. 4.1).

The goal in phototherapy is to maximize the therapeutic dose with an acceptable skin redness. To achieve this, we need to know how effective different wavelengths of UV radiation are in causing erythema, relative to their ability to heal disease. This can be summarized as follows.

	Heals	Burns
UVC	No	Yes
UVB	Yes	Yes
UVA	No	No

HISTORICAL PERSPECTIVE OF PHOTOTHERAPY

Sunlight has been used empirically in the treatment of skin disease for thousands of years. The ancient Egyptians used a substance presumed to be psoralen extracted from plants in combination with exposure to sunlight to treat vitiligo. It is only in the past century that alternative sources of ultraviolet radiation have been developed to allow treatment of patients in a controlled environment that does not rely on sunlight.

The first clinical use of UVA in combination with psoralen was reported in 1947. El-Mofty (1968) performed extensive work, which defined the use of 8-methoxypsoralens (8-MOP) and 5-methoxypsoralens (5-MOP), which were administered topically and orally for vitiligo.

In 1974 Parrish developed high-intensity UVA fluorescent bulbs and reported complete clearance of psoriasis in 21 patients and in 1978 Fritsch et al reported that a combination of oral retinoid and PUVA enhanced efficacy of treatment for psoriasis by increasing the clearing rate and decreasing the total UVA dose.

Development of machinery and fluorescent tubes is ongoing and accurate knowledge of

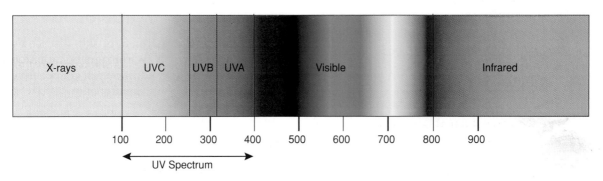

Figure 4.1 The ultraviolet spectrum.

long-term side effects, especially the incidence of cutaneous carcinoma, is continually changing.

The 1990s saw a new form of phototherapy UVB treatment called narrowband UVB (TLO1 Philips lamps). More recently, the use of high-intensity visible light in combination with a photosensitizer, called photodynamic therapy (PDT), has been introduced. This is useful for some forms of skin cancer and may have a place in the treatment of psoriasis.

EFFECTS OF UV LIGHT ON THE SKIN

The skin reacts in a predictable way following exposure to ultraviolet radiation (UVR) and these effects can be divided into acute and chronic reactions.

Acute effects

Erythema

There is an initial flushing of the skin following exposure to UVR, which soon subsides. This is followed by a second erythemal response 6–12 hours later which is more prolonged and is caused by blood vessel damage and inflammation secondary to cell damage and death.

Sunburn

This results in more severe cutaneous damage and is primarily caused by UVB. There is cell damage and death in the epidermis and blood vessel damage in the dermis. Delayed erythema is followed by oedema of both the dermis and epidermis and then blistering. The skin is very tender, dead cells are shed and several days later the skin peels. Topical steroids can reduce this reaction and may provide symptomatic relief.

Thickening

For those who do not tan, this is the main form of cutaneous protection from sunlight. Repeated sun exposure leads to increased epidermal cell division, causing thickening of the epidermis. This forms a physical barrier to UVR, which allows for more prolonged sun exposure without burning.

Sebaceous glands

The sebaceous glands tend to atrophy with chronic sun exposure, leading to dry skin. Atrophic follicular cavities can dilate to form senile comedones.

Carcinogenesis

Prolonged exposure of the epidermis to UVR can cause epidermal dysplasia, which may lead to epidermal malignancy. Premalignant skin tumours include solar keratosis, actinic keratosis, porokeratosis and Bowen's disease. Basal cell carcinomas (BCC) are the commonest skin cancer but are locally invasive and never metastasize. Squamous cell carcinomas (SCC) may rapidly grow and metastasize. Malignant melanoma may occur in much younger patients and is still relatively rare but, due to its capacity to metastasize, deserves special vigilant attention.

Tanning

UVA is primarily responsible for immediate tanning which is caused by the darkening of preformed melanin precursors and occurs within minutes, peaks at 1 hour and then slowly declines over 12 hours. Delayed tanning is caused by UVB, which stimulates melanocytes to produce melanin, which is distributed to the epidermal cells. This starts 10–12 hours following exposure to UVB and can persist for weeks. A deep tan can reduce by 90% the amount of UVR reaching the basal epidermis.

Chronic effects

The extent of UV-induced skin damage depends upon the actual protective responses of the skin (i.e. skin tanning type) and the degree of UV exposure.

Epidermis

Thinning of the epidermis occurs with chronic UV exposure, with flattening of the basal layer.

Dermis

Long-term exposure of UVR results in changes to the dermal connective tissue with degeneration of both collagen and elastic fibres. New elastotic tissue grows but in a disorganized fashion, resulting in solar elastosis. This is characterized by yellowish, leathery thickening of the skin. These changes lead to a loss of the normal mechanical properties of the skin with increased wrinkling and telangiectasia caused by poor support of dermal blood vessels.

Melanocytes

Damaged and inactivated melanocytes can lead to areas of cutaneous hypopigmentation. Some melanocytes can enlarge and produce excess pigment, leading to the formation of solar lentigos.

TYPES OF UV MACHINES AND LIGHT SOURCES

Phototherapy and PUVA are complex. Equipment available in a busy phototherapy unit may include one or more PUVA cabinets, a canopy, a pair of hand-and-foot units, a phototherapy comb and separate UVB cabinets and canopies which may be broadband or narrowband or may be combined UVA and UVB machines with radiometers for UVA and UVB. The photodynamic equipment may vary in size, shape and treatment abilities. The list is endless and appropriate equipment should be selected for safe, effective treatment of patients.

Artificial sources of UVR can cause injury to the skin and the eyes. Safety in the therapeutic use of UVR should be paramount.

1. Goggles must always be worn by patients receiving phototherapy. UVB radiation is potentially more dangerous than UVA. Patients receiving systematic PUVA should wear UVA-resistant glasses for 24 hours following oral administration of psoralens.
2. Male patients should protect genitalia with appropriate clothing as male genitalia are particularly susceptive to the carcinogenic effects of PUVA.

3. Patients, especially PUVA patients, should minimize direct exposure to sunlight during the course of UV treatment.

Other safety measures, including the accurate calibration of machines, dosimetry and record keeping, are all essential in patient radiation protection.

Protection of visitors and staff

Phototherapy machines should be adequately shielded; drawn curtains are sufficient. Staff must protect their eyes if directly exposed to UVR, especially when using unenclosed hand-and-foot units and when performing MED testing (see p. 72). All exposed skin, e.g. arms, neck and face, should be adequately protected by clothing, high-factor sunscreen or face shield. The level of UVB in a phototherapy room is very low as radiation is well contained within the cabinets when doors are fully closed.

PHOTORESPONSIVE DISEASES

Some of the more common conditions treated by UVB or PUVA are shown in Table 4.1.

Indications for treatment

Although it is not understood exactly how phototherapy and photochemotherapy work, there is no doubt about their efficacy in a range of conditions. That, coupled with the freedom from unpleasant topical treatment, accounts for their increase in popularity.

PUVA or UVB may not always be the most suitable treatment for the conditions as shown in Table 4.1 and they have been known to exacerbate the condition rather than help it.

It is important that any patient suspected of having one of the conditions in Table 4.2, especially solar urticaria, should have an extensive and detailed history taken, including monochromator phototesting in a photobiology unit. This will ascertain which wavelength of light is causing the problem.

Table 4.1 Skin conditions treated with UVR

Skin condition	Use/benefits	Type of UVL
Psoriasis	Poor response to topical treatments Chronic plaque Guttate psoriasis Palmo/plantar psoriasis	NBUVB BBUVB PUVA
Eczema	Topical steroid sparing Additional treatment	NBUVB BBUVB PUVA
Mycosis fungoides	Palliative rather than curative PUVA used for thicker lesions	PUVA favoured but UVB can be used Photopheresis (also see Chapter 12)
Vitiligo	Most effective for those affected on face, neck and trunk Skin types IV and V are most likely to benefit Long courses required, usually 50 treatment sessions or more	PUVA
Pruritus	May be beneficial for itch in liver disease, kidney disease or associated with malignancy May be beneficial for itch with no proven cause	BBUVB NBUVB
HIV pruritus	May be beneficial for itch	BBUVB NBUVB PUVA Photophoresis

BBUVB = broad band UVB
NBUVB = narrow band UVB
PUVA = psoralen and UVA
Not all phototherapy units have photopheresis; therefore it is not always an option.

Table 4.2 Some photodermatoses treated with UVB or PUVA

Skin condition	Use/benefits	Type of UVL
Polymorphic light eruption (PLE)	As a desensitization programme Usually given in the springtime or just before the usual onset time	NBUVB BBUVB PUVA It is important to find out which wavelength of light causes the problem
Chronic actinic disease (CAD)	As a desensitizer Patient usually has multiple allergies Most patients respond to sun avoidance Usually found in older men	NBUVB BBUVB PUVA It is important to find out which wavelength of light causes the problem
Actinic prurigo	If unresponsive to conventional treatments Treat as PLE	NBUVB BBUVB PUVA
Solar urticaria (SU)	Detailed phototesting assessment essential to determine initial wavelength Careful screening and observations (advantageous if patient is hospitalized) Treatment for whole surface area of body could be dangerous, therefore should be treated in specialist units. May treat habitually exposed areas only	NBUVB BBUVB PUVA It is most important to find out which wavelength of light causes the problem

Absolute contraindications

The conditions in Box 4.1 should never be treated with UVL as this can and will provoke the condition, which could become life threatening. (These conditions are also provoked by natural daylight.)

Relative contraindications

There are rules that may be broken in certain circumstances. This particularly applies to patients who must be treated where there is no satisfactory alternative. For example, whilst it is recommended not to treat under the age of 16 years, the potential adverse effects in, say, atopic eczema must be weighed against those of the alternative treatment of high-dose systemic steroids.

The suggested lower age limits are only guidelines. PUVA should be considered for children with severe dermatoses unresponsive to safer treatment. The reason behind these guidelines is a child's presumed greater susceptibility to long-term ocular and cutaneous damage.

Box 4.1 Contraindications to therapy are divided into absolute and relative

Absolute	Relative
Xeroderma pigmentosum	**Major**
Gorlin's syndrome	Pregnancy
Hereditary dysplastic naevus syndrome	Porphyria
Lactation	Young age (less than 5 years)
Systemic lupus erythematosus	Previous or current non-malignant melanoma
Dermatomyositis	Previous exposure to arsenic or ionizing radiation
Trichothiodystrophy	
Bloom's syndrome	Current premalignant skin lesion
Cockayne's syndrome	Non-compliant patient
Previous malignant melanoma	
Albinism	**Minor**
	Less than 16 years of age
	Cataracts
	Bullous pemphigoid
	Pemphigus
	Previous or concomitant treatment with methotrexate
	Significant hepatic dysfunction
	Previous internal malignancy

Skin typing

No single treatment protocol is ideal for all patients. Accurate skin assessment must be carried out before every treatment in order to determine the next incremental dose. If the patient states they always burn in the sun you may assume they are type I but they may sometimes tan, in which case they would be type II. As a rule, skin types V and VI are based on pigmentation (Table 4.3).

Skin typing is not a precise method of determining UV dosages and subsequent increments. Patients with the same skin type can react quite differently to the same dose.

An MPD test (see p. 74) should always be performed prior to commencement of PUVA. There are, however, times when this is not possible, e.g. when the skin condition is too extensive or for vitiligo patients. Skin typing and the increment guide then aid assessment (see Increments, p. 74).

Erythema grading

An erythema grading system (Table 4.4) should be used to assess accurately the patient's skin response to therapy, which is then documented at each visit (see Documentation, p. 78).

The system grades the different degrees of pinkness/redness from 0 to 4. This system is particularly important and useful when there is more than one nurse responsible for delivering the UV therapy. Further increments are based on the degree of erythema following the previous UV therapy session; therefore, if it has not been assessed and documented fully, the patient may receive too high a dose. The aim of each session is for the skin to respond at either grade 1 or grade 2 (see Table 4.4).

Table 4.3 Skin typing

Skin type	History
I	White skin, always burns, never tans
II	Usually burns, sometimes tans
III	Sometimes burns, always tans
IV	Never burns, always tans
V	Moderately and heavily pigmented
VI	Black African skin

Table 4.4 Suggested erythema grading

Grade	Erythema
0	No erythema
1	Barely perceptible – faint pink
2	Well-defined asymptomatic erythema – marked
3	Fiery erythema with oedema – red and very sore
4	Severe, fiery erythema with oedema and/or blistering

Table 4.5 PUVA- and UVB-induced erythema

	PUVA	UVB
Onset	12–36 hours	2–6 hours
Normal peak	48–96 hours	12–18 hours
Normal duration	One week	24–48 hours
Extreme peak	Over 96 hours	14–20 hours
Extreme duration	3–6 months	1–2 months

Always ask the patient how they are feeling. Is their skin itchy or sore? Press the skin to assess if there is any blanching and/or pain. It is also helpful to look at untreated skin, e.g. under their pants, if worn, to compare affected and non-affected skin.

The onset and duration of PUVA-induced erythema is quite different from that of UVB (Table 4.5).

UVB PHOTOTHERAPY

UVB is phototherapy which consists of exposing the skin to short-wave ultraviolet radiation. There are two forms of UVB currently in use: broadband (290–350 nm) and narrowband (311–313 nm).

The rationale behind selective UVB is that all wavelengths emitted by broadband are therapeutically important but some of these wavelengths contribute unwanted effects.

Indications for UVB

The range of conditions which respond to UVB is similar to those listed for PUVA. It is primarily used for psoriasis. It is also used when topical treatment fails to adequately control a patient's skin disorder or the patient requires potent topical steroids over an extended period. UVB has no systemic effect so pregnant women/nursing mothers and children can be treated safely. UVB is the therapy of choice before moving to PUVA.

Advantages

UVB therapy compared with PUVA

1. No oral or topical medication.
2. No eye protection necessary following therapy.
3. The incidence of side effects is lower, e.g. nausea.
4. Can be used during pregnancy.
5. Shorter irradiation times (unless bath PUVA).
6. Probably safer than PUVA for children.
7. Possibly less photocarcinogenic.

TLO1 compared with broadband UVB

1. Reduced incidence of burning episodes.
2. Longer remission.
3. Increased efficacy.

Disadvantages

UVB therapy compared with PUVA

1. Given three times weekly (PUVA twice weekly).
2. Remission may in some individuals be shorter with UVB than PUVA.

TLO1 compared with broadband UVB

1. Longer exposure times.
2. Long-term photocarcinogenic effects not known.
3. Safe maximum number of treatments is not yet known.

Many units are using the PUVA guidelines until proven. It is as safe as broadband UVB.

Treatment protocols

The procedure for initiating a course of UVB is similar to that used for PUVA. The patient has a course of treatment prescribed by the consultant dermatologist, a consent form is completed and the patient attends the unit for counselling and explanation of the treatment and routine procedures of the unit.

Minimal erythema dose (MED)

Before treatment is started, a test dose, termed an MED (minimal erythema dose), is performed to determine the correct starting dose for each patient (Box 4.2). This avoids the risk of under- or overdosage at the start of the course of UVB. Underlying photosensitivity which was not identified in the dermatology clinic can be determined.

The MED is performed on the lower back or buttocks. A template is affixed and each square is exposed to a different dose of radiation.

The selection of doses is based on skin type. Six or eight doses may be given.

Box 4.2	Dosages for UVB treatment

Narrowband UVB

Skin types I and II	100	140	200	280	390	550 mJ/cm²
Skin types III and IV	140	200	280	390	550	770 mJ/cm²
Skin type V	280	390	550	770	1100	mJ/cm²

Broadband UVB

| Skin types I and II | 5 | 10 | 15 | 20 | 25 | 30 mJ/cm² |
| Skin types III and IV | 25 | 30 | 35 | 40 | 45 | 50 mJ/cm² |

UVB doses can be measured in time or millijoules per cm² (mJ/cm²). Millijoule dosing (Table 4.6) is preferred as this unit of energy is constant whereas time is directly related to the energy output of a light cabinet. The energy varies as the tubes in the machine get older. The output, which is measured in milliwatts per cm² (mw/cm²), reduces and therefore time needs to increase accordingly.

Narrowband UVB treatment

Psoriasis, eczema, nodular prurigo and urticaria

1. MED is performed and read in 24 hours.
2. Initial dose 70% MED.
3. UVB 3 times weekly, 48-hour minimal interval between each dose.
4. Skin is assessed before each treatment, i.e.:
   - no erythema – 20% increase on previous dose
   - grade 1 (mild erythema) – repeat dose then 10% increase on subsequent visits
   - grade 2 (moderate erythema) – miss one treatment, repeat previous dose then 10% increments thereafter
   - grades 3 and 4 (severe erythema) – reviewed by doctor. May need to stop course or reduce increments as instructed.
5. Course of treatment continues 4 past clearance:
   - About 20 for psoriasis
   - About 30–40 for eczema and nodular prurigo.

Photodermatoses, e.g. polymorphic light eruption (prickly heat) and actinic prurigo

1. MED read in 24 hours.
2. Initial dose 30% MED.
3. UVB three times weekly.
4. Increments 14% each visit.

Skin desensitization or hardening is the aim. Erythemal response is not therapeutic in these conditions.

Adverse events for broadband and narrowband UVB

- If patient cancels/misses one or two treatments, repeat previous dose.
- If patient cancels/misses three treatments, treat with penultimate dose.
- If patient cancels/misses four or more treatments, check dose with doctor.

Table 4.6 Protocols for broadband UVB

Skin type	Initial dose (mJ/cm²)	Subsequent dose (mJ/cm²)
I	5–10	5
II	15–20	5–10
III	25–30	10–15
IV	35–40	15–20
V	45–50	20–25
VI	55–60	30–35

- If patient develops itch, encourage use of prescribed topical steroids and emollients.
- If patient develops facial erythema or unacceptable facial pigmentation, a face shield or sunscreen can be applied before each treatment.
- It is very important to maintain consistency throughout the course of treatment.

Documentation

- It is important to document previous phototherapy or PUVA history, including sunbed usage.
- Current medication.
- Sun exposure history and occupation (i.e. outdoor workers).
- Family history of skin malignancy.
- Skin type and MED result.
- Skin assessment for erythema and response.
- Improvement – slow or rapid.
- Worsening or no change should be noted. Each dose, increment and output of cabinet.

PUVA THERAPY

Mechanism of action of PUVA therapy

We do not know for sure how PUVA therapy works. The aim is to deliver the treatment, obtaining all the benefits, without exposing patients to undue risks from the side effects. PUVA can also be given with retinoids and is then called re-PUVA. Retinoids can make the skin more susceptible to UVL, as do many other systemic treatments.

Psoralen compounds

Psoralen is a substance that sensitizes the patient's body surface area to ultraviolet light (UVL) for up to 24 hours after ingestion, less if applied topically. It is imperative that the patient does not expose any of their skin to any other form of UVL during this period, other than the prescribed amount of UVA when they visit the hospital. (This includes natural daylight.)

Systemic psoralens

The doctor initiating the treatment plan prescribes the appropriate dose of psoralens. Psoralens taken by mouth are distributed more or less evenly throughout the body, including the eyes.

Topical bath/soaks

Topical bath PUVA is only suitable for large areas of skin involvement, preferably the whole body and generally only those parts which can be immersed in bath water.

Emulsion, paints or gels

Applying these to the affected skin is easy but almost impossible to repeat consistently from one treatment to another. There is only a very low risk of systemic absorption with the topical treatments compared with oral psoralens. The selected topical treatment is applied and left in situ for a determined amount of time prior to exposure to the correct dosage of UVA.

This form of PUVA therapy avoids most of the unwanted side effects of systemic PUVA, e.g. nausea and the need for eye protection. The amount of nursing time taken to treat patients with topical psoralens should not be underestimated.

Mechanism of action

Systemic psoralen compounds are absorbed unchanged through the gastric mucosa and are gradually absorbed and excreted by the liver over a period of 12–24 hours. Topical psoralen is absorbed locally through the epidermis.

Psoralen dosages

Psoralens can be prescribed either by:

- finding out the patient's body surface area and calculating the required dose of psoralen or
- weighing the patient and calculating the amount of psoralen required per kilogram of weight. For MPD, see page 74

Adverse effects

Common acute effects

- *Nausea and/or vomiting* – this is more common with 8-MOP than 5-MOP (psoralens).
- *Excessive erythema* – can be minimized by careful assessment of the patient's skin prior to each treatment.
- *Pruritus* – this is a common symptom of dry skin conditions. Encourage frequent liberal applications of an appropriate emollient.
- *PUVA itch* – described as a deep burning sensation, a feeling of insects crawling under the skin. The common sites are upper chest, outer aspects of the arms and thighs, breasts and buttocks. PUVA is either stopped for 1–2 weeks or until the itch is resolved. Occasionally the treatment ceases altogether.

Less common acute effects

- *Friction blisters* – this can happen when the patient's treatment dose is close to their erythema threshold and their clothing rubs their skin (or skin folds rub), causing blistering.
- *Herpes simplex* – these may occur in patients with a preexisting history.
- *Photoonycholysis* – painful white or yellow discoloration of one or more nails.

Chronic effects

- *Ocular damage* – proper eye protection should be worn (see below).
- *Skin cancer* – treatment doses and cumulative doses should be kept to a minimum. The importance of not using sunbeds should be stressed to the patient, especially whilst receiving UVB or PUVA therapy as this will increase the cumulative dose, which in turn could lead to skin cancer.

Contraindications

There are rules that may in special circumstances be broken. This applies to patients who must be treated when there is no other satisfactory alternative.

Eye and skin protection

The psoralen is distributed around the tissues of the body, including the lens and cornea of the eyes. For this reason, it is imperative that from the time the psoralens are ingested and for the following 24 hours, UV safety glasses are worn (except when sleeping). The glasses should be a recommended pair, with UVL side filters, provided by the hospital. The patient may remove the glasses if there is no UVA present. They must bear in mind that a small amount of UVA is emitted from fluorescent tubes and sunbeds and not just by natural daylight.

Treatment

Minimal phototoxic dose (MPD)

Using a template on a small area of unaffected skin, usually on the back or the buttocks, the skin is irradiated with 6–8 different doses of UVA 1–2 hours after psoralen ingestion and the result read 72 hours later. An MPD is the lowest dose of UVA which provokes a barely perceptible erythema on the skin. Except in exceptional circumstances, an MPD should always be performed.

Increments

The initial dose is 70% of the MPD followed by increments of 10%, 20% or 40% of the previous dose, at every treatment, alternate treatments or weekly, dependent on skin condition and skin type.

When not using MPD testing, a guide to starting doses and subsequent increments can be based on skin type, as in Table 4.7.

These are guidelines only; the patient's response to the previous dose will determine the next dose.

Table 4.7 Guidelines for starting doses and increments

Skin type	Starting dose (J/cm²)	Increment (J/cm²)
I	0.5	0.5
II	1	1
III	1.5	1.5
IV	2	2
V	2.5	2–2.5
VI	3	2.5–3

Protocols for specific conditions

Psoriasis. The aim is to clear the psoriasis as quickly as possible, reaching the highest dose necessary with the minimum of treatments. (Too slowly and the patient will have a higher treatment number and higher cumulative dose.)

Vitiligo. Treat as skin type I because you are treating areas of skin with little or no pigmentation.

Mycosis fungoides. Start at $0.5–1 \, J/cm^2$, depending on skin type. An MPD is used when possible. PUVA therapy can be given on the same day as local radiotherapy.

Atopic eczema. Both adults and children can be treated with PUVA. If a child is to commence PUVA therapy they and their parent(s) will require pretreatment counselling and orientation by the nursing staff to discuss the general precautions and the instructions for PUVA.

Polymorphic light eruption (PLE). As a guideline, PUVA is an effective prophylactic treatment, usually given in the spring. Exposed sites only or complete body PUVA therapy can be given for this condition. Starting doses can be initiated in one of two ways:

1. an MPD and increasing by 10% at every visit or
2. starting at $0.5 \, J/cm^2$ and increasing by 40% increments.

The patient's skin should be assessed at every visit to check for any evidence of the condition erupting. These are guidelines only as each patient differs.

PHOTODYNAMIC THERAPY

In 1903, von Tappeiner and Jesseiner used eosin as a photosensitizer with natural and artificial light.

Those treating patients with skin cancer, lupus of the skin and condylomata of the female genitalia reported that it was an oxygen-dependent process and coined the term photodynamic therapy (or PDT for convenience).

PDT uses a combination of:

- a photosensitizer, generally a porphyrin derivative, and
- a light source, emitting radiation in the absorption spectrum of the photosensitizer.

The photosensitizer is introduced into the tissues being treated, either systemically or topically, and excited by the electromagnetic radiation from the light source to bring about the therapeutic effects from the photochemical reactions.

How it works

PDT works by generating photosensitized molecules by the action of light of certain wavelengths (usually around 630–700 nm) causing energy-dependent cytotoxicity, leading to destruction of the dysplasia. PDT is being used by surgeons to treat bladder, oesophageal, stomach and early-stage lung cancers, which are usually treated intraluminally by lasers, which is the most common source of light for the photoactivation of photosensitizers in PDT.

Dermatologists are also interested in PDT for the treatment of superficial skin carcinomas, precancerous lesions and psoriasis.

Effectiveness

Trials have shown that:

- treatment of Bowen's disease using 5-amino laevulinic acid (ALA) has a 90–100% complete response rate and recurrence of 0–9% after 14–18 months
- treatment of superficial basal cell carcinoma (BCC) has 87.6–100% complete response rate and recurrence of 2–43% after 12–17 months
- treatment of nodular BCC has a complete response in 35% of cases, 85% for BCCs less than 1 mm thick and 50% for those more than 1 mm thick.

Procedure

Equipment required will normally include:

- a dressing pack
- normal saline for washing off scale
- opaque dressings (gauze is adequate)
- eye protection for patient and staff against the wavelengths being used

- photosensitizer (usually 5-ALA)
- cotton buds for topical application of preparation
- Micropore tape or similar, for fixing dressings to the surrounding skin
- Melolin/Telfa/nonadherent dressings
- radiation source (such as Waldmann PDT 1200 or similar high-power radiation source).

Patient instruction and information should be given verbally and in writing, for the patient to take home and read carefully, and comprises at least the following two phases.

Advice relating to the treatment period

The patient should be informed that:

- the procedure is non-invasive
- the ALA occasionally stings on application
- the lesion(s) should not be exposed to light once the ALA has been applied
- the procedure may be uncomfortable, but most patients can tolerate PDT without the use of a local anaesthetic but this will be made available if needed (plain lignocaine should be used)
- depending on its type, the light source may feel hot, sometimes described as the feeling of sunlight through a magnifying glass on the skin
- the lesion starts to smart and feel 'burning' within a couple of minutes but this remains more or less constant during the treatment, so if it can be tolerated for the first few minutes, a local anaesthetic will probably not be required
- the discomfort settles shortly after the light source is switched off.

Advice relating to the postprocedural period

The patient should be informed that:

- the lesion may blister and ooze for a few days
- the surrounding skin may become quite red
- a crust will form 7–10 days after the procedure, which will then fall off after 1–3 weeks, depending on the site of the lesion
- once the crust has come away, new skin will be revealed underneath.

Method

The procedures must be explained carefully to the patient (and carer, if appropriate) and the patient should give signed consent to the treatment, with an opportunity to ask questions.

The lesion should be prepared, debriding as much as possible using forceps and washing off with sterile saline. The photosensitizer is applied, covering the lesion completely with a margin, and rubbed in gently with a cottonbud. The area is then covered with Tegaderm and opaque dressing for 4 hours (solar keratoses or Bowen's lesions; up to 6 hours for BCCs).

When the patient returns to the clinic for the radiation part of the treatment, the source needs to be positioned carefully about 10–20 cm from the lesion (or as appropriate for the light source characteristics) and the output checked with a meter calibrated for use with the source wavelengths.

The exposure time is computed in the same way as for UV therapy and the timer set. The patient's healthy skin should be covered as far as possible and a portable fan may be switched on to keep the area cool. When all is set up and the patient is relaxed and comfortable, the light source can be switched on. Some patients may require a local anaesthetic (3–10 ml of 1% lignocaine).

Calculation of the exposure time

$$\text{Time (in seconds)} = \frac{\text{required dose (in millijoules/cm}^2)}{\text{output (in milliwatts/cm}^2)}$$

For example, if the patient is to be given a total dose of 150 J/cm^2 to the lesion, the exposure time using a 100 mW/cm^2 lamp will be given by:

$$\frac{150\,000}{100} = 1500 \text{ seconds}$$

(÷ by 60 to obtain exposure in minutes = 25 minutes)

For a higher powered source, a treatment time of 12–20 minutes is typical, depending on the patient's tolerance. Note that a lower output from the source will result in less discomfort but a longer time in the treatment position, which may be uncomfortable in itself.

Advice on discharge from the clinic

The patient should be advised:

- to keep the lesion clean and dry
- to apply a little Vaseline around the area
- not to apply dressings unless the lesion is oozing plasma
- to bathe and shower normally (and to ensure that the treated area is carefully and thoroughly dried afterwards)
- that the discomfort will stop as soon as the light source is switched off but it may linger for 24 hours or so. Paracetamol can be taken as required to relieve the discomfort.

Patient review

It is important to ensure that the patient is seen by the clinic or GP:

- at 1 week, to ensure there is no postprocedural infection
- at 1 month, to ensure that the wound has healed correctly and to check for retreatment, if necessary
- at 6 months, to check for any need for retreatment
- and at 1 year, to ensure that all traces of the lesion have been removed.

Advantages of PDT

1. Convenient
2. Specific, and several lesions may be treated at one session
3. Non-invasive, and only diseased tissue is destroyed
4. Suitable for elderly patients, and gives good results in poorly vascularized skin
5. At least as effective as cryotherapy
6. Generally well tolerated

Limitations of PDT

Optical penetration of 630 nm radiation (red visible light) is of the order of 1–5 mm, so the criterion for treatment of superficial BCCs is that they should be less than 1 mm thick, demonstrated by a 3–4 mm punch biopsy.

Some patients cannot tolerate the burning sensation caused by the photoactivation of the ALA during treatment.

RESPONSIBILITIES OF THE NURSE

- It should be the doctor's responsibility to explain the treatment and the adverse effects and to obtain written consent.
- Following this initial consultation with the doctor, the nurse should conduct a pretreatment interview with the patient, including a nursing assessment. This is to ensure that the patient fully understands the treatment, possible adverse effects and the precautions needed during therapy.
- Present medication and any new medication started during the course of treatment, including over-the-counter products, should be documented. There are a number of oral drugs and topical treatments that can cause photosensitivity.
- A demonstration of the machines and orientation of the unit, including meeting other members of staff, will help to alleviate anxiety for the patient.
- The patient should be instructed as to the correct dosage of psoralens and what time to take them, including the wearing of eye protection.
- The patient should be advised to avoid alcohol on the days of treatment.
- Stress the importance of avoiding other forms of sun exposure, i.e. sun bathing or using sunbeds, during treatment courses.
- Advise on protecting the skin with clothing, i.e. long sleeves, trousers, hats and gloves. Loose-weave clothes allow UVA to penetrate.
- Advise the patient on general topical skin care.
- Keep the machines clean between each patient.
- Document and sign for every treatment, informing the doctor of any problems.
- On completion of the course, a clinic appointment should be made for review by the doctor so the course can be documented in the medical notes and progress monitored.

The maximum number of treatments a patient can receive is 200 which may only be up to 10 courses in a patient's lifetime. Psoriasis is often troublesome as it may need more than the restricted one course per year, so patients should be advised to use this precious treatment wisely.

STAFF TRAINING

The main aim of the phototherapy unit is to give safe and effective treatment to all patients and therefore maximize benefits and minimize adverse effects. Nurses undertaking this role should ensure that they have been properly trained and have the necessary knowledge and skills before starting treatments. This will help to ensure the minimum standards of nursing care and satisfy the UKCC *Scope of professional practice* and the RCN *Standards of care for dermatology nursing*. An appropriately trained and experienced person, who provides a formal structured programme, should facilitate this training.

The level of ultraviolet radiation in the phototherapy room is very low as the radiation is well contained within the cabinets when the doors are fully closed. It is therefore safe for staff to operate the machines without the need for eye protection. However, staff should wear eye protection, sunblocks and protective clothing when checking that all the lamps are functioning.

Nurses must take responsibility for their own practice, ensuring that the treatment given is research based and follows established guidelines and/or protocols which are current and updated. Nurses should be both competent and confident, especially if working in a nurse-led clinic with little access to a doctor's opinion. They must also ensure that the equipment used is regularly serviced and calibrated and meets health and safety guidelines.

DOCUMENTATION

Maintaining accurate and legible documentation is the responsibility of both the doctor and the nurse working in a phototherapy unit. The doctor is responsible for the initial referral, the pretreatment assessment, updating of medical and PUVA notes and written instructions for any changes in the treatment plan.

The nurse's responsibilities are for ensuring that the PUVA notes contain all the necessary information to provide safe and effective treatment. The nurse has a legal responsibility to provide a comprehensive picture of care delivered, associated outcomes, pertinent information regarding the patient and the measures taken to respond to identified needs. All entries must be relevant, accurate, legible, dated and signed.

A record book should be kept of all incidents, including those that happen to patients, relatives and staff, so that the phototherapy unit can be seen to be safe, effective and efficient.

Records should also be kept of equipment used, when and how serviced and maintained. Recorded in this book should be the readings of the lamp intensity, which must be checked and recorded regularly.

CONCLUSION

The main aim of ultraviolet light treatment is to obtain the benefits that derive from the appropriate therapies without exposing the patient to undue risks from unwanted side effects. This is difficult and sometimes we have to accept a compromise, as in most medical interventions. An ongoing and cumulative dose should always be documented, as any one patient can only have a limit of 1000 J/cm^2 of PUVA in a lifetime. There is at present no documented information as to the amount of UVB one can safely receive during a lifetime but the ongoing and cumulative dose should always be recorded.

REFERENCES

El Mofty A M 1968 Vitiligo and psoralens. Pergamon Press, Oxford

Fritsch P, Hönigsmann H, Jeschke E, Wolff K 1978 Photochemotherapie bei psoriasis: steigerung der wirksamkeit durch ein orales aromatisches. Retinoid Dtsch Med Wochenscher 103: 1731–1736

Parrish J A, Fitzpatrick T B, Tanenbaum L, Pathak M A 1974 Photochemotherapy of psoriasis with oral methoxsalen and longwave ultraviolet light. New England Journal of Medicine 291: 1207–1211

FURTHER READING

Abel E A 1992 Phototherapy in dermatology. Igaku-Shoin, New York & Tokyo, pp 289–308

British Photodermatology Group 1994 British photodermatology guidelines for PUVA. British Journal of Dermatology 130: 246–255

Collins L, Anstey A Protection against ultraviolet radiation in the workplace. Training Manual for Phototherapists. Glan Hafren NHS Trust, Royal Gwent Hospital, Wales

Dermatology Nurses' Association 1994 Phototherapy core curriculum. ICN Pharmaceuticals, California

Diffey B L 1982 UV radiation in medicine (MPH). Adam Hilger

Drake L A et al 1994 Guidelines of care for phototherapy and photochemotherapy. Journal of Academic Dermatology 31: 643–648

Drugs that cause photosensitivity 1995. Medical letter 37: 35–36

Hawk J M L 1982 Responses of normal skin to ultraviolet radiation. In: Regan J D, Parish J A The science of photomedicine. Plenum Press, New York, pp 219–260

Kligman L H, Kligman A M 1986 The Nature of photoageing: it's prevention and repair. Photodermatology 3: 215–227

McClelland P 1991 PUVA staff training manual – a practical guide for professionals. ICN Pharmaceuticals, California

Morrison W L 1991 Phototherapy and photochemotherapy of skin disease, 2nd edn. Raven Press, New York

Roelandts R 1991 The history of photochemotherapy. Photodermatol Photoimmunol Photomed 8: 184–189

Royal College of Nursing 1995 Standards of care for dermatology nursing. RCN, London, pp 17–18

Stern R S et al 1990 Genital tumors among men with psoriasis exposed to psoralens and ultraviolet A radiation (PUVA) and ultraviolet B radiation. New England Journal of Medicine 322: 1093–1097

UKCC Administration of Medicines

UKCC Exercising Accountability

UKCC Standards of Records and Record Keeping

Van Weelden H et al 1990 Comparison of narrowband UV-B phototherapy and PUVA photochemotherapy in the treatment of psoriasis.

5

Dermatological surgery and cryosurgery

Fiona Pringle

Surgical procedures and interventions form an increasingly important part of dermatology practice in both primary and secondary health-care settings. The range of surgical procedures is wide and can vary from the diagnostic biopsy used to establish or confirm a diagnosis to Mohs' micrographic surgery for the excision of invasive basal cell carcinomas (BCC). It has been estimated that up to 40% of dermatology referrals to consultant dermatologists are surgically related (BAD 1994).

SURGERY

Skin cancer is the most common form of cancer and accounts for 0.46% of all deaths. Whilst every year 40 000 people in the UK contract skin cancer, the surgical removal of malignant lesions only accounts for a small proportion of all lesions treated.

Skin cancers can be divided into three groups: benign, premalignant and malignant. The most common conditions requiring surgical intervention are shown in Table 5.1.

Types of surgical procedure

Surgical procedures of differing complexity will require facilities of different standards. Diagnostic biopsies, curettage and cautery and other procedures where no suturing is involved may take place in a clinic or designated biopsy room, provided adequate arrangements are made to provide a clean area in which to work.

Table 5.1 Common lesions requiring surgical removal

Lesion group	Type of lesion	Features
Benign lesions	Dermatofibroma	Pink-brown colour, nodular, asymptomatic
	Seborrhoeic warts	Variably hyperpigmented warty plaques with greasy surface. Sharply demarcated edges
	Viral warts	Commonly found on face, hands, knees and feet
Premalignant lesions	Actinic keratosis	Itchy, scaly, pink-grey hyperkeratosis on sun-exposed areas. Common in elderly fair-skinned people
	Bowen's disease	Pink, scaly, crusted lesion with slow growth pattern
	Lentigo maligna	Flat brown lesions. Irregular pigmentation
Malignant lesions	Basal cell carcinoma	*Morphoeic* – waxy, indurated plaques. Indistinct borders *Nodular* – raised with translucent pearly borders. May ulcerate in centre *Superficial* – spreading flat, red, scaly patches
	Malignant melanoma	Irregular pigmentation, asymmetric borders. Diameter greater than 4 mm
	Squamous cell carcinoma	Indurated, expanding nodule usually on preexisting damaged skin

However, full-thickness skin excisions for diagnostic or curative purposes, which are repaired with layered suturing, should ideally only take place in a fully equipped sterile operating theatre. A quality service should include:

- a specified dermatology operating theatre, equipped with appropriate instruments and facilities
- a defined caseload
- trained nursing staff, accustomed to assisting with dermatological procedures or trained to carry out some procedures themselves (BAD 1994).

One of the most important issues in dermatological surgery is the good practice of sending all specimens for histological examination. It may appear unnecessary to send all specimens to histopathology but, unless they are, a melanoma may be missed, to the patient's detriment (Lask & Moy 1996).

Equipment

Skin biopsy packs will vary from department to department depending on the type of surgery performed and the preference of the clinician. The basic biopsy pack should contain the following instruments (Heard 1998):

- sharp scissors

- skin hook
- scalpel handle
- suture holders
- mosquito forceps
- sterile towel
- gauze.

In addition, the following will be required:

- skin cleanser
- a sterile no. 10, 15 or 22 scalpel blade
- a selection of sutures.

Local anaesthesia

In cutaneous surgery most local anaesthesia is produced by direct infiltration into the skin. Field blocks, peripheral nerve blocks and topical anaesthesia are also used. As with the administration of all drugs, there is a small risk that the patient may suffer an allergic reaction to the anaesthetic (Auletta 1994).

Methylparabens is used as a preservative in the multidose vials of lignocaine and may cause allergic reactions in PABA-sensitive individuals. The early symptoms of an anaphylactic reaction are: pruritus, urticaria and erythema, nausea, vomiting, abdominal cramps, diarrhoea, coughing, wheezing, dyspnoea, cyanosis and laryngeal oedema. The immediate treatment is adrenaline 0.2–0.5 mg by subcutaneous injection.

Lignocaine

Lignocaine 0.5–2.0% is the most important local anaesthetic. It is available with or without adrenaline 1/80 000 to 1/200 000. In addition to its anaesthetic action, it causes mild vasodilatation and adrenaline counteracts this. The maximum safe adult dose is 200 mg (or 3 mg/kg) for plain lignocaine and 500 mg (or 7 mg/kg) for lignocaine with adrenaline (Erksson 1979).

Achieving haemostasis

Haemostasis starts with the preoperative assessment and accurate recording of the patient's medical history. Any bleeding tendencies and drugs such as aspirin or warfarin should be taken into consideration when planning surgery and, if necessary, the operation should be delayed until the effect of any drugs has worn off. Local anaesthetics containing adrenaline are very useful in controlling general ooze but at least 5 minutes must elapse after injecting the local anaesthetic to allow time for vasoconstriction to occur.

Intraoperative haemostasis may be achieved using light pressure. This clears pools of blood away from the operating field and is often all that is necessary to control small vessel bleeding.

It may be necessary to clamp larger vessels if the bleeding persists. Vessels over 1 mm in diameter should be ligated with an absorbable suture such as a 3/0 Vicryl tie.

Diathermy

This is used as either unipolar or bipolar.

Unipolar. The circuit is made from the machine through a single wire to the patient. Usually forceps are used to conduct the current. The return to the machine is via a pad usually strapped to the patient's leg.

Bipolar. With this method the current passes down one limb of a forceps across the intervening gap if it is filled by a conducting medium and up the other limb of the forceps to return to the machine. Thus, only the material grasped between the tips of the forceps is cauterized, so minimizing tissue damage.

Electrocautery

This is the use of a high-amperage, low-voltage electric current to heat wire or a filament which causes thermal damage. The current does not pass through the patient. The advantages of electrocautery are that it is self-sterilizing and safe to use with electronic equipment such as pacemakers.

Topical haemostatic agents

These can be divided into agents such as Oxycal and Gelfoam which cause no necrosis and are slowly absorbed but which may lead to increased risk of infection, and caustic agents such as Monsel's solution and aluminium chloride, which probably act as protein-precipitating agents. The caustic agents should not be used in wounds to be sutured as they may cause excessive necrosis. They are most useful for wounds left to heal by secondary intention, e.g. shave biopsy wounds. Silver nitrate sticks are also useful in this context but may cause tattooing if they are enclosed within a wound.

Postoperative pressure

Manual pressure over the wound for 20 minutes after surgery is very useful in preventing haematomas. This can be combined with elevation of the treated part. If the part is accessible, a pressure bandage for 24 hours is helpful and, in some sites such as ears, is mandatory.

If bleeding occurs postoperatively, elevate the affected part and apply pressure for 30 minutes without interruption. If bleeding still persists the wound must be explored, the bleeding vessel ligated and the haematoma removed.

Postoperative dressings

The purpose of a dressing is threefold.

1. To immobilize the wound and stabilize the skin edges.
2. To prevent the formation of oedema and haematoma.
3. To keep the wound clean and to prevent infection.

In general, a dressing suitable for an elliptical excision may consist of a small strip of dressing gauze directly over the wound and the whole clean area covered with a transparent semipermeable membrane such as Tegaderm or Op-site. This type of dressing enables observation of the area around the wound without disturbing it. However, there are no hard and fast rules and individual preference for dressings will develop (Burge et al 1996).

Punch biopsy

Diagnostic biopsies are performed to establish or confirm a diagnosis. When the full thickness of the skin needs to be assessed, a punch or incisional biopsy is performed. Incisional biopsies can be performed using a sterile no. 15 scalpel blade. Punch biopsies are disposable circular blades which come in a variety of sizes, from 2 to 7 mm diameter. The punch is placed on the anaesthetized area and downward pressure applied. The punch is rotated to ensure the cutting action before being removed from the skin. The section of tissue can then be removed using a skin hook or forceps. It may be necessary to use a sterile blade to cut the base of the specimen away from the site.

Curettage

Curettage is well established as a diagnostic and therapeutic technique and is often used for the removal of seborrhoeic warts and verrucas, leaving a wound similar to a deep graze. The conventional instrument used is the sharp spoon curette (Fig. 5.1). Seborrhoeic warts typically appear as if stuck on the skin and it is easy to lift them off with a curette. The skin surrounding the lesion is held taut between the fingers of one hand and the curette should be held firmly in the other hand as if holding a racket handle. A quick striking movement across the skin will often cause the wart to separate (Motley 1997).

However, there are several disadvantages inherent in the spoon curette. The curette should be capable of cutting cleanly but if not regularly sharpened, becomes blunt and then does not

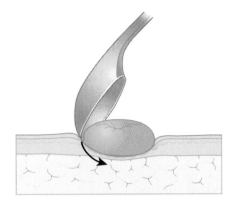

Figure 5.1　Spoon curette in action.

function effectively. A blunt spoon curette is generally distressing and unpleasant for the patient because of the pressure that must be exerted on the skin. Consequently, the wound does not heal as readily and the quality of any tissue samples obtained is poor (Breuninger 1996).

A more modern alternative to the spoon curette has now been developed, the disposable ring curette, which is available in two sizes (4 mm and 7 mm). The ring curette is a circular blade with a sharp cutting edge. The excellent cutting properties of the ring curette allow it to be used for indications other than those for which a sharp spoon was previously used; for example, the debridement of necrotic tissue from a leg ulcer or for performing shave excisions.

Shave excision

Tangential (shave) excisions are an ideal method for removing raised lesions such as seborrhoeic warts or skin tags. The lesion is excised using a scalpel or razor blade held parallel to the skin (Fig. 5.2). Single-edged razor blades have been developed for this purpose. The resulting wound is similar to that of a graze.

Excisional biopsy

Excisional biopsies are necessary if the lesion to be removed is too large for a punch biopsy. To ensure an acceptable cosmetic result, fusiform elliptical excisions are the preferred method of

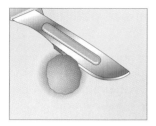

Figure 5.2   Tangential excision using a razor blade.

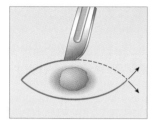

Figure 5.3   Elliptical excision.

removal. The area to be removed should be marked using a skin marker, taking into consideration the relaxed tension lines so that the line of the sutured wound runs along them. Before attempting to operate on any area of the skin, the clinician should consider the underlying structures, especially those arteries and nerves close to the skin surface.

The skin is cut in the shape of an ellipse, with a length-to-width ratio of 3:1. The scalpel is held so that the point is vertical as it enters the skin at the apex of the ellipse (Fig. 5.3). The skin is cut to the other apex and then repeated on the other side of the wound. The specimen is then lifted using a skin hook to prevent the tissue being crushed and the base cut square across. The resulting wound is then sutured.

Mohs' surgery

Mohs' micrographic surgery was first developed in 1932 by Dr Frederic Mohs as a technique for removing skin cancers which enables the surgeon to immediately evaluate the extent of tumour spread by microscopic examination of the tissue margins (Coleman et al 1983). Mohs'

surgery can be time consuming and difficult to perform so patients need to be carefully selected prior to undergoing this type of surgery.

The main indications for using Mohs' micrographic surgery as opposed to simple excision are as follows.

- Recurrent skin tumour
- Large tumour
- Tumour present in a young adult
- Location of tumour in an area of high recurrence (e.g. lip, ear, nose)
- Location of tumour on or adjacent to a critical functional or cosmetic structure (e.g. eyelid, nasal folds)
- Indistinct clinical borders
- Aggressive growth pattern

(Ratner & Grande 1994)

There are several steps involved in performing the procedure.

1. Under local anaesthesia, the tumour is debulked using a curette. This defines the gross margins of the tumour. Tumour tissue is softer and more friable than normal tissue and a gentle scraping of the lesion is usually sufficient to remove the bulk of the tumour and to give an approximation of its extent.
2. The tumour is excised in a saucer-like configuration. A reference map is drawn showing the anatomical locations and configurations of the specimen (Fig. 5.4).
3. The specimen is then divided into sections and numbered on the map (Fig. 5.5).

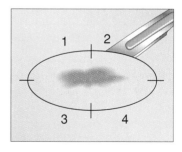

Figure 5.4   Reference map for anatomical location and configurations (reproduced with the permission of St John's Institute of Dermatology).

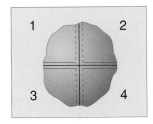

Figure 5.5 Numbering of sections.

4. The edges of two or more adjacent sides of each section are dyed. These are then indicated correspondingly on the reference map.
5. In the laboratory the technician freezes the excised tissue and horizontal cuts from each of the sections are taken. Once stained, the frozen sections can be examined microscopically. This process takes approximately 45–60 minutes.
6. Any residual tumour found on microscopic examination can be localized with reference to the dyed edges and the exact location can be plotted on the reference map (Fig. 5.6). The areas of remaining tumour are located on the wound itself, marked and removed (Allen 1990) (Fig. 5.7). The entire process is repeated until no more tumour is found.

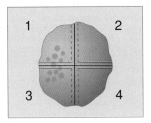

Figure 5.6 Plotting the location of residual tumour.

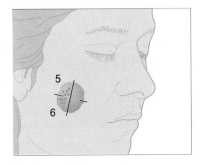

Figure 5.7 Removal of remaining tumour.

Nursing care of patients undergoing surgery

The role of the nurse in caring for patients undergoing any type of skin surgery is vital preoperatively. The patient must be prepared both physically and psychologically for the procedure. The patient's level of anxiety may be significantly reduced by a comprehensive explanation of what will be involved, including the fact that the patient will be awake during the procedure.

Preoperative nursing role

For patients undergoing extensive surgery such as Mohs' surgery, a full nursing assessment should be made and preoperative vital signs recorded. In most cases of simple shave excisions and punch biopsies, formal documentation is unnecessary. However, it is vital that any allergies or use of anticoagulant therapy are documented. Prior to undergoing any surgery, however minor, the nurse must assess the patient's readiness for surgery and ensure that they fully understand the procedure to be performed (Whyte 1994) (Table 5.2).

Communication is vital, both verbal and written. Unlike many surgical procedures where the patient is given a general anaesthetic and wakes up with a neat incision in an area that can most often be covered with clothing, removal of a skin cancer by Mohs' surgery often requires long periods of waiting, repeated layers of tissue removal and periods of discomfort. The entire procedure is performed under local anaesthesia and so the patient can become anxious. Recognition and relief of tension can be accomplished through the relationship developed with the patient and their family throughout the procedure.

Perioperative nursing role

During the procedure the nurse is required not only to assist the medical team but also to monitor the patient and ensure that they are comfortable and stable.

Immediately before the surgery commences, the consent form should be checked to ensure

Table 5.2   Preoperative nursing care

Nursing action	Rationale
Ascertain whether preoperative education has been assimilated by patient	To determine whether the patient understands the reasons for surgery
Assess anxiety levels and ability to tolerate procedure	Anxious patients may not be able to tolerate procedure under local anaesthetic and may require a sedative
	Physical disabilities such as hearing loss or arthritis may impair patient's tolerance of procedure
Record patient's vital signs and assess mental status	Is the patient alert and fully aware of the procedure they are to undergo?
Review and document medical history, especially in relation to:	
Diabetes	Consider time of day procedure is to take place in relation to meals, so that food intake and drug regimen can be modified if necessary
Heart disease	If recent MI then defer operation for at least 6 months. If pacemaker fitted then consider type of diathermy used
Epilepsy	Lignocaine may need to be limited
Record any history of allergies or allergic reactions	It is essential to check whether patients have an allergy to topical or systemic medicaments, in particular antibiotics and local anaesthetics, as well as sensitivities to Elastoplast or latex
Assess patient for history of healing and scarring	Discuss likelihood of formation of keloids and length of healing. Severe cases may require referral to plastic surgeon for reconstruction
Assess social history	Does patient live alone? Need for district nurse input postoperatively? Transport to and from hospital?
Ensure written consent has been obtained	Patient must be fully informed about procedure. Written consent is required from a parent or guardian for patients under the age of 16

that it has been correctly filled in and signed by both doctor and patient and any questions the patient may have answered and anxieties allayed. If the patient is very anxious it may be necessary to give a mild sedative such as diazepam. Any medication currently being taken should be documented. The surgical tray should be checked for any extra instruments that may be needed and cautery and suction obtained. The patient may be required to change into a theatre gown. This not only reduces the risk of infection but prevents their own clothes from being damaged by blood spills.

Throughout the operation the patient is monitored for side effects of the local anaesthetic and to ensure that they are comfortable and free from pain. Verbal communication with the patient during the procedure is im-portant so that the patient is aware of what is happening.

The nurse will also assist the doctor in circulating and gathering necessary supplies and equipment, providing haemostasis and assisting with the closure of the wound.

Postoperative nursing role

Depending on the type of wound closure, for example whether the wound is sutured or left to heal by secondary intention, the wound will need dressing. The skin will need cleansing using sterile saline to remove any blood and then a dressing applied. Many factors will influence the choice and size of dressing, the need for non-adherent dressings, antibiotic ointments and the use of pressure dressings.

Once the dressing has been completed, the patient should be given written as well as verbal wound care instructions (Box 5.1). If the dressing needs to be replaced at home then adequate supplies of dressings should be given to the patient. It may be necessary to arrange for a district nurse to change the dressings initially. The patient should be made aware of the signs and symptoms of postoperative complications such as infection and given the contact telephone number of the department in case of problems. It is important that the patient has adequate postoperative analgesia to take home with them.

A follow-up appointment should be scheduled to assess the rate of healing and to change the dressings. The timing of this will depend on individual departments' preferences. On discharge home, a letter should be sent to the patient's GP informing them of the surgery undertaken and the postoperative dressing regime.

Box 5.1   Sample of postoperative patient information sheet

Following your minor operation:

Please contact your General Practitioner's Surgery to have the stitches removed in .... days.

Wound care
1. You are advised to keep the initial dressing dry and do not remove for 24–48 hours.
2. After this, you can either leave the wound open to the air or re-cover the wound with either a waterproof plaster or a dry gauze dressing.

Washing
1. You can get the wound wet but do not soak it.
2. Pat the area dry thoroughly after washing.

If the wound is on your upper body, do not do any energetic exercise and be careful not to do any vigorous movement which might tear out the stitches.
   If, following the operation, the area is uncomfortable then you may take a painkiller such as paracetamol, but do not exceed the recommended dose.
   If the wound becomes red, warm or painful then contact the department.
   If you have further questions or problems then please telephone the dermatology department (Tel. No.....................).

CRYOSURGERY

Cryosurgery is a relatively quick and simple technique that uses liquid nitrogen to destroy unwanted tissues. Liquid nitrogen is the cryogen of choice as it has the lowest boiling point ($-196°C$) of all available refrigerants.

The basis of safe practice is the initial diagnosis of the lesion. A biopsy should always be taken and sent for histopathology prior to treatment of the lesion with cryosurgery.

Spray technique

Liquid nitrogen spray equipment has become increasingly dominant over other methods. The most popular units used are small, metal or plastic vacuum flasks with a screw-on top and a spray release valve. Most flasks have a capacity of no more than 500 ml. The most widely used flasks (Brymill Corporation Cryospray range) have a range of four screw-on brass spray tips with diameters of 1 mm down to 0.375 mm, labelled A–D respectively. In general, spray tips B and C are the most commonly used.

For the majority of benign lesions, the field to be treated is marked, allowing a margin of approximately 1–2 mm beyond the visible pathological margin. If premalignant or malignant lesions are to be treated then margins of up to 1 cm of clinically normal skin may be included.

Spot freeze method

The spot freeze method was developed in an attempt to standardize cryosurgery treatment so that:

- medical personnel of limited experience could use the method in exactly the same way and obtain the same success rates as more experienced practitioners
- accurate knowledge could be obtained regarding the relative sensitivity or resistance of different lesions to cryosurgery
- if treatment should fail, one could exactly repeat or lengthen the second spray (Dawber et al 1997).

The liquid nitrogen spray tip is held approximately 1 cm from the skin over the centre of the area to be treated. Spraying is commenced and the white ice spreads outwards, forming a circular icefield. When the ice has developed within the desired field the spray is maintained with sufficient pressure to keep the field frozen for the length of time considered adequate. This timing can vary from 5 to 30 seconds depending on the pathology of the lesion.

The spot freeze method is only satisfactory for fields up to 2 cm in diameter. If the lesion to be treated is greater than 2 cm then the field is divided into overlapping circles of 2 cm diameter which are each treated separately. Beyond 2 cm, the temperature of any ice seen to form is greater than −15°C and therefore not low enough to reliably kill cells.

If a second freeze is required, as it is with most malignant lesions, then complete thawing is important after the initial freeze. This can be judged as the time at which the ice has disappeared and can no longer be felt on palpation. This stage is usually more than three times the duration of the freeze time after ice formation. Much of the cellular injury occurs during the thaw phase (Colver & Dawber 1991).

Cottonwool bud technique

This is the simplest method of applying liquid nitrogen to skin lesions. Despite the introduction of the cryospray, this technique is still widely used, especially in primary care for the treatment of warts and solar keratoses. As its name suggests, the treatment involves dipping a cottonwool bud into the liquid nitrogen and firmly applying it to the lesion until a narrow halo of white ice forms around the bud. For larger lesions, redipping and reapplication of the bud may be necessary.

Benign lesions

Most benign lesions are amenable to treatment with cryosurgery. However, as keratin is an excellent insulator, it may be difficult to achieve subzero temperatures at the base of the lesion without first debulking it using a curette or scalpel blade.

Seborrhoeic keratoses appear to sit on the skin and a good result is possible with very little inflammation of the surrounding tissue. Some viral warts, depending on the subtype of human papilloma virus producing the lesion, have a deeper component and considerable swelling and tissue damage may accompany successful treatment.

In some individuals blistering is seen after short and superficial freezes, whereas others may tolerate more prolonged or deeper freezes with only minimal oedema. As there is such a variation in individual reactions, it is wise to freeze cautiously at the first visit and record accurately, in the patient's notes, the duration of freeze (Kuflik 1994).

Common benign lesions that are amenable to cryosurgery include:

- cutaneous horn
- dermatofibroma
- granuloma annulare
- haemangioma
- keloid
- seborrhoeic keratosis
- skin tags
- solar keratosis
- spider naevi
- tattoos
- warts – common, plane, periungal, filiform, genital, plantar, mosaic

(Dawber et al 1997).

Premalignant and malignant lesions

Whilst both premalignant and malignant lesions are amenable to cryosurgery only an experienced practitioner should undertake the treatment of such lesions. Initially, it is important to select the right lesions for cryosurgery. Whilst it is safe to undertreat a benign skin lesion, the degree of freeze given to a malignant lesion is crucial. There are several reasons why freezing may be the treatment of choice.

- All ages can be treated, even elderly patients in poor health.
- Caucasians respond well because hypopigmentation and hypertrophic scar formation are less of a problem.

- Patients on anticoagulants and those allergic to local anaesthetics can be treated safely.
- Lesions on skin which has previously undergone irradiation will heal satisfactorily.

If malignant lesions are to be treated then the following types are likely to do well.

- Superficial basal cell carcinoma
- Nodular or ulcerated basal cell carcinoma
- Basal cell naevus syndrome
- Small, well-differentiated squamous cell carcinoma
- Tumours under 2 cm in diameter
- Tumours with definable margins
- Tumours overlying cartilage and bone
- Infected tumours
- Recurrent tumours from previous radiotherapy

(Sinclair & Dawber 1995)

Side effects

As with all surgery, cryosurgery is not without side effects. These can be divide into groups (Dawber 1990) (Box 5.2).

Pain

All patients will feel some degree of discomfort or pain when local anaesthesia is not used. As pain is subjective, this varies from patient to patient. However, even the shortest cottonwool bud freeze gives a perceptible sensation of heat or burning. Pain during the thaw phase, particularly after prolonged freeze times required for treating malignant lesions, may last for many minutes and can be intense. Certain anatomical sites are more likely to produce pain, particularly fingers, helix of the ear, lips, temples and the scalp.

Oedema

Oedema occurs to some degree with every patient, the amount of oedema relating directly to the severity of the treatment carried out. The severest oedema is typically seen in lax skin sites – eyelids and lips. Oedema of the periorbital tissue may occur following aggressive freezing of lesions on the temple.

Blistering

Blister formation relates to the dermoepidermal split produced by the freeze schedules whilst oedema relates to dermal and subcutaneous swelling. If sufficient capillary and venular damage occurs then haemorrhagic bullae may develop within 12–24 hours. These blisters are often painless and they heal rapidly without scarring (Figs 5.8 and 5.9). The degree of inflammation can be minimized by a twice-daily application of clobetasol propionate cream (Dermovate) for 5 days following treatment.

Within a week of aggressive cryosurgery treatment, it is not uncommon for the treated field to become cyanosed, with subsequent necrosis and sloughing of the dead tissue. This is probably due to delayed thrombosis of capillaries and venules and may be an important part of tumour death (Shepherd & Dawber 1984).

Box 5.2 Cryosurgery side effects

Immediate	Delayed	Prolonged but temporary	Prolonged but permanent
Pain	Postoperative infection	Hyperpigmentation	Hypopigmentation
Headache	Haemorrhage	Milia	Ectropion and notching of eyelids
Haemorrhage	Granulation tissue	Hypertrophic scars	Notching and atrophy of tumours overlying
Insufflation of	formation	Nerve-ending damage	cartilage
subcutaneous tissue		Bone necrosis	Atrophy
Oedema			Hair and follicle loss
Syncope			
Blister formation			

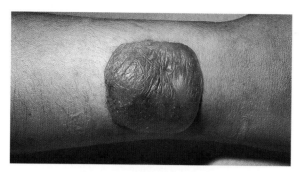

Figure 5.8   Haemorrhagic blister (reproduced with the permission of St John's Institute of Dermatology).

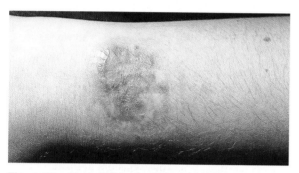

Figure 5.9   Healed blister (reproduced with the permission of St John's Institute of Dermatology).

Patient information and nursing care

Before starting treatment, consent should be obtained from the patient or guardian in the case of a child. It is important to explain:

- the aims of treatment
- the possible side effects from the treatment, such as swelling, pain and blistering
- the subsequent changes and care of the treated area
- the probable cosmetic outcome of treatment
- the follow-up arrangements.

If malignant lesions are to be treated, the reaction of the malignant and surrounding tissues is considerable and complete healing takes several weeks. Before treatment, it is therefore most important to give a through explanation of all the possible side effects and the subsequent care required of the treated lesion. The advice is ideally reinforced by an information sheet which the patient can take home and refer to. The information sheet should contain advice on wound care and healing (Box 5.3).

Box 5.3   Sample of information sheet

WHAT IS CRYOSURGERY?
Cryosurgery is a method of freezing which uses liquid nitrogen. The liquid nitrogen is sprayed onto the area of skin requiring treatment using a special flask.

WHAT CONDITIONS CAN BE TREATED?
Freezing treatment can be used for a number of different conditions, such as warts (verrucas) and solar keratosis.

Your treatment may be carried out by a doctor or a nurse.

WILL IT HURT?
The procedure is very simple but may be a little uncomfortable as the temperature of your skin will drop to −50°C.

If you are bringing a child for treatment then the doctor may give you a local anaesthetic cream to put onto the area 2 hours before the appointment.

WHAT WILL HAPPEN AFTERWARDS?
Depending on the length of time of freezing treatment, the skin will become red and may form a blister or the area may become weepy. **This is normal.**

If a blister forms then simply let out fluid and keep repeating this process until the blister no longer reforms.

Once the area has stopped weeping a blackish scab will form. This will take about 3 weeks to drop off leaving a pinkish coloured area underneath which gradually fades.

The healing process may take up to 6 weeks.

If you have received a long freeze then you may be given some ointment to put on the area. The ointment will need to be put on twice a day for 5 days. The nurses will show you how to apply it correctly before you go home.

You can wash the treated area but do not soak it and we advise you not to go swimming until the area has scabbed over.

If, following the treatment, the area is uncomfortable then you may take a painkiller such as aspirin or paracetamol, but do not exceed the recommended dose.

WHAT DO I DO IF I'M WORRIED?
If changes occur that have not been explained to you then please contact your doctor or nurse on (Tel no.............................).

The doctor performing your cryosurgery today was:

The nurse looking after you was:

Cryosurgery is an easily learned technique and its relative low cost makes it suitable for use in primary care as an extension of minor surgical procedure (Jackson 1991).

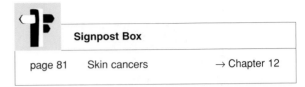

	Signpost Box	
page 81	Skin cancers	→ Chapter 12

REFERENCES

Allen B 1990 Mohs' surgery: nursing responsibilities, efficiency, and accountability. Dermatology Nursing 2(3): 154–157

Auletta M K 1994 Local anaesthesia for dermatologic surgery. Seminars in Dermatology 13: 35–42

BAD 1994 Quality in the dermatological contract. British Association of Dermatologists, London

Breuninger H 1996 The use of the ring curette in dermatology. Der Deutsche Dermatologe 44(4): 366–369

Burge S, Colver G, Lester R 1996 Simple skin surgery. Blackwell Science, Oxford, pp 1–10

Coleman W, Maloney S, Davis R S 1983 Preoperative preparation and anaesthesia. In: Coleman W, Colon G, Davis R S (eds) Outpatient surgery of the skin. Medical Examination Publishing, New York, pp 7–8

Colver G, Dawber R 1991 Malignant spots: spot freezes. In: Robins P (ed) Surgical gems in dermatology. Igaku-Shoin, New York, p 53

Dawber R 1990 Complications, contraindications and side-effects. In: Breitbart E W (ed) Advances in cryosurgery. Elsevier, New York, pp 108–114

Dawber R, Colver G, Jackson A 1997 Cutaneous cryosurgery: principles and clinical practice, 2nd edn. Martin Dunitz, London

Erksson E (ed) 1979 Illustrated handbook of local anaesthesia. Lloyd-Luke, London

Heard R 1998 How to assist during a skin biopsy. British Journal of Dermatology Nursing 2(1): 8–9

Jackson A 1991 Treatment of skin cancers in general practice. British Journal of General Practice 41: 213

Kuflik E G 1994 Cryosurgery updated. Journal of the American Academy of Dermatology 31: 925–944

Lask G P, Moy R L 1996 Principles and techniques of cutaneous surgery. McGraw Hill, New York, pp 235–238

Motley R 1997 Seborrhoeic warts. Dermatology in Practice 5(3): 6–7

Ratner D, Grande D J 1994 Mohs' micrographic surgery: an overview. Dermatology Nursing 6(4): 269–273

Shepherd J P, Dawber R 1984 Wound healing and scarring after cryosurgery. Cryobiology 21: 157

Sinclair R, Dawber R 1995 Cryosurgery of malignant and premalignant diseases of the skin: a simple approach. Australasian Journal of Dermatology 36: 135–142

Whyte A 1994 Pre and postoperative evaluation of patients undergoing cutaneous surgery. Dermatology Nursing 6(4): 248–250

6

Psychosocial issues in dermatology

Ray Jobling

The Ancient Greeks used the term *stigma* to refer to bodily signs exposing something unusual and bad about the *moral* status of the person. Such signs advertised that the individual was a blemished person, ritually polluted, to be avoided, especially in public places. Centuries later in the Christian world, layers of metaphor were added. Some skin eruptions were taken to be signs of holy grace but ultimately, they came to be seen as the surface indications of underlying physical disorder.

Today the word 'stigma' would be used to indicate *disgrace*, rather than bodily evidence of it. Stigma implies that an individual or group has allegedly shown evidence of undesirable attributes. The stigmatized are not only different in some way, their difference is undesirable. They are reduced in our minds from whole, usual, normal persons to tainted, discounted and discreditable ones. Their undesirable attribute has flooded out other features of their personality and reputation, no matter that they may be in other respects positive. The point is that there is something about the person concerned which is potentially obtrusive and destructive to interaction and relationships. It demands attention and cannot be ignored.

Normal people will, of course, seek to justify and explain their reactions and reasoning, constructing a *stigma theory* to warrant their strongly felt sense of the potential danger represented by those they stigmatize. Such theories may, paradoxically, include not only a wide range of supposed imperfections based on the original one but also sometimes exceptional, desirable attributes.

Thus stigmatization begins with perceived difference which is then, in a complex set of social and psychological processes, elaborated and socially and culturally represented in ways which are bound to have serious consequences for the well-being and quality of life of those subjected to it. Those with psoriasis, or indeed any major skin disorder, are indisputably different. Their affected skin is not only different when viewed through the microscope or inspected at cellular level – it simply feels and looks different in everyday life. Moreover, the scales which the psoriasis sufferer sheds, for example, leave a visible mark upon the environment in a way which evidently distinguishes them from those with a normal skin. These features are drawn together in a fashion which adds connotational meanings of larger significance than could be justified in biological or physical terms alone. It is indeed in the psychological and social spheres that psoriasis has been seen to have its most notable effects.

To continue with the example of psoriasis, it can be distressing. It harms affected individuals and those who care for them because of its consequences for self-image and self-esteem. It is, moreover, relevant to intimate, interpersonal encounters or contacts with strangers, where there is an ever-present anticipated threat of unwanted attention, enquiry or rejection. It has been said that psoriasis imprisons those afflicted by it, leading to restricted social life, occupational choice and so on. More importantly, the disorder can impact upon longer term relationships, and where this is so the hurt is deeper, more substantially etched into the identity, life pattern and well-being. Feelings of shame and guilt become a powerful reality.

Stigmatization can be so pronounced as to make obvious nonsense of the assertion that a skin complaint is but a trivial 'cosmetic' disorder, with little by way of essential consequences for the affected individual. It is not easy to ignore, nor is it a simple matter to learn to live with it. On the contrary, it can demand the acquisition of quite complex psychological and social skills, learned

and practised not only individually but also in partnership with sympathetic supporters and helpers. Such social manoeuvring is characteristic of all skin disorders. Psoriasis is not common on the face but those with facial acne or eczema feel, of course, even more pressure and stress.

Sadly, however, the usual public response to skin disease and its problems is not one of recognition, understanding and readiness to offer assistance. At a general level it is hard to point to unambiguous evidence of systematic rejection, although there is well-documented prejudice and discrimination which deserves further investigation, study and action. More commonly, it is a matter of disinterest. To quote a leading dermatologist:

… It is a mortal disease, not any old disease of mortals, that races the public pulse; the swift termination of life will always be seen as more horrific than survival with an emotionally disabling but physically minor disorder. (Shuster 1993)

Professor Shuster goes on to chastise his colleagues in dermatology:

Nor is anyone fooled by our new-found, but long overdue, recognition of the profound depression of self-image and well-being created by skin disease – the new band-wagon which both academics and the industry are more than pleased to power-push. These embarrassing attempts to gain quick growth in stature deserve the failure they will ultimately be seen to achieve.

Those with psoriasis, for example, are therefore not just different. They are different in ways which provoke stigmatizing reactions. They face problems which impair their functioning in key areas of life. Psoriasis can affect individual adjustment to the world in fundamental ways, all the more so since the unsophisticated can react to, and against, that difference, making successful adjustment difficult. Psoriasis is interpreted, understood and labelled (however imperfectly, irrationally and falsely) in ways which cannot be ignored or avoided. Sociologists and social psychologists would say that the difference has been socially transformed into (alleged) *deviance*. There is a real sense in which psoriasis thus constitutes a socially constructed *disability* and those who have it are to some extent *disabled*. They find that there are barriers to their full involvement in the world as ordinary normal people.

The disabled are victims of their difference and many would argue that their incapacity and dependence stem directly from the character of that difference. Medical professionals address this problem by seeking to eliminate or, if that is not possible, to modify the manifestation of differentness at the level of the afflicted individual. They seek to bring it under management and control. To bring it to order, they require the compliance of their patients with regimens justified by that objective; and attitudes, demeanour and discipline believed to be appropriate to their dependent patient status. It is not just the disease or the 'case' but also the patient who is being managed. Yet paradoxically those very therapies may themselves mark the patient off as different and impair physical, psychological and social functioning. The form, content and interpreted meaning of treatments potentially impact upon self-esteem and social reputation, just as much as the original disorder. They can shackle patients physically and psychologically, by their very nature reinforcing and exaggerating the effects of the problem they are supposed to solve. To undergo apparently exceptional treatment for an exceptional disorder is to be doubly at risk of stigmatization.

In the case of psoriasis, it is important to recognize that popular (or folk) knowledge and interpretations of it have been formed and articulated on the basis of supposed information and evidence of its meaning and implications, which have developed over generations. It is psoriasis as a concept, construct or, as the social psychologists would put it, as a *social representation* which forms the grounding for individual adaptation and social interaction. If the disorder has a 'bad press' then the problems facing the sufferer must be all the more difficult. Images do not, of course, simply emerge in a fortuitous way. They may be drawn from the collective folk memory in an unreflective fashion. However, they can be, and are, deliberately constructed.

This is to argue that physical attributes and differences are subjectively (phenomenologically) experienced. They have social and cultural meanings within a framework of social meanings and values. They bring advantage or disadvantage in different settings, groups and societies at one historical moment and not another Why do some manifestations of difference excite emotion, prejudice, avoidance, disrespect and stigma in an enduring fashion?

In the case of skin disorder in general and psoriasis in particular, there is a problem to be faced. Major skin conditions can provoke negative reactions and judgements based upon beliefs and perceptions so deeply implanted in our culture that they are difficult to eradicate. They are perceived to be not merely unattractive in a physical sense but somehow seem to imply carelessness at best and, at worst, evil intent on the part of those afflicted. A disordered skin is suggestive of deeper disorder and disorderliness, danger way beyond the ordinary. Skin diseases elicit distrust as easily, perhaps more easily, than sympathy and understanding. To have a blemished skin is to suffer damage to the reputation in a deeper way. A blemished skin implies a blemished character. A disordered skin has become a metaphor for weakness, wilfulness and wickedness frequently deployed by novelists and journalists alike.

What lies behind these stigmatizing processes? The human body is more than just a biological organism or physical object to be regarded objectively and neutrally. It engenders feelings both positive and negative as we scrutinize and evaluate our own bodies and those of others. The body is the bearer of psychological, social and cultural meaning. It is a signifier of symbolic value. Body size, shape, colour, movement and performance characteristics are important to reputation. The skin is the largest, most visible and most commonly obtrusive organ of the body. Arguably, along with the eyes, it is the most important to social interaction. It has exceptional significance in displaying and conveying who we are and how we are to be regarded.

Our social reputation rests upon numerous building blocks, among which is the evident state of our body – the state into which we have moulded it in deliberate fashion (working, of course, within the genetic limitations) or into which we seem to have carelessly and culpably allowed it to fall. It is the skin (including the hair) which is most immediately the self which we see in the mirror and offers up the image of ourselves which we present to the world. It works for us, and of course potentially against us, in social encounters. A disordered skin can put us at a disadvantage, spoiling our image and putting at risk our reputation and the respect which we seek from others. In consequence, we are self-conscious, low in self-esteem, indeed humiliated. The American writer John Updike has put it powerfully.

Strategies of concealment ramify, and self examination is endless. You are forced to the mirror, again and again: psoriasis compels narcissism, if we can suppose a Narcissus who did not like what he saw ... One hates one's abnormal erupting skin but is led into a brooding, solicitous attention towards it ... Only Nature can forgive psoriasis; the sufferer in his self-contempt does not grant to other people this power. (Updike 1989)

Those with such a physical problem must to a greater or lesser degree accept that potentially it has a social dimension requiring attention and work. In some cases the burden can be considerable, not least because the physical signs can be so magnified in the mind's eye as to damage self-esteem and to generate persistent anxiety about the anticipated threat of adverse social judgement and rejection. Updike's imagery when writing about psoriasis is always vivid, dramatically expressing the ever-present sense of self-attributed fault, personal vulnerability and social rejection that it evokes. He says, 'Spots, plaques and avalanches of excess skin ... expand and migrate across the body like lichen on a tombstone' and goes on, 'The name of the disease, spiritually speaking, is humiliation' (Updike 1976).

Skin disorders do seem to be socially significant. They have carried connotations of disgrace and danger for centuries and in many cultures. Skin complaints stigmatize. A notable component of the process is the connotation of *dirtiness* which in particular attaches to them. It is because this notion is so persistent and widespread that those seeking to counter stigma, and to normal-

ize interactions between those with skin problems and those with whom they mix, announce so loudly that conditions like acne, eczema and psoriasis are not the result of poor hygiene. Nor, it is said, is it a matter of infection or contagion – both apparently inextricably bound up with the notion of dirtiness.

But there is a confusion at the heart of such campaigning. Dirtiness has more to it than alleged individual laxness of hygiene. It was Sigmund Freud who first taught us that weeds are no more than flowers out of place and, in an important sense, out of control (Freud 1959). So too is 'dirt' merely matter out of place. Our bodies are organic matter and they generate waste. Those waste products must be managed and controlled, kept in their place and disposed of discreetly, screened out of public view and encounters. In an important but neglected study Hirt et al, in empirically testing ideas formulated by Kubie (1937), invited respondents to rank bodily waste products on a clean–dirty scale (Hirt et al 1967, 1969, Kurtz et al 1968, Ross 1968). They found that human milk, blood and tears emerged at the cleanest end of the scale. The 'dirtiest' of all were blackheads, 21st out of 21 products. Skin products (excepting hair) clustered together at the dirty end of the scale. Interestingly, dandruff and dry skin from between the toes were rated 'dirtier' than menstrual discharges, urine or even faeces.

A disorder involving excessive and difficult-to-manage (over-) production of skin waste, most obviously psoriasis, must therefore carry a risk of being seen as 'dirty'. Bits or flakes of skin should be controlled or at the very least discreetly kept from view, as they are for the most part in conditions of bodily normality. Obtrusive bodily waste is matter out of place, out of control, hinting strongly of individual neglect, carelessness and culpability. Supposed culpable responsibility invites blame on the one side and shame and guilt on the other. Messy evidence of a disordered or disorderly skin suggests a disorderly person. Such people are dangerous.

A sense of shame and guilt can therefore nag away at the unfortunate victim, perhaps in a barely conscious and ill-understood fashion or, in the worst case, to a degree which is psychologically disabling. Shame and guilt were pervasive, for example, in the autobiographical self-reflections of the British writer Dennis Potter who suffered grievously from chronic and disabling psoriatic arthritis. His *Singing detective* is plagued by guilt (Potter 1986). It is evident, too, in what the American author John Updike wrote about the experience of psoriasis in his literary work. Updike himself had the condition for most of his life. Another contemporary writer, Bernard MacLaverty, has, more gently than either Potter or Updike but nonetheless tellingly, dealt with feelings of shame and attendant social shyness in his short story about a boy with psoriasis (MacLaverty 1989). As he puts it in the title, there is a real risk of suffering 'More than just the disease'. Skin disorder spoils identity.

Further illumination of the psychosocial significance of the skin, both normal and disordered, comes from social psychological work on body consciousness and body imagery. Most prominent in this field have been Seymour Fisher and Sydney Cleveland (Fisher & Cleveland 1958). Fisher's research has concentrated upon the problem of perceptions of the body's boundary in psychologically well and sick respondents.

Each individual has to develop confidence that the walls of his body can adequately shield him from all of the potentially bad things out there ... some people clearly visualize their bodies as possessing a boundary, or border, that separates them from what is out there and is capable of withstanding alien things that might try to intrude upon them. But there are others who have trouble perceiving their bodies as separate or possessed of a defensible border. They feel vulnerable. (Fisher 1976)

Fisher goes on to suggest, on the basis of his own and others' researches, that, '... the greater a person's uncertainty about the protection provided by his own body, the more he will seek compensatory ways of reaffirming that border' (p. 22). Such persons employ:

... a thousand rituals to provide awareness of their borders. They rub themselves with lotions and oils, apply hot and cold to their surfaces, and massage their muscles. They put on tight garments that articulate large body segments. One of the rewards

that may drive people to expose themselves mercilessly to the sun's rays may be the boundary reinforcing effect of feeling the sun's rays over a wide body area not to mention the visual reinforcement of seeing the skin darkened and more vivid because of its changed appearance. (p. 23)

There are social strategies too which are protective for such individuals: 'The amount of distance between ourselves and others may well announce how secure our borders feel. Those with shaky boundaries are inclined to keep their distance' (p. 24).

All this is highly relevant to the situation of the skin disordered, particularly the psoriasis sufferer who is all too aware that his body boundary is constantly crumbling away. The rituals of topical psoriasis therapy no doubt constitute an attempt to handle this problem in the ways described by Fisher.

Fisher & Cleveland did in fact venture into psychosomatics in a study of rheumatoid arthritis. Many psoriasis sufferers, particularly those with the most unpredictable, unstable form, develop arthritis. Fisher found that arthritics were greatly concerned with their bodies and gave TAT and Rorschach responses emphasizing the protective boundary-defining qualities of the periphery of percepts. They concentrated on the hardness or protective insulation value of the periphery, especially of the body periphery, which they saw as a hard defensive wall. Alongside this, one must set their findings of the difficulty arthritics had in expressing anger. They rarely lost their temper and indeed remained affable even under conditions of extreme frustration. Fisher & Cleveland state their 'hard' psychosomatic thesis plainly.

One could conceive of the arthritic as a person who has certain unacceptable impulses over which he is fearful of losing control that he has found it necessary to convert his body into a containing vessel whose walls would prevent the outbreak of these impulses ... (he is) utilizing a particular layer of his body (striate musculature) to achieve a protective wall about himself. His muscle stiffness seemed to be equated with inhibition and making the body exterior tough and resistant. (Fisher & Cleveland 1958, p. 56)

They argue that it is not simply a reaction to having lived with symptoms but body image difficulties playing an aetiological role in the choice of symptom site.

> The skin and striated musculature constitute the part of the individual most directly in contact with reality … emphasis on the body-image boundary is a reflection on a style of life based on an unusually strong definition of self-identity and an active self-expression aimed at setting up a stable, controlling, relationship with the environment. (p. 91)

Reflecting on these insights, it may be the case that the psoriasis sufferer, in experiencing problems in his relationship with the world, seeks to strengthen the defences of his base of operations (i.e. the boundary of his body) by excessively producing skin. Such an individual is genetically predisposed. An acute attack or episode must be *triggered* and the argument here might be that the trigger is a (perceived) threat or insult in interpersonal interaction and relationships. Having manifested itself as the symptoms of psoriasis, the problems are in fact multiplied. Seeking further to protect themselves and simultaneously keep in anger, some sufferers may reinforce their boundaries via stiffening of the muscles and joints (psoriatic arthritis).

An argument similar to this has been advanced in relation to psoriasis by Sadie Zaidens (1951).

> … the skin may also serve symbolically as a protective layer, covering up that patient's inadequacy, immaturity, failure or inability to cope with everyday problems. This symbolic representation is frequently seen in patients who have psoriasis. Most psoriatics present a calm and benign façade to the outer world which is in keeping with their thickened scaly skin. Such patients attempt to repress or cover up their psychological difficulties and try to give the appearance of acceptance. However, under the placid façade frequently lie volcanic rumbles of resentment, aggression or hostility which occasionally erupt …

Zaidens has in this way emphasized the skin as a barrier, a defensive wall behind which the psoriatic seeks protection. But one might equally argue that the contrary is true. The psoriatic receives no protection from his skin. It crumbles and disintegrates before his eyes, peeling away in layers or eroding into fine dust. It allows the deeper body elements to be exposed and lost through exudation and bleeding. Bleeding has been shown to prompt feelings of shame, guilt

and felt stigma among psoriasis sufferers. In psoriasis the physical boundaries of the body itself are shown, dramatically, to be impermanent. The psoriatic cannot even keep 'body and soul' together. His own negative reactions are reinforced by those of others (in his mind's eye, at least), further serving to deepen his sense of insecurity. Seen psychosomatically, in psoriasis, far from offering a reinforcement of one's defences, the thickened but crumbling skin demonstrates that the defensive possibilities of the outer perimeter are weakened.

The social anthropologist Mary Douglas has taken us beyond the insights of individual psychology and psychosomatic medicine and into the realms of wider cultural symbolism, social order and control (Douglas 1966, 1973). Following her lead, one might begin to see how, given the power of the bodily system as a metaphor for the social system, obvious disorder of the body's boundaries, i.e. the skin, represents a significant symbolic threat to public order.

Douglas argues that the conception of dirt as matter out of place implies only two conditions – a set of ordered relations and a contravention of that order. Dirt is a catch-all category for all events which blur, smudge, contradict or otherwise confuse accepted classifications. The underlying feeling is that a system of values which is habitually expressed in a given arrangement of things has been violated. Pollution prohibits physical contact, and this applies to physiological pollutions in particular because they represent symbolic expressions of other undesirable contacts, which might have repercussions for the structure of the social order. Anything crossing or blurring significant margins or boundaries is seen as dangerous and demands control. Rituals of transition are expressions of these fears and of the urge to impose control. All margins (hence all marginal persons) and boundaries which are used in the ordering of experience and relations are potentially dangerous and polluting.

In obtrusively breaking the rules and pattern of bodily order, the signs of skin disease threaten the fundamental system of categorization we employ to order all things. They dirty the pattern. Only clear controls, physical and social, will suffice to restore 'good order' and normality. Accordingly treatment, again both physical and social, may well be strict and ritualized, authoritarian and arguably even punitive (Jobling 1988). The role of strict ritual in the management of 'offenders' is given clear recognition in the biblical discussion of the purification of unclean 'leprosy', which was of course psoriasis and not modern-day leprosy, Hansen's disease.

It is obvious that treatment, especially long-term continuous treatment which involves the application of topical agents rather than oral medication, constitutes important experience for all concerned. It has phenomenological reality and impact interacting with the experience of the physical disorder itself. Both disease and treatment call up responses from sufferers and those who observe and judge them alike. All treatments have psychosocial side effects. Some represent an insult to the patient in that domain, if no other. Like the diseases they are designed to confront, treatments may not necessarily be neutral, let alone unambiguously positive in their moral impact. They can affect reputation.

Treatments which appear extraordinary and which involve exceptional effort or cost to those adopting them are bound to influence the sufferer's social position (Jobling 1992). In the case of psoriasis, steroids under whole-body suits of polythene, as seen in the 1960s, offer one example. Even PUVA raises questions.

Complementary or alternative therapies on the 'fringe' are of considerable interest. It is inevitable that a difficult condition, notably unresponsive to treatment (except in terms of short-term results), will attract the attentions of those who have unusual treatments to offer: treatments which, whilst purporting to deal with physical symptoms, are probably more intriguing and important for their relevance to the deeper cultural and psychosocial 'meanings' of the disease. Therapies which are so evidently different and, indeed puzzling, esoteric and mysterious further serve to set the disease apart and to make the sufferers into something more than merely 'patients'. What are the reputational effects at an individual or collective level of press and media coverage of the 'doctor fish of Kangal' in Turkey,

which nibble at the skins of those who travel to that remote place, ostensibly for physical benefits? What sense does the public make of people who subject themselves to 30 minutes in an electric chair delivering low-voltage currents to the body, in an effort to alleviate psoriatic symptoms? This is to say nothing of weird and wonderful diets, mud baths and the like. What, for that matter, do people make of the therapeutic interest shown by psychologists, sociologists and psychiatrists? To be treated so differently sits ill with the attempt to depict psoriasis as just another physical disorder and psoriasis sufferers as normal people who only have a commonplace medical problem.

When treatments fail to live up to expectations, clearance is difficult to achieve or is short-lived, what then? Many therapeutic innovations and options promise much on first adoption. When they do work they can prompt unrealistic euphoria. Hopes can be dashed among the unwary, to be followed by depression and distress, if not anger. But even a treatment for a chronic disorder which is apparently 'working' can represent a challenge and a source of anxiety. John Updike, following a PUVA regimen, reported that he worried about his psoriasis and the underlying flaw fleeing into deeper tissue, waiting there for rebirth in some more threatening, loathsome and even devilish form. He probably had in mind a risk of cancer. A clearance offered by new products and procedures may be persistently uncertain and ambiguous. There is an accompanying anticipated threat of a relapse sooner or later. This is subjectively felt to be all the worse for the widespread acclaim being awarded to the so-called therapeutic breakthrough. To be a PUVA failure was, according to Updike, to be a leper among lepers.

Whilst a new treatment is apparently working, of course, the patient is in a sense a 'new' person. To be so transformed after a lifetime of adjustment to the disease, its treatment, its psychological implications and its social reception is not necessarily easy. One is not any longer the person one believed oneself to be. Paradoxically, clearance can potentially disrupt identity. Attention to this dimension is important to the therapeutic intervention. Much more than the skin is under transformation.

Finally, it must be said that there is a possibility of secondary gains in all this. Even morbid experience can contribute to individual personal growth and offer opportunities for concern and care for others (Jobling 1999). It can enhance life rather than totally blighting it. Major skin disorder makes one sensitive not just to one's own feelings but, by extension, to those of others. Sympathetic social support and quite elaborate psychosocial work can often accompany the routines of treatment. Bernard MacLaverty's psoriatic boy is helped by the insight and kindly concern of an old lady who guides him to think about his disorder and to get it into proportion (MacLaverty 1989). She counsels him to watch out that he doesn't impose needless suffering upon himself. Take care, she says, that you don't suffer more than just the disease.

Those who work in a professional capacity with skin disorders do not yet enjoy the rewards of a high reputation among their peers. To an extent, of course, they suffer from *stigma fallout*. Their reputation is affected by the low public regard in which their patients are held. The treatments they offer can seem superficially simple, even crude. And yet, as outlined here, they are working on problems of considerable complexity, dealing with issues of major significance in psychological, social and cultural terms. Their role is subtle and sophisticated. Given contemporary debates concerning resources and rationing, of who should have what and why and who might seem to deserve less or even nothing at all,

they are also currently at the sharp end of the politics of health care (Jobling 1999). In conditions of supposed resource scarcity, is it right that what many would see as 'merely cosmetic' problems should deny others with what are said to be more fundamental difficulties? By way of response, both professionals and their patients can testify that quality of life is at issue.

Dermatology and specialist dermatological nursing are complex professional fields. The essential skills must include psychosocial assessment and sophistication in interpersonal work and counselling, perhaps long term (Jobling 1978). The practitioners ought also to have a community orientation in their work, in which they act, inform, educate and, where possible, promote cultural change. Skin disorders imply a risk of disability. Rather than slavishly following the medical model, in dermatology if in no other field, there is an opportunity to break free from sole attention to individual 'difference' and its elimination. It is the social perception and reception of skin lesions which handicap and disable. They require attention too. Socially and culturally constructed images and prejudices must be a central focus of professional activity in dermatology.

REFERENCES

Douglas M 1966 Purity and danger. Routledge and Kegan Paul, London

Douglas M 1973 Natural symbols. Penguin, London

Fisher S 1976 Body consciousness. Fontana, New York

Fisher S, Cleveland S 1958 Body image and personality. Van Nostrand, Princeton, New Jersey

Freud S 1959 Character and anal eroticism. In: Strachey J (ed) The standard edition of the complete psychological works of Sigmund Freud. Hogarth, London

Hirt M, Ross W D, Kurtz R 1967 Construct validity of body-boundary perception. Proceedings of the 75th Annual Convention of the American Psychological Association, pp 187–188

Hirt M, Ross W D, Kurtz R 1969 Attitudes to body products among normal subjects. Journal of Abnormal Psychology 74: 486–489

Jobling R 1978 Nursing with and without professional nurses – the case of dermatology. In: Dingwall R, McIntosh J (eds) Readings in the sociology of nursing. Churchill Livingstone, Edinburgh, pp 181–195

Jobling R 1988 The experience of psoriasis under treatment. In: Anderson R, Bury M (eds) Living with chronic illness. Unwin Hyman, London, pp 225–245

Jobling R 1992 Psoriasis and its treatment in psychosocial perspective. Reviews in Contemporary Pharmacotherapy 3(7): 339–345

Jobling R 1999 The patient's perspective. In: Griffiths C, Barker J (eds) Key advances in the effective management of psoriasis. RSM Press, London, pp 9–12

Kubie K 1937 The fantasy of dirt. Psychoanalytical Quarterly 6: 388–424

Kurtz R, Hirt M, Ross W D 1968 Investigations of the affective meaning of body products. Journal of Experimental Research in Personality 3: 9–14

MacLaverty B 1989 More than just the disease. In: The Great Profundo and other stories. Penguin Books, London

Potter D 1986 The singing detective. Faber and Faber, London

Ross W D 1968 The fantasy of dirt and attitudes towards body products. Journal of Nervous and Mental Disease 146: 303–309

Shuster S 1993 A misdiagnosed case of Cinderella syndrome. Dermatology International 3: 6

Updike J 1976 From the journal of a leper. The New Yorker July 19: 28–32

Updike J 1985 At war with my skin. The New Yorker September 2: 49–57

Updike J 1989 At war with my skin. In: Self consciousness: memoirs. André Deutsch, London

Zaidens S 1951 The skin – psychodynamic and psychopathologic concepts. Journal of Nervous and Mental Disease 113: 388–394

7

Age-specific issues in dermatology nursing

Julie Van Onselen

INTRODUCTION

The aim of this chapter is to consider the nursing care and treatment of age-related skin conditions. The practical aspects of skin care will focus on healthy skin care in childhood, pregnancy and the elderly and the dermatology nursing care of skin conditions specific to age but will not include age-specific presentations, treatment and nursing care of common skin conditions (psoriasis, eczema, acne, skin cancer) as they are covered in the individual chapters.

CHANGES IN HEALTHY SKIN OVER THE LIFESPAN

Infancy and childhood

The embryonic skin formed 4 weeks after conception is a rudimentary structure of a periderm over a basal cell layer. The role of the periderm is the secretion and absorption of fetal nutrients. At 8 weeks' gestation an intermediate layer develops between the basal cells and periderm and stratifies up to 24 weeks' gestation to form the epidermis, when the periderm ceases to exist (Weston & Lane 1991). Between 14 and 24 weeks' gestation, the basal cell layer develops the hair follicles, sebaceous and sweat glands (Higgins & du Vivier 1996). Additional developments include Langerhans cells for immuno-regulatory function from 6 weeks' gestation, melanocytes by 12 weeks' gestation and Merkel cells, which are thought to be primitive nerve cells, by 18 weeks. Nails are formed by 20 weeks' gestation.

The skin is fully formed by 30 weeks' gestation. Infants born at full term have smooth, fully formed skin. Premature babies have fragile skin which is susceptible to trauma, so require very gentle and careful handling. Post term babies are likely to have dry and peeling skin, particularly on their hands and feet (Mackie 1992). The skin of premature babies additionally has poor barrier properties and is vulnerable to infection (Higgins & du Vivier 1996). Newborn epidermal, hair, sweat and sebaceous structures are fully mature. However, the nails of a newborn infant, especially on the fifth finger and toes, can appear to be curved but will straighten out by 6 months of age (Mackie 1992). Infants generally have soft downy hair at birth and those infants born with thick dark hair often shed their first growth and become temporarily bald for a few weeks. The newborn dermis is less mature with less organized vascular and nerve structures, collagen and elastic fibres. The adult form of the dermis is not fully developed until 2 years of age (Weston & Lane 1991).

Adolescence

From the age of 2 to 11 years there are no physiological changes in the development of healthy skin. Skin changes occur again in adolescence with the hormonal changes of puberty. The increase in the hormone androgen leads to the stimulation of the sebaceous glands, which have lain dormant since birth. Consequently, the skin becomes greasy from the sebum which may lead to development of closed comedones (whiteheads) and open comedones (blackheads), papules and pustules causing acne. Sebaceous glands are present in large numbers on the face and scalp and in smaller numbers on the chest and back. The hair in the teenage years can also become greasy and lank as a result of increased sebaceous activity (Mackie 1992). The apocrine glands in the groin and axilla areas are activated in adolescence, after lying dormant in the childhood years. Perspiration interacting with normal skin flora may cause body odour.

The ageing skin in adulthood

Skin shows the outward signs of ageing and changes are more apparent in sun-damaged skin. Wrinkles increase in number, depth and prominence but normal fine markings in the skin actually decrease with age. The stratum corneum changes little in thickness but the corneocytes (horny cells) increase their surface area and the rate of renewal of the stratum corneum is altered as the loss of corneocytes decreases with age.

The epidermis becomes thinner and the epidermal cells shrink. The young adult mean epidermal thickness of limb and trunk skin is 35–50 µm; at 70 years it has reduced to a mean thickness of 25–40 µm. The renewal time of the stratum corneum increases and epidermal cell production decreases.

HEALTHY SKIN CARE IN INFANCY, CHILDHOOD AND ADOLESCENCE

Infancy

The skin of a newborn infant is delicate and skin irritation is common as the immune response is gradually developing.

Washing and cleansing

The infant's skin needs to be treated carefully as many external factors can make the skin vulnerable. Soaps, cleaners and shampoos used must be formulated for the infant's skin. If dry skin is a problem, a soap substitute must be used. Remember that detergents will irritate and damage the infant's skin, so restrict the use of bubble baths and use non-biological washing powders for clothing, bedding and nappies.

Napkin care

It is important to advise parents of newborn infants on the prevention of napkin dermatitis.

- Decreasing moisture and friction – keep the nappy area dry. Change the nappy frequently and ideally immediately after urination or defaecation (2-hourly when the child is awake and once during the night). Leave the nappy off for a period during the day. Avoid rubber and plastic pants over cloth nappies and use super-absorbent disposable nappies. Apply a barrier cream to reduce friction.

- Reduce washing of the nappy area and allow it to dry. Use aqueous cream to cleanse.
- Continue breastfeeding as breast milk produces stools with a lower pH.

Prickly heat

Newborn infants are unable to regulate their temperature efficiently. Heat rash or prickly heat is common in infants and consists of areas of small raised papules on the stomach and back.

- Remove the infant's clothing and keep cool.
- Use a simple moisturizing cream (e.g. aqueous cream) to cool and soothe.

Sun care

Sun protection for infants and children is discussed in Chapter 12.

Childhood

The growing child's skin is less vulnerable than the infant's but allergic responses to environmental factors can be a problem for children with atopic disease. Children commonly present with problems of skin infection and infestation. Play can lead to cuts and bruises with the risk of infection.

Cuts and abrasions

1. Cleansing the skin with a mild antiseptic following injury is essential.
2. Keep the wound clean and dry and cover with a plaster or simple non-stick dressing.
3. If the wound does not heal, becomes red and tender with discomfort and pain for more than 48 hours, medical advice should be sought.

Adolescence

Physical skin changes in adolescence can be confusing for the teenager. Body image becomes very important. Most teenagers will take an active interest in skin care as their appearance matters. Teenagers will often ask the nurse for advice on acne and general skin care.

Teenage skin care

- Bath or shower daily. Use a frequent-use shampoo if washing hair daily.
- Use a deodorant or antiperspirant daily.
- Use oil-free cosmetics and remove make-up at night with a cleanser or moisturizer.
- Wash face with a soap free facial wash.
- Avoid picking and squeezing spots.
- Eat a balanced diet and exercise regularly.

Adolescent striae

Striae (stretch marks) caused by growth spurts are a common physiological occurrence in adolescence. Boys tend to have striae on their lower back and girls on their upper arms and thighs, especially if they are obese.

Acne and fungal infections

Acne is almost universal in the teenage years. Fungal infections are also extremely common. These are discussed in Chapters 11 and 13 respectively.

COMMON SKIN CONDITIONS IN CHILDHOOD

Transient cutaneous conditions in the newborn

The majority of newborn infants have a transient skin condition that appears and disappears during the first few days to months of life. Table 7.1 outlines the most common transient cutaneous conditions in the newborn.

Seborrhoeic dermatitis (cradle cap)

Seborrhoeic dermatitis (Fig. 7.3) is a form of eczema, occurring commonly on the face, scalp

Table 7.1 Transient cutaneous conditions in the newborn

Condition	Appearance	Course	Treatment and nursing care
Acne neonatorum	Transient facial pustules	May persist up to 8 months	
Cutis marmorata (mottling) (Fig. 7.2)	Blue/purple mottles, predominant on limbs	Usually fades on warming (normal physiological response to lower temperatures)	Parental reassurance but persistent mottling in older children may suggest connective tissue disorder or hypothyroidism
Erythema toxicum neonatorum	Erythematous macules on trunk	Very common condition affecting 50% of full-term babies. Fades within 2–3 days	A normal response that needs only parental reassurance
Neonatal erythema	Generalized erythema	Fades within 48 hours of birth	A normal response that needs only parental reassurance
Neonatal pustulosis	Sterile pustular eruption	Resolves in several months; may leave pigmented macule	Commoner in black children. Parental reassurance
Milia	Small keratin cysts within the dermis	Spontaneous rupture of cysts within 6 weeks	Parental reassurance
Miliaria (Fig. 7.1)	Vesicular eruption due to retention of eccrine sweat	May develop at any age, common in infants	Avoid excessive heat which predisposes to condition
Sebaceous gland hyperplasia	Transient papules, especially over nose	Resolves within a few weeks. Secondary to maternal androgens	Parental reassurance
Subcutaneous fat necrosis	Rare disorder with granuloma of the subcutaneous fat. Thickened plaques within the subcutaneous tissue of the buttocks, thighs and back	Present at birth but may develop up to 6 weeks later. Lesions resolve slowly over several months. Residual atrophy may occur	Observe for signs of hypercalcaemia: vomiting and failure to thrive

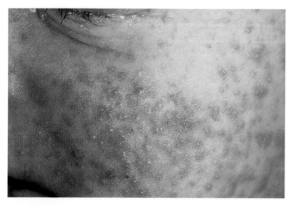

Figure 7.1 Milaria (reproduced with the permission of St John's Institute of Dermatology).

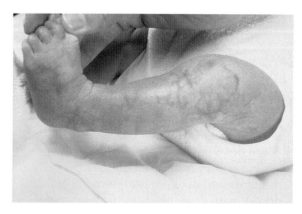

Figure 7.2 Cutis marmorata (reproduced with the permission of St John's Institute of Dermatology).

and flexures, which is self-limiting and usually resolves over several weeks.

The onset of seborrhoeic dermatitis is early, usually before the age of 3 months. It presents with yellow scales and erythema but the condition is not itchy and the baby is happy and not bothered by their skin condition. The condition may be complicated by fungal infection with candida and in Afro-Caribbean children, hypopigmentation may occur.

Nursing advice and skin care

- Cradle cap – use a mild shampoo daily and massage the scalp regularly with aqueous cream, aveeno cream (thick scales) or coconut oil (mild scaling). Massage with a very gentle circular motion and encourage scales to lift.
- Body – daily emollient bath with soap substitutes.
- Any erythematous areas can be treated with Daktacort or 1% hydrocortisone cream.

Napkin dermatitis

Napkin dermatitis is the most common form of napkin eruption and is commonly seen in the first year of life and is rare after 12 months. The nappy area is affected with a glazed erythema and the skinfolds are commonly spared.

Napkin dermatitis is an irritant contact dermatitis caused by many exogenous factors including occlusions and moisture (plastic pants), friction, urine and ammonia, faeces,

Candida albicans (fungal), *Staphylococcus aureus* (bacterial) and infant susceptibility (Wahrman & Honig 1997).

Nursing advice and skin care

- Advise parents on the preventive measures outlined in the section on healthy skin care (pp. 104, 105).
- Decrease skin inflammation by using 1% hydrocortisone cream twice daily for 3–5 days.
- Treat for fungal infection if skin is erythematous and glazed and if rash has been present for 72 hours. Canesten HC or Daktacort is ideal if inflammation is severe. Canesten or Daktarin can also be used.
- Treat bacterial infection if there is crusting or excoriation/weeping. Fucidin H is very useful.
- Decrease the pH of the nappy environment. Urine can be acidified by giving the child over 9 months 60–80 ml of cranberry juice daily.

Juvenile plantar dermatosis

Juvenile plantar dermatosis is a form of dermatitis which was identified during the 1970s. This exclusively childhood condition (age 8–14 years) is one of erythema and fissuring on the plantar forefoot only (Fig. 7.4). It is believed to be a form of irritant dermatitis related to modern footwear made of synthetic materials which causes sweating, friction and occlusive conditions. The skin around the ball of the foot becomes painful and fissured with a glazed red appearance.

Nursing advice and skin care

- Use copious emollients, especially at night, on foot area.
- Wear cotton socks.
- Change to alternative footwear, leather shoes or, in the summer, open-toed sandals until condition has resolved.

Juvenile spring eruption

This is an uncommon self-limiting condition, similar to polymorphic light eruption. Boys are more likely to be affected and the condition causes blisters on the ears with general pruritus,

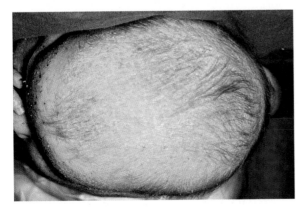

Figure 7.3 Seborrhoeic dermatitis (cradle cap).

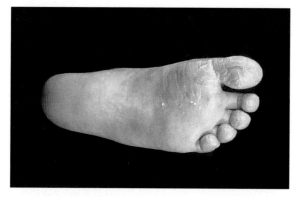

Figure 7.4 Juvenile plantar dermatosis (reproduced with the permission of St John's Institute of Dermatology).

occurring in the spring. There is no treatment and the condition will resolve spontaneously.

Bacterial infections

Impetigo contagiosa

Impetigo contagosia is, as its name suggests, a highly infectious bacterial skin infection which is common in childhood. The infection is largely due to *Staphylococcus aureus*, especially when blisters are present. However, group A streptococci are often responsible for non-bullous infections. Impetigo starts as small vesicles which blister and erode with a honey-coloured crust (Fig. 7.5). Children who have an impaired skin barrier, have a poor standard of hygiene, are malnourished or who live in warm humid climates are predisposed to impetigo.

Nursing advice and skin care

- Impetigo is extremely contagious and requires prompt treatment to stop the spread of infection. Topical antibiotics (fusidic acid is ideal and non-staining) are used alone only for minor cases and in combination with oral antibiotics (oral flucloxacillin) for more widespread cases.
- The family needs to be careful with hygiene and the child should use separate face cloths and towels until the infection has resolved.
- If the child has recurrent episodes of impetigo, the whole family should have nose, axilla and groin swabs to detect the carriage of

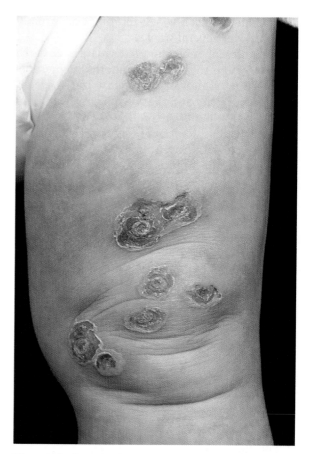

Figure 7.5 Impetigo (reproduced with the permission of St John's Institute of Dermatology).

Staphylococcus aureus. Any staphylococcus carriers need to be treated with antiseptic baths (chlorhexidine), topical antibiotics and nasal ointment (mupirocin).

Cellulitis

Cellulitis is commonly caused by a streptococcus and isolated to a localized area. This is a deep bacterial infection of the dermis and subcutaneous tissues. The affected area is well demarcated, inflamed and very tender. The child feels unwell and is often febrile.

Nursing advice and skin care

- Swab the area, as systemic antibiotics are required depending on the bacteriology result.

- The child needs to rest with their temperature controlled.
- The affected limb requires elevation.

Staphylococcal scalded skin syndrome (SSSS) or Ritter's disease

This is a rare and serious bullous bacterial infection which occurs in children aged 6 years and under. Without prompt treatment, the mortality rate is 50%, especially in children under 1 year and those who have greater than half the skin surface affected. The causative bacterium is a *Staphylococcus aureus* of phage group 2 and generally the child has a focus of preceding infection, usually the ear, eye or umbilicus, and is febrile. Large areas of skin become inflamed and tender; there may be a few patches or the entire body may be involved. The skin then blisters as the epidermis is stripped (Fig. 7.6). The skin heals in 1–2 weeks.

Nursing advice and skin care

- The child is usually hospitalized and needs acute care with special attention to fluid balance, temperature control and protein loss.
- Systemic antibiotics are used (flucloxacillin or cephalosporin).
- The child's skin is fragile and sore so needs gentle and careful handling, pressure relief and care of the blistered areas.
- In the recovery phase, copious emollients should be applied as the skin will be extremely dry.

Table 7.2 outlines some other bacterial infections seen in children.

Fungal infections

Common fungal infections in infancy include candida infections and in childhood and adolescence, dermatophyte infections (e.g. Tinea corporis, Fig. 7.12).

Tinea capitis (scalp ringworm)

Tinea capitis is one of the most common fungal infections in children from infancy to 14 years of age, with a predominance in African and Afro-Caribbean races. The most common mode of

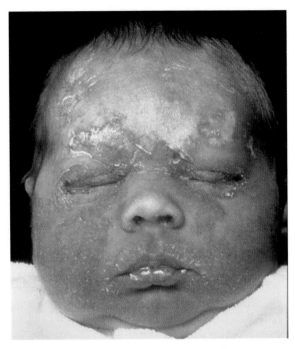

Figure 7.6   Staphylococcal scalded skin syndrome (reproduced with the permission of St John's Institute of Dermatology).

transmission is by human-to-human spread of anthropophilic dermatophytes (e.g. *Trichophyton tonsurans*). Transmission is encouraged by the communal use of brushes, combs and hats. This fungus is generally endothrix (invading the hair shaft without destroying the cuticle).

Other modes of spread are from animal to human (*Microsporum canis*). The fungus involved here is ectothrix (invading the outside of the hair shaft and destroying the cuticle) (Winsor 1998). Diagnosis is made by mycological examination of the hair and skin scale.

The child can be an asymptomatic carrier or present with alopecia, which may be inflammatory, diffuse or patchy scaling (Fig. 7.7). Severely affected children will have follicular pustules and kerion (a painful, crusted suppurative lesion) formation.

Nursing advice and skin care

- Treatment is with systemic antifungals, with griseofulvin (10 mg/1 kg body weight) being currently the only drug licensed for children.

Table 7.2 Other bacterial infections seen in children

Skin condition	Appearance	Treatment and nursing care
Ecthyma – deep necrotic infection secondary to injury/*Staph. aureus*	Induration, ulcer, crust	Remove crust, clean with saline, non-adherent dressing, oral antibiotics
Folliculitis – infection of hair follicle due to *Staph. aureus*. Pseudomonas more likely with occlusion	Yellow pustules around hair follicle, erythema, deep painful abscesses	Swab for microscopy, oral antibiotics, incise and drain boils, exclude diabetes, screen family for *Staph. aureus.*
Lyme disease – arthropod infection from ticks, common in forests	Annular rash 1–2 weeks. Occasional associated lymphadenopathy	Amoxycillin or phenoxymenthyl penicillin. Severe complications include meningitis, myocarditis, arthritis
Kawasaki disease – mucocutaneous lymph node syndrome; an acute, rare vasculitic disease of young children (affects under-5s, peak incidence between 12 and 24 months). No causative organism,? superantigen stimulating massive immunological response	Acute pyrexial stage 10–14 days followed by subacute phase 25 days and several weeks' convalescence. General erythema with desquamation, dry red lips, inflamed palms and soles, conjunctival congestion, cervical lymphadenopathy	Intravenous gammaglobulin (reduces risk of cardiac complications). Aspirin and reduce fever. Cardiac complications may develop in acute and subacute phase, including coronary artery aneurysms, myocardial infarction, myo- and pericarditis, pericardial effusions and tamponade. Endocardiology at 4 weeks and after diagnosis (to assess for and monitor cardiac symptoms)
Scarlet fever – systemic group A streptococcus infection spreading to tonsils	Incubation period 2–5 days, blotchy erythema, bright red mucous membranes	Systemic penicillin, early referral for renal and cardiac complications
Swimming pool granuloma – mycobacterial infection acquired through grazed skin in swimming pools and by cleaning fish tanks	Indurated erythematous papules which enlarge and ulcerate	Culture of skin biopsy at low temperatures. Co-trimoxazole (young children), tetracycline (teenagers). Inform local public health authorities to investigate swimming pools

The duration of treatment is on average 8 weeks. Treatment should be preferably in conjunction with mycology. Children and parents need to be advised to continue with treatment and informed that there may be some mild side effects (headaches, skin rashes and gastrointestinal disturbances).

- All family members and friends must be screened.
- Antifungal shampoos must be used at least once weekly for the whole family. The shampoos will decrease shedding of the infective spores and help reduce transmission to close contacts.
- Preventive measures include:
  1. screening and treating close family members
  2. notification to the school or nursery about infected individuals
  3. health education for all health-care professionals and those who care for children
  4. discouraging the sharing of hats, caps, brushes, combs and towels
  5. the continued use of antifungal shampoos
  6. prompt referral, diagnosis and treatment.

Viral infections

Common viral infections in infancy, childhood and adolescence include common warts, herpes simplex and molluscum contagiosum.

Erythema infantum

This is a viral infection caused by the human parvovirus B19, causing a bright red erythema on the face with a slapped cheek appearance. The condition is also known as slapped cheek syndrome and fifth disease (Fig. 7.8). The viral infection is spread by droplet (incubation period 7–14 days) and will occur in epidemics, usually in the spring. The erythema will erupt from the face to the trunk and limbs and then fade after 1 week (Higgins & du Vivier 1996).

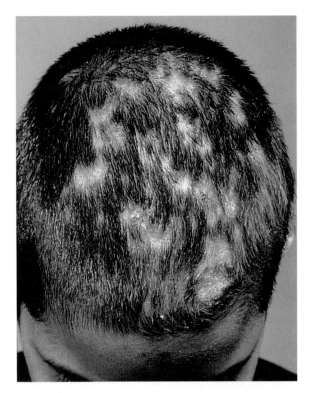

Figure 7.7   Tinea capitis (reproduced with the permission of St John's Institute of Dermatology).

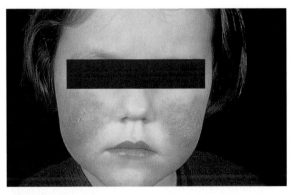

Figure 7.8   Erythema infantum (slapped cheek syndrome) (reproduced with the permission of St John's Institute of Dermatology).

Nursing advice and skin care

- Parents and children should be reassured that the erythema will fade within a week.
- If the skin feels hot, aqueous cream can be applied.

- The child needs to be off school for 1 week.
- Avoid the child getting overheated (hot baths, overexertion and excessive exposure to the sun) during the course of the infection and for several weeks after the rash has faded.
- Pregnant women should avoid exposure as the parvovirus can cause transplacental infection.

Infestations

Scabies

Occurs in all ages and spreads rapidly throughout families and close contacts. Infants will need their entire body to be treated (see Chapter 13).

Head lice

Head lice (pediculus humanus capitis) infestation is extremely common, particularly in children of primary school age. Head lice infestation is a very emotive issue, causing much anxiety for parents and children. This is due to negative reactions and the erroneous belief that head lice infestation is caused by bad hygiene. Head lice are best regarded as a nuisance which can become widespread in a child population. Parents and children need consistent advice and reassurance from well-informed health-care and educational workers.

Head lice infestation should be the responsibility of the whole community and parents need to be given precise instructions on the effective control of head lice (Simmons 1999).

Nursing advice and skin care

- Head lice facts – ensure that parents and children are aware of the following.
  1. Head lice are tiny, flat, wingless insects measuring 2–3 mm in length. They are unable to fly, hop or jump between heads and are only transmitted by prolonged head-to-head contact.
  2. Head lice live close to the scalp as they require surface temperatures of greater than 31°C to live. The eggs are glued to the hair. They hatch in 7–10 days and live for 20–30 days (Burgess 1995). Head lice which are found on pillows or hats are not viable and will not transfer to another

head. Black particles that fall from the hair during brushing or combing are lice faeces.

3. Head lice infestations generally produce no symptoms. Itching can be a problem due to an allergic reaction to the louse's saliva.

4. Treatment must only be commenced when live lice have been detected. Evidence of nits, which are empty egg shells, is not an indication for active treatment (Simmons 1999).

- Teach parents to diagnose the presence of live head lice by using a plastic detection comb on wet hair. The hair should be combed and any lice or debris removed onto a white tissue.
- Active treatment depends on the local public health department policy due to combating resistance to insecticides. First-line treatment often involves malathion lotion, with at least 50 ml of lotion applied to the scalp and hair at the base of the hair shaft and left for a minimum of 12 hours. The hair should then be washed and 10 days later the scalp rechecked. If live lice continue to be present, this treatment should be repeated.
- All family members and school friends should be checked and treated if live lice are present.
- If after the second treatment live lice are still present, another preparation such as permethrin can be used in the same procedure. If live lice are still present, the public health department will need to be contacted.
- Preventive measures for the community can include Bug Busting, which is organized by a charity called Community Hygiene Concern. This procedure involves the following routine: hair is washed and rinsed and conditioner applied but not rinsed out. Using the fine-toothed bug-busting comb, the hair is combed. The hair is rinsed and combed again. If head lice are found, the combing must continue on every fourth day until the life cycle of the head lice is halted (Duncan 1997).

Vascular lesions and naevi

Vascular lesions and naevi, commonly known as birthmarks, affect up to 40% of all infants (Atherton 1992). There are three classifications:

1. telangiectatic naevi (salmon patches) – a transient cutaneous condition in the newborn, which will gradually fade and resolve within six months
2. haemangiomas (capillary or strawberry, cavernous, mixed, verruccous and neonatal)
3. vascular malformations (port wine stains).

Haemangiomas

A haemangioma is a benign proliferation of the vascular endothelium (Mackie 1997a) (Fig. 7.9). The most common type is the capillary haemangioma (referred to as a strawberry mark), which one child in 10 will develop. The most common site for a capillary haemangioma is the head and neck (60%), then the trunk (25%), with the remainder appearing on other body sites.

Capillary haemangiomas appear within the first few weeks of life, undergo rapid growth for the first 3 months and will have reached their maximum size when the infant is 6 months old. The capillary haemangioma will generally remain static and then slowly fade and disappear by 5 years of age (Syed & Harper 1996). Complications due to capillary haemangioma generally occur due to the site, e.g. the eye, impairment of vision, or the lip, feeding difficulties.

Nursing advice and skin care

- Generally no treatment is needed. Parents will be very anxious so will need lots of reassurance that spontaneous resolution with a good cosmetic result will occur.

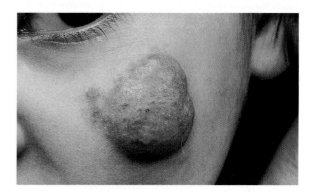

Figure 7.9 Haemangioma (reproduced with the permission of St John's Institute of Dermatology).

- Occasionally, haemangiomas in complicated sites require treatment. First-line treatment is oral prednisolone (2 mg/kg), reducing slowly. Second-line treatment is with the pulsed dye laser if the lesion is ulcerated and/or telangiectasia remains after the haemangioma has resolved (Syed & Harper 1996).

Port wine stains

A port wine stain is a pink to deep red to purple vascular malformation of developmental origin with ectasia of superficial dermal capillaries (Fig. 7.10). Port wine stains are unilateral and commonly affect the face. They are present at birth and, without treatment, will persist throughout life. Females are more commonly affected, with an incidence of three in every 1000 births.

Nursing advice and skin care

- Treatment is by pulsed dye laser, which is safe and effective. Children treated at the youngest possible age (3 months to 6 years) generally have the best response to treatment, so early referral to a specialist centre is essential.
- Children with port wine stains around the eye are more susceptible to developing glaucoma so regular ophthalmological review is essential.
- Psychological support is essential as parents and children will often be devastated by port wine stains, especially if they occur on the face.
- Cosmetic camouflage techniques can be taught to parents and children for any areas still visible after laser treatment.

Genodermatoses

Ichthyosis

Ichthyosis is a genetically determined (autosomal dominant or sex-linked recessive) condition of keratinization. The skin is extremely dry and very scaly, with rough and horny papules (Fig. 7.11). Ichthyosis will mainly present in infants and children but occasionally adolescents may acquire it.

Autosomal dominant ichthyosis is more common, affecting one in 250–300 children (Mackie 1997b). Children with this form of ichthyosis will become affected early in childhood and generally improve as they grow older. Sex-linked recessive ichthyosis is much rarer and in the fully developed form is only seen in males. This form of ichthyosis produces greasy yellow and brown scales and is unlikely to resolve.

Nursing advice and skin care

- Liberal emollients (bath oils, soap substitutes and moisturizers) with descaling properties or salicylic acid.
- Urea-containing emollients are helpful but can cause stinging.

Epidermolysis bullosa

This condition is discussed fully in Chapter 14.

Dermatitis artefacta

This is a condition defined by self-induced or aggravated bizarre skin lesions, which generally

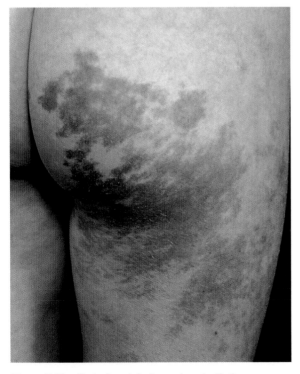

Figure 7.10 Port wine stain (reproduced with the permission of St John's Institute of Dermatology).

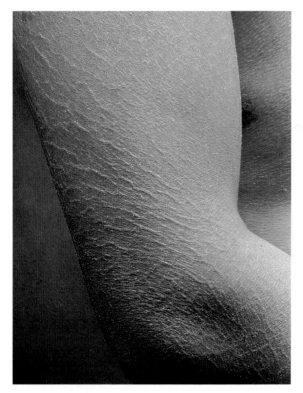

Figure 7.11 Ichthyosis (reproduced with the permission of St John's Institute of Dermatology).

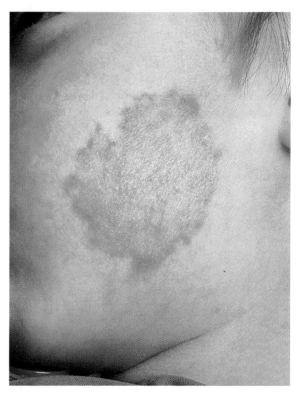

Figure 7.12 Tinea corporis in a child (reproduced with the permission of St John's Institute of Dermatology).

are unusual shapes on any body site. The skin lesions have been deliberately initiated or are existing lesions which have been aggravated by the patient. This condition is rare and affects all age groups but may be particularly seen in children and teenagers who have psychological difficulties. The children and teenagers are likely to be quiet and withdrawn and when confronted about the skin lesions, will get upset.

Nursing advice and skin care

- Understanding and emotional support.
- Occlusion of the lesions with bandages and dressings.

PREGNANCY

There are several significant skin changes in pregnancy which are a normal physiological response. There are some skin conditions that occur only in pregnancy. Existing chronic skin conditions can change in nature and appearance during the antenatal and postnatal periods. A nursing assessment of any skin changes in pregnancy needs to include:

1. parity and stage of pregnancy in which the manifestation first occurs
2. past history of skin conditions
3. description of the lesions
4. duration of symptoms
5. events which have precipitated an outbreak (e.g. delivery, menstruation or the use of contraceptives)
6. a comprehensive skin assessment (Zellis & Pincus 1993).

Pregnancy-related skin changes due to physiological response

Melasma (chloasma)

The normal physiology of hormonal changes (increase in oestrogen and progesterone) in pregnancy influences melanin pigmentation. This causes an increase in the pigmentation of the skin of the pregnant female known as melasma or chloasma. The precise cellular action of the melanocytes in pregnancy is unknown but in some way the melanocyte-stimulating hormone stimulates melanocyte activity which causes changes in skin pigmentation (Liskay & Heer Nicol 1998).

Melasma is a common, inevitable pattern of pigmentation in pregnant females. There are variations in the pattern and extent of melasma, which most commonly affects the cheeks and centre of the face. Other areas of skin affected are the midline of the abdomen, genitalia and nipple areolae. The pigmentary changes consist of darkening of the skin, exacerbated by sun exposure. These pigmentary changes can also affect moles, which can darken and enlarge, and new moles can also appear in pregnancy (Callan 1984).

These pigmentary changes will fade after delivery but may take some time to disappear and may be permanent.

Nursing advice and skin care

- Avoid sun exposure and wear sunscreen and a hat when outdoors.
- Reassurance that pigmentary changes will fade after delivery but complete disappearance may take some time.

Increase in hair growth during pregnancy and hair loss in the postpartum period

During pregnancy, there is an increase in androgens and normal hair loss diminishes and the hair becomes healthy, shiny and thick. There is also an increase in facial hair growth.

In the postpartum period there is an increase of telogen follicles which causes hair loss for a maximum of 90 days after delivery (Rotstein 1993). The hair will recover fully within a few months.

Nursing advice and skin care

- Reassurance that hair growth will recover fully within a few months.

Vascular changes

There is increased cutaneous blood flow in pregnancy and, together with the increase of oestrogen activity, various vascular changes occur. Many females experience degrees of oedema and varicose veins worsen. Spider naevi appear, generally on the face, upper trunk and arms. Palmar erythema is a common occurrence in pregnancy, the palms becoming redder and warmer. All these symptoms fade and disappear after delivery.

Nursing advice and skin care

- Reassurance that vascular changes are likely to fade after delivery.
- Referral to dermatologist for laser treatment.

Striae distensae (stretch marks)

Striae distensae are caused by skin stretching and disrupting the dermal connective tissues, resulting in thinning and loss of elasticity in the dermis. They are characterized by linear lines of atrophy, which are initially bright red and raised, then purple and after pregnancy fade to pale depressed shiny lines on the skin. In pregnancy they occur over the lower abdomen and breasts during the third trimester (Marks 1993).

Nursing advice and skin care

- Regular moisturizing.
- Advise gradual and moderate weight gain in pregnancy.
- Dermatology referral for laser treatment in severe cases.

Skin diseases unique to pregnancy – autoimmune bullous diseases and non-bullous diseases

Generalized pruritus in pregnancy (prurigo gravidarum)

Pruritus is very common during pregnancy, especially during the last trimester, and peaks in the last month. Prurigo gravidarum produces small grouped pruritic pustules on the limbs and trunk. Pruritus is known to occur in 14% of all pregnancies (Dacus 1990) and is thought to be due to cholestasis, induced by oestrogens, which leads to biliary retention. The pruritus will cease after parturition but is likely to reoccur in subsequent pregnancies.

Nursing advice and skin care

- Stop using soap in the bath, add bath oils and use soap substitutes.
- Use moisturizers regularly to soothe, hydrate and provide comfort.
- Emollients with added menthol may be helpful in soothing the itch.
- Occasionally systemic antihistamines may be prescribed in severe cases.

Polymorphic eruption of pregnancy

This skin condition is relatively common, affecting one in 200 pregnancies (Holmes & Black 1993). Polymorphic eruption of pregnancy occurs only in primigravidae and in the last trimester (after 34 weeks). The symptoms start with pruritus, erthyema and papules, starting in striae distensae on the abdomen, with the umbilicus spared and progressing to the inner arms, thighs and buttocks (Zellis & Pincus 1993). Occasionally the urticarial papules can be so severe that the appearance resembles a drug reaction. The eruption remains during pregnancy and then disappears postpartum.

The cause of polymorphic eruption of pregnancy is non-specific, but immunofluorescent tests are carried out to exclude herpes gestationis. The fetus will not be affected. The treatment is generally conservative and aimed at controlling the pruritus and itching, using emollients, antihistamines and topical steroids. If the pruritus is intolerable, oral prednisolone may be considered (Alcalay 1990). This condition was previously known as PUPP (pruritic urticarial papules and plaques of pregnancy).

Nursing advice and skin care

- Advise on total emollient therapy.
- Monitor and teach patient correct application techniques for topical steroids.
- Monitor patients on systemic steroids.

Herpes gestationis

Herpes gestationis is a rare autoimmune bullous disease of pregnancy, affecting approximately 1:60 000 pregnancies (Alcalay 1990). The name of the condition causes confusion as the condition has no relation to the herpes virus but comes from the Greek word *herpes* meaning 'to creep'. It is a skin eruption, consisting of erythematous papules and plaques with vesicles and blisters extending widely. The upper and lower extremities of the body are affected and the face is generally spared. The blisters can appear on normal-looking skin and intense pruritus is very disabling.

Herpes gestationis is most common in the second and third trimesters in a multigravida. The condition will often disappear towards the end of the pregnancy and then may flare up during delivery. Occasionally, herpes gestation is will occur just after delivery or in the first 6 weeks of the postpartum period.

Herpes gestationis is a genetic condition with a HLA histocompatibility complex located on chromosome 6. This antigen combination is only seen in 3% of women and produces an immune response. Herpes gestationis may affect the fetus; there is evidence of low birth weight babies in term pregnancies and 10% of the newborn infants suffer a mild and transient skin eruption which resolves within a few weeks (Alcalay 1990).

Treatment is with oral steroids, with 40 mg/day needed to adequately control the symptoms. The fetus will need to be carefully monitored during treatment for herpes gestationis.

Nursing advice and skin care

- Advise on total emollient therapy and control the pruritus.
- Monitor and teach patient the correct application techniques for topical steroids.
- Monitor patients on systemic steroids.

Table 7.3 outlines skin conditions unique to pregnancy.

SKIN CONDITIONS IN THE ELDERLY

Skin conditions unique to the elderly can be caused by:

- intrinsic effects of ageing (normal ageing)
- extrinsic effects of ageing
- external signs of internal problems.

Table 7.3 Skin conditions unique to pregnancy

Skin condition	Gravidae	Trimester	Recurrence in subsequent pregnancies
Pruritus gravidarum	Primi/multigravidae	Third trimester	Yes
Polymorphic eruption of pregnancy	Primigravidae	Third trimester	No
Herpes gestationis	Multigravidae	Second and third trimesters	Yes

Intrinsic effects of ageing are normal effects of the ageing process. The individual onset of the ageing process of the skin is genetically determined. The common features of ageing on the skin are dryness (xerosis), decreasing elasticity, thinning skin and prominent blood vessels. The skin also ages as a result of the extrinsic effects of ageing, namely sun exposure. Sun exposure causes pigmentary changes, dryness, textural changes (rough and leathery skin) and wrinkling.

Intrinsic effects

Dryness (xerosis)

General advice on maintaining healthy and supple skin includes the avoidance of soaps, detergents, perfumes and irritating fibres such as wool and the regular use of unscented moisturizers. Hormone replacement therapy provides some protection against ageing drying skin.

Skin that becomes extra dry will benefit from total emollient therapy. Moisturizers containing lactic acid are useful for intensive hydration and dissolving scale. If the skin becomes inflamed, mild to moderate topical steroids can be used for short periods.

Solar lentigines (liver spots)

These are benign and only require investigation if they thicken or crust.

Xanthelasma

These are fat deposits in the skin appearing as raised yellow plaques, commonly around the eyes. Xanthelasma are caused by raised lipid levels. Treatment is to lower lipid levels by diet and medication.

Skin tags (acrochordons)

Skin tags are common in people who are obese. They are pedunculated papules found in areas subjected to friction (neck, axillae and groin). Skin tags require no treatment but some people will ask for them to be removed for cosmetic reasons. Skin tags can be removed by snipping or cryosurgery.

Facial leisons

Telangiectasias, cherry angiomas, are vascular lesions which can be treated for cosmetic reasons with laser.

Sebaceous hyperplasia are enlarged sebaceous glands of the face, 1–3 mm in size, usually combined with oily skin. They do not require treatment.

Senile purpura

Collagen degeneration due to capillary fragility.

Extrinsic factors

Elastolysis (wrinkling)

Mid-dermal elastolysis is deep wrinkling caused by overexposure to ultraviolet light and smoking.

Seborrhoeic keratoses

These are benign, non-pigmented, brown or black papules and nodules, solitary or numerous which have a characteristic appearance of being stuck on the skin. They are seen in the over-60s on sun-exposed skin. The surface of seborrhoeic keratoses is greasy, waxy or scaly. The most typical sites are the face (forehead and nose), backs of hands and on the bald scalp.

Seborrhoeic keratoses should be removed as they are premalignant. Cryotherapy may be used or a topical cytotoxic drug (Efudix) is applied carefully to the lesion; an inflammatory reaction will be provoked and the lesion will clear in a few weeks.

Skin diseases common in the elderly

Skin cancer

Basal cell and squamous cell carcinomas are more common in the elderly. Basal cell carcinomas are slow growing and usually occur on the face. Bowen's disease is a term used to describe carcinoma in situ (slow growing but will progress to squamous cell carcinoma), presenting as thickened red scaly patches, often seen on the lower legs or trunk of the elderly. Bowen's disease can also present as raised ulcerated lesions and non-healing leg ulcers can warrant biopsy. Squamous cell carcinomas are related to cumulative sun exposure and occur typically in sun-exposed areas, face and backs of hands. Malignant melanomas become more common after the age of 40 but affect all age groups (Marks 1999).

Asteatotic eczema

Asteatotic eczema is also known as eczema cracqelée, which aptly describes the crackled, 'crazy paving' type appearance of the eczematous skin, which is scaly, fissured and itchy (Fig. 7.13). Asteatotic eczema is more likely to occur on the lower limbs and trunk. The condition is associated with overuse of soaps, overheating and low

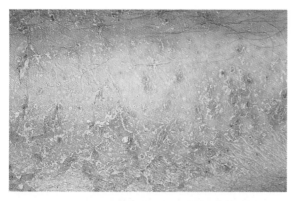

Figure 7.13 Asteatotic eczema (reproduced with the permission of St John's Institute of Dermatology).

humidity. It usually occurs in the winter and exclusively in older patients (Peters 1998).

Nursing advice and skin care

- Liberal emollients, with care taken with bath oils.
- Increase humidity and reduce heat.
- Moderately potent steroids may be necessary if the skin is irritated by dryness and itching.
- Cotton clothing.

Gravitational eczema

Gravitational eczema is also referred to as venous eczema, varicose eczema or statis dermatitis. It occurs on the lower limbs of patients suffering from venous hypertension and follows an eczematous pattern on one or both lower limbs. The skin becomes dry, flaky, itchy, red and irritated, is more prone to damage and can break down easily, leading to venous leg ulcers. In a small number of patients, the eczema generalizes to the rest of the body. The condition tends to remit and relapse. Middle-aged and elderly adults are affected and it is more common in females.

Nursing advice and skin care

- Prevent dry, flaky skin by using a moisturizer on the lower legs twice a day.
- Avoid washing with soap and perfumed products, which will cause dryness and irritation.
- Use potent steroids on the inflamed areas and reduce to lower potencies and emollients only when the eczema resolves.
- Wear support stockings, which need to be removed at night and applied before getting out of bed.
- Advise patients to improve circulation by taking regular walks, avoiding standing for long periods and when sitting with elevated legs. Protect skin from damage and if the skin breaks, seek nursing assistance immediately.

Intertrigo

Intertrigo is a frictional disorder, common in the elderly and obese patient. It is an inflamed and macerated lesion caused by friction seen in the skinfolds of the groin, abdomen, breasts and axillae. Flexural psoriasis (sharply demarcated area with fine scale) and seborrhoeic dermatitis (maceration not always present) are frequently misdiagnosed as intertrigo. Intertrigo is often infected with yeast and bacteria.

Nursing advice and skin care

- Swab the area and treat any fungal or bacterial infection present.
- Wash area with very dilute potassium permanganate solution and dry very thoroughly.
- Separate skinfolds with butter muslin to prevent friction.

Pruritus and nodular prurigo

Pruritus with dry skin is a common problem in the over-70s. It is extremely important to exclude all other causes of itching including scabies and other internal disorders which may manifest as an itch in the skin, e.g. hyperthyroidism, renal failure, obstructive jaundice. Nodular prurigo is characterized by generalized pruritus which leads to papules and nodules, which are often excoriated.

Nurses need to be aware that pruritus is similar to pain and is thus an individual experience. Pruritus, like the itch of eczema, is a diffuse intense itch, deep within the skin and impossible to relieve (Perkins 1996).

Nursing advice and skin care

- Liberal emollients, with care taken with bath oils.
- Occlusion of prurigo nodules with potent steroids under Duoderm (left in place for 1 week) can be helpful in reducing the number of nodules.
- Psychological support in understanding the effects of itch on the patient.
- Sedating antihistamines at night, if sleep is disturbed.

Herpes zoster

Herpes zoster, more commonly known as shingles, is a debilitating viral infection. The varicella zoster virus remains in the dorsal root ganglia

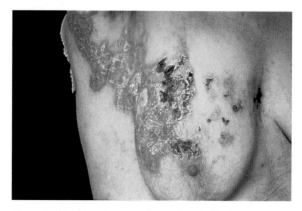

Figure 7.14   Herpes zoster (reproduced with the permission of St John's Institute of Dermatology).

after an episode of chickenpox in the younger years. The viral infection can manifest after many years, when host defences are weakened, typically in the elderly. The trunk is the area of the body commonly involved as the virus manifests with discomfort, paraesthesia and pain as a papulovesicular rash from a single dermatome. The rash then becomes crusted, erythematous, swollen and necrotic (Fig. 7.14), causing more pain and distress. Postherpetic neuralgia can persist for years (Ahmed & Berth-Jones 1999).

Nursing advice and skin care

- Ensure early treatment within the first few days of the rash appearing with antiviral agents (aciclovir or famciclovir) to shorten the duration of illness.
- Pain control with regular analgesia. Neuralgic pain may be additionally helped with amitriptyline or carbamazepine.
- Non-adherent dressings for areas of skin breakdown.
- Rest and general nursing care.

Bullous pemphigoid (see Chapter 14)

External signs of internal problems

There are many systemic diseases where skin changes are the first sign. The nurse needs to be vigilant with skin assessment in the elderly and report changes.

Signpost Box

REFERENCES

Ahmed I, Berth-Jones J 1999 Recognise skin conditions in the elderly. Practice Nurse 18(1): 44–49

Alcalay J 1990 Skin diseases unique to pregnant women. Dermatology Nursing 2(3): 148–150

Atherton D J 1992 Naevi and other developmental defects. In: Champion R H, Burton J L, Ebling F J G (eds). Textbook of dermatology. Blackwell Science, Oxford, pp 445–526

Burgess I F 1995 Human lice and their management. Advanced Parasitology 36: 243–271

Callan J P 1984 Pregnancy's effect on the skin. Postgraduate Medicine 75: 138–145

Dacus J V 1990 Pruritus in pregnancy. Clinical Obstetrics and Gynaecology 33: 728–745

Duncan C 1997 Bug busters. Nursing Times 93(49): 46–47

Higgins E, du Vivier A 1996 Skin diseases in childhood. Blackwell Science, Oxford

Holmes R C, Black M M 1993 The specific dermatoses of pregnancy. Journal of the American Academy of Dermatology 8: 405–412

Liskay A, Heer Nicol N 1998 Anatomy and physiology of the skin. In: Hill M (Ed) Dermatologic nursing essentials: a core curriculum. Anthony J Jannnetti, New Jersey

Mackie R 1992 Common skin conditions. Oxford University Press, Oxford

Mackie R 1997a Clinical dermatology, 4th edn. Oxford University Press, Oxford, pp 172–173

Mackie R 1997b Clinical dermatology, 4th edn. Oxford University Press, Oxford, pp 68–70

Marks R 1993 Roxburgh's common skin diseases. Chapman and Hall, London

Marks R 1999 Skin disease in old age. Martin Dunitz, London

Perkins P 1996 The management of eczema in adults. Nursing Standard 10(35): 49–53

Peters J 1998 Eczema in adulthood. Primary Health Care 8(5): 17–22

Rotstein H 1993 Principles and practices of dermatology. Reed International Books, Sydney

Simmons R 1999 The management of head lice: the East Kent experience. British Journal of Dermatology Nursing 3(3): 5–7

Syed S, Harper J 1996 Vascular birthmarks in children and treatment with the pulsed dye laser. Maternal and Child Health Care 2: 44–47

Wahrman J E, Honig P J 1997 The management of diaper dermatitis – rational treatment based on specific etiology. Journal of Dermatologic Therapy 2: 9–17

Weston W L, Lane A T 1991 Color textbook of pediatric dermatology. Mosby, St Louis, pp 223–230

Winsor A 1998 Tinea capitis – a growing headcount. British Journal of Dermatology Nursing 2(3): 10–12

Zellis S, Pincus S H 1993 When the pregnant woman experiences itching. Dermatology Nursing 5(5): 380–383

PATIENT SUPPORT GROUPS

Ichthyosis Support Group
National Contact (People with Ichthyosis and Carers)
16 Cambridge Court
Cambridge Avenue
Kilburn
London NW6 5AB
Tel 020 7461 0356 (after 8pm)

ISG Secretary (Medical Professionals)
2 Copnor
Woolton Hill
Newbury
Berkshire RG20 9X4
Tel 01635 253829

8

Care of the acutely ill dermatology patient

Jane Watts

INTRODUCTION

Dermatology is usually a speciality which deals with problems which may be debilitating and cause discomfort and mental anguish but are not life threatening. Although this is the general rule, we should not forget that some dermatological conditions can cause a patient to be acutely ill and have significant mortality attached to them. Knowledge of the structure and functions of the skin enables us to understand why serious skin disease can cause other organs and systems to fail.

It is essential to understand from the beginning that nursing care plays a large part in the management of acutely ill dermatology patients and has an effect on the outcome of the disease.

GENERAL ISSUES

The concept of acute skin failure

Although the consequences of liver, kidney and heart failure are well recognized it may not be as easily understood that the largest organ in our body, the skin, may also fail. The concept of acute 'skin failure' may help us understand both the severity and serious consequences of extensive skin disease (Roujeau & Revuz 1990, Irvine 1991), where large amounts of skin will slough off, leaving large, open, raw areas. It has now been recognized that these patients suffer a clinical course similar to that of extensive second-degree burns.

Consequences of extensive skin loss

As a barrier between our internal organs and the outside world, the skin prevents loss of body fluids and the entry of harmful elements from the environment. The barrier function is mainly located within the lipid structure of the stratum corneum and is altered by skin diseases which affect its quality or quantity (Blank 1987).

Fluid loss and the catabolic state

Fluid is normally lost through our skin in the form of perspiration. However, when the stratum corneum is damaged a much greater amount of fluid will be lost. The total daily cutaneous fluid loss in an adult patient with toxic epidermal necrolysis (TEN) involving 50% of their body surface area is on average 3–4 litres (Roujeau & Revuz 1990). If a disease has blisters as a component or feature, there will not only be loss of electrolytes and fluid but also protein. The loss of fluid, electrolytes and protein will lead to a reduction in the intravascular volume which must be corrected in order to prevent acute renal failure and so reduce the risk of septic shock.

The metabolic response to injury is one of marked catabolic hormonal predominance resulting in hypermetabolism and protein wasting. Energy expenditure increases with increasing severity of injury and reaches a maximum of twice resting energy expenditure when 50% of total body surface area is burned (Pasulka & Wachtel 1987). This can be likened to skin loss due to skin disease.

Infection

Infection is a big problem in damaged skin and is the main cause of death in exfoliative dermatitis, autoimmune blistering disorders and TEN (Revuz et al 1987, Murphy et al 1997). The skin lesions are usually first colonized by *Staphylococcus aureus* but may later be colonized by bacteria from the digestive tract. The use of steroids and broad-spectrum antibiotics can cause unusual pathogens to colonize, such as *Candida albicans*. Great care should be taken with any catheters or intravenous lines as they all carry a risk of introducing systemic infection. They should not be inserted near or through lesional skin, whenever possible.

Temperature regulation

Our skin plays a large part in regulating our body temperature; extensive skin damage will cause this mechanism to fail. Excessive amounts of heat will be lost through the skin and, even without infection, patients will usually have a fever and shiver. Shivering demonstrates the high level of muscular activity required to keep up the body's core temperature. The skin may feel 'hot to touch' but fanning or trying to cool the patient will further reduce the core temperature, which should remain above 37°C in order to maintain vital functions. In most patients, extensive skin loss will produce a fever. However, if hypothermia occurs there may be severe infection and irreversible septic shock.

Increased penetration of topical application

With the barrier function of the skin failing it must be remembered that applications to the skin will penetrate more easily and may produce systemic side effects.

Immunological function

The skin is an outpost of our immune system and with the skin damaged, the body's defence against microbial antigens and other organisms is reduced. This again increases the risk of septic complications.

Increased blood flow through the skin

An erythrodermic patient has a greatly increased cutaneous blood flow. This can increase the cardiac index and produce high-output cardiac failure (Fitzpatrick et al 1997). This is most likely in susceptible patients, such as the very old, the very young and those with previous heart disease.

Increased energy expenditure

Patients with large areas of skin loss due to extensive disease have been likened to patients with burns. In burns it has been demonstrated that energy expenditure rises with the extent of skin involvement (Gamelli 1988). Low environmental temperature (below 25°C) will also increase energy expenditure, as does protein loss from exudative skin lesions.

Glucose and energy expenditure

With extensive skin loss various neurologic and humoral factors are relayed through the hypothalamic pituitary axis, mediating a biphasic action.

In the first few hours, there is a decrease in cardiac output and energy expenditure; however, over the next few days, a hypermetabolic phase begins with an increase in the metabolic rate, cardiac output and oxygen consumption.

In the initial phase insulin secretion is diminished but later increases, even to above normal levels. The concomitant increase in catecholamine leads to lipolysis (fat breakdown) and insulin resistance. The blood glucose may be high but glucose utilization for energy production is suppressed at a time when the patient's catabolic state requires increased energy production.

Box 8.1   Consequences of extensive skin lesions

1. Loss of barrier function
   - Fluid loss
   - Infection
   - Impaired thermoregulation
   - Increased penetration of local applications
2. Increase in cutaneous blood flow
3. Alterations in immunological function
4. Increase in energy expenditure

DERMATOLOGICAL DISEASES WHICH CAN CAUSE THE PATIENT TO BE ACUTELY ILL

Eczema herpeticum

It needs to be remembered that a condition as prevalent as eczema can cause a dermatological emergency. Eczema herpeticum can occur when a patient with atopic eczema comes into contact with the herpes virus. Herpes simplex virus I is the most common cause of eczema herpeticum in patients with preexisting disease like atopic eczema. The virus remains latent in the sensory nerve ganglia after the primary infection and can be reactivated when triggered by sun exposure, local trauma, hormonal changes or stress. The virus can be life threatening in the immunocompromised or a person with established skin disease. Transmission is by close person-to-person contact and all patients with atopic eczema should be warned to keep away from others with active herpes infections (cold sores). Health professionals with herpes infections should keep away from the immunocompromised and those with active skin disease.

The disease starts with vesicles 1–3 mm in size developing in areas of eczema and on normal skin. They can spread rapidly over large areas of skin, becoming pustular, and then crust over within several days. The patient usually feels very unwell with fever, dehydration, electrolyte imbalance and localized or generalized lymphadenopathy. If areas around the eyes are affected, an ophthalmic opinion must be sought immediately to reduce the risk of permanent eye damage. Antiviral therapy and good supportive care have reduced the mortality rate from 50% to 10% for the severe forms of the disease (Strong 1998). With swift recognition of the disease and commencement of intravenous antiviral therapy the patient may only need 3–4 days of inpatient treatment, in a side room on a general dermatology ward. On discharge home, the course of antiviral treatment can be continued orally.

Psoriasis

Psoriasis is another common condition which rarely may prove fatal. The two types of psoriasis which can make a patient acutely ill are:

1. erythrodermic psoriasis
2. pustular psoriasis.

Erythrodermic psoriasis

This is a rare, very active form of psoriasis. In many cases, there are no known precipitating factors. However, it may be sparked off by the irritant effects of tar or dithranol or by a drug eruption or the withdrawal of potent topical or systemic steroids. The skin becomes red all over with variable scaling. It feels hot and uncomfortable and the patient will shiver and feel very unwell. There is often lymphadenopathy.

This type of psoriasis can take weeks to clear and/or revert to a lesser form of psoriasis. Treatment is slow and cautious to allow the active psoriasis to calm down. Plenty of emollients should be used plus a weak topical steroid. Systemically, an agent such as methotrexate or a retinoid will be given.

Generalized pustular psoriasis

This again is a rare form of psoriasis and, as with erythrodermic psoriasis, it may be started by irritant treatments or withdrawal of potent topical or systemic steroids or can be triggered by an infection in some patients (Ohkacuara et al 1996). There is a sequence of burning erythema followed by the appearance of tiny non-follicular superficial pustules that usually become confluent, forming lakes of pus. If the skin peels off, it leaves superficial oozing, erosions and then crusting. The lesions appear anywhere on the body but especially in flexural areas. The lesions can appear in waves and as one set of pustules dries, another one can develop. The patient will have a fever, generalized weakness, severe malaise and a leucocytosis.

Topical therapy is usually kept very bland, consisting of emollients, mild antiseptics and/or bacterial agents. Systemically retinoid or methotrexate therapy may be given. Other symptomatic treatment is given as necessary.

Autoimmune blistering disorders

Autoimmune blistering disorders are serious conditions. Pemphigus has a mortality rate of 5–10% (Bystryn 1984) and is a more aggressive disease than pemphigoid. However, the mortality rate of pemphigoid is higher, at around 20% of patients at 1 year since the onset of the disease (Savin 1987). Even if most deaths are related to the older age of the patients it is argued that pemphigoid should be considered the more severe of the two diseases (Roujeau & Revuz 1990). In both disorders high doses of systemic steroids are needed to get the disease under control. The patient is most at risk of death when erosions and blisters remain despite high doses of drugs.

Pemphigoid

Bullous pemphigoid is a chronic, autoimmune disorder caused by antibodies to the basement membrane and presenting as a chronic blistering eruption. Bullous pemphigoid is the most common immunobullous disease in Western Europe. In France and Germany the incidence is approximately 6–7 cases per million of the population per year (Wojnarowska 1998). It is usually a disease of the elderly, the average age of onset being between 60 and 80 years. It presents with bullae arising from normal skin or on an urticated base (Fig. 8.1). The blisters arise subepidermally which explains why the serum-filled bullae are tense and usually seen intact (Fig. 8.2). Nikolsky's sign is negative (Nikolsky's sign is dislodging of the epidermis by finger pressure in the area of a lesion, leading to erosion or extension of a blister). The flexures are often affected but the mucous membranes are not. Pemphigoid can be a self-limiting disease and often the treatment can be stopped in 1–2 years. The disease is diagnosed by clinical presentation and by skin biopsies for histology and immunofluorescence.

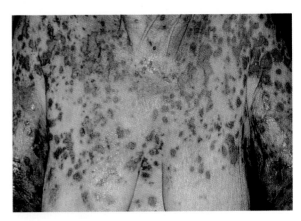

Figure 8.1 Bullous pemphigoid on the chest.

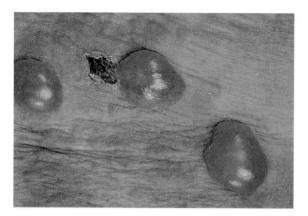

Figure 8.2 Pemphigoid blisters.

Treatment is with high-dose oral steroids, often with other immunosuppressants. The aim is to reduce the doses when possible and end up on a lower maintenance dose until treatment can be stopped.

Pemphigus vulgaris

This is another serious, acute or chronic bullous disorder, characterized by acute exacerbations and remissions. Pemphigus vulgaris has a worldwide incidence of approximately 0.5–3 per 100 000 per year and onset is usually between the ages of 40 and 60 years. The blisters arise from normal or erythematous skin and form intraepidermally (Fig. 8.4A). This gives rise to flaccid blisters which rupture easily and leave large erosions (Fig. 8.3). The skin and mucous membranes are affected; many patients have lesions in the mouth first. Nikolsky's sign is positive. Patients usually feel

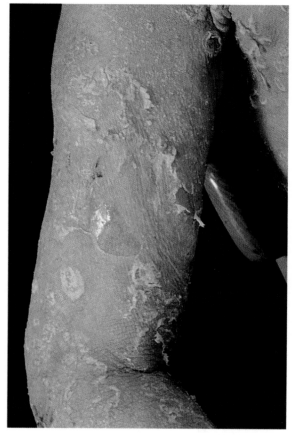

Figure 8.3 Pemphigus vulgaris.

unwell with malaise, weakness and weight loss. Even with treatment, the course of the disease is long with continued exacerbations and remissions. Diagnosis is made by the clinical picture and skin biopsies for immunofluorescence and histology.

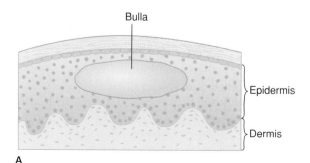

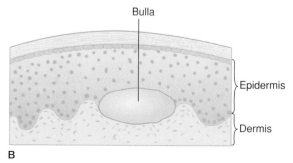

Figure 8.4 **A:** Intraepidermal bulla, as in pemphigus. **B:** Subepidermal bulla, as in bullous pemphigoid.

Treatment, as for pemphigoid, is with high-dose oral steroids and steroid-sparing drugs such as azathioprine. Topical steroids will also be applied to the affected areas. In these conditions the topical steroids can be applied to the open lesions, as they will reduce the disease process and inflammation, thus promoting healing.

Case study 8.1 A patient's perspective on pemphigus vulgaris

Since 1995 I've had PV and although it's been fairly volatile, it was relatively well controlled. I was used to minor flares and crises and thought I'd learned to live with its ups and downs but I don't think I'd realized just what could happen till early this year when lesions in my mouth and throat went completely crazy. I had about 5–6 mouth lesions but nothing too bad. Then within only 4 days, I suddenly deteriorated to the point where mouth, palate and throat were completely lesioned and I had to be hospitalized with complete dysphagia, unable even to swallow my own saliva. Everyone was marvellous and pulled me through but what was so frightening was realizing that despite being controlled, the PV could become life threatening so quickly and with no prior warning. I couldn't help thinking that if I hadn't had access to such a good medical team and the necessary drugs, then I'd have died within weeks. It's the *speed* of deterioration that's terrifying.

There are other things that are also hard to deal with. The pain of oral lesions is really intense and you have to live with that constantly to one degree or another. Although medical books often don't mention it, body lesions can itch and burn continuously. It's very hard to put up with. PV patients really rely on nurses to help with the pain and the itching and burning.

The other thing that often gets forgotten is how rotten you can feel on the drugs, not just with long-term problems like osteoporosis but daily problems like exhaustion and nausea.

Erythema multiforme

Erythema multiforme is usually brought about by a reaction to the herpes simplex virus or to a drug. Typically, lesions are preceded by symptoms of an upper respiratory tract infection. Annular, non-scaling plaques then appear on palms, soles, face, arms and legs. The lesions enlarge but clear centrally, giving the typical 'target' in presentation (Fig. 8.5). New lesions will continue to appear for 1–2 weeks or until the precipitating factor has been removed.

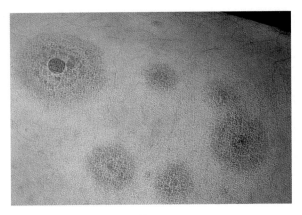

Figure 8.5 Erythema multiforme.

Erythema multiforme minor is not life threatening and resolves with the removal of the cause. It may only need symptomatic treatment such as emollients and antihistamines for itching.

Erythema multiforme major involves mucous membranes and is more extensive and severe and lesions can become confluent and bullous with positive Nikolsky's sign. Involvement of mucous membranes can cause complications with the eyes, mouth and genitalia. With this form of the disease, the patient will feel generally unwell and have a fever.

Stevens–Johnson syndrome (SJS) and toxic epidermal necrolysis (TEN)

SJS and TEN have often been linked into the erythema multiforme spectrum of disease (Wolkenstein & Revuz 1995). However, the spectrum of SJS–TEN and that of erythema multiforme can now be distinguished (Bastuji-Garin et al 1993). The clinical features of the two conditions are different, with SJS patients having widely distributed purpuric macules and blisters on the trunk and face, rather than the target lesions of erythema multiforme on the extremities (Wolkenstein & Revuz 1995).

Nearly all cases of TEN and SJS are related to pharmaceutical agents; much less commonly they have also been linked to viral, bacterial and fungal infections and neoplastic disease (Murphy et al 1997). Both SJS and TEN tend to be induced by the same drugs. Drugs often implicated are

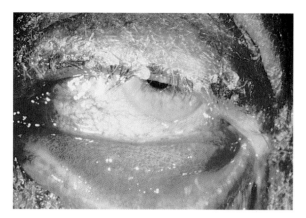

Figure 8.6 Stevens–Johnson syndrome.

sulphonamides, anticonvulsants and non-steroidal antiinflammatory drugs (Roujeau & Revuz 1990). The similar histopathological findings and causative drugs for both SJS and TEN suggest that SJS is a mild form and TEN is a severe form of the same spectrum (Roujeau 1994).

Stevens–Johnson syndrome

This is characterized by skin tenderness, erythema of the skin and mucosa, blistering and extensive cutaneous and mucosal exfoliation. SJS always involves the mucous membranes and there is severe blistering and erosion of the lips, eyes (Fig. 8.6) and genitalia. In SJS there is usually less than 10% of epidermal detachment.

Toxic epidermal necrolysis

This is the most severe acute blistering disease with a death rate of around 30% (Roujeau & Revuz 1990). It occurs in all age groups, including babies, but the incidence increases sharply among the elderly (Wolkenstein & Revuz 1995). In TEN more than 30% of the epidermis will be detached from the dermis. The mucous membranes are involved in almost all cases. Patients will experience fever and flu-like symptoms 1–3 days prior to the onset of the lesions. The skin will become tender and there may be conjunctival burning or itching. The lesions then develop quickly with a widespread sheet-like loss of the

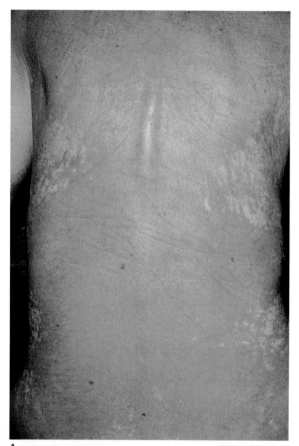

A

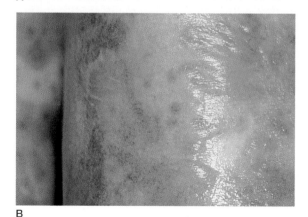

B

Figure 8.7 **A&B:** Toxic epidermal necrolysis.

epidermis, leaving a dark-red oozing dermis. The entire skin surface may be involved with up to 100% of the epidermis sloughing off (Fig. 8.7).

The histology of an advanced lesion shows necrosis from the basal cells spreading to the whole of the epidermis. It is recommended that a skin biopsy be taken to confirm the diagnosis in all cases in which drugs may be involved as this will avoid any subsequent controversies (Roujeau & Revuz 1990).

Severe involvement of mucous membranes is seen in virtually all patients with TEN. In order of frequency, the most common surfaces involved are the lips, buccal mucosa, tongue, conjunctiva, urethral meatus, vagina and anus. The severity of the oesophageal involvement usually parallels the severity of the skin lesions. With urethral involvement, retention of urine can be a complication. The incidence of occular complications in TEN is from 50% to 100% (Born & Zawada 1989).

TEN has a less favourable prognosis than burns of the same extent because of systemic involvement. Half the patients will have liver changes and stress and infection can lead to glycosurea. Haematological abnormalities are present in almost all patients. The most serious systemic complication is lung involvement and 10–20% of patients may need artificial ventilation. Infection is the main cause of death in patients with TEN. Treatment is mainly symptomatic, with fluid replacement, antibacterial therapy and nutritional management.

NURSING CARE

Treatment of life-threatening dermatology conditions involves intensive nursing care. This is not only vital for the comfort of the patient but also, by keeping the patient free of infection or by monitoring and acting on early signs of infection or change in status, nurses can make a difference to the patient's outcome. The lack of skilled nursing care can have a negative impact on patients' survival (Murphy et al 1997).

Every patient with a life-threatening dermatosis will present with an individual set of symptoms and problems. Nursing care will therefore be different for each one, although principles remain the same (see Box 8.2). The areas outlined below should all be taken into consideration

***

Box 8.2 Points to consider when treating patients with acute skin failure

1. Fluid replacement
2. Electrolyte balance
3. Nutrition
4. Treatment of infection
5. Environmental temperature
6. Anticoagulant therapy
7. Pain relief
8. Bed (reduce pressure to skin)
9. Dressings
10. Psychological effects
11. Exercise (physiotherapy)
12. Care of relatives

***

when planning the patient's care. Relevant areas can be identified for each patient.

Environment

A seriously ill dermatology patient needs to be cared for in a well-staffed and well-equipped area. This is usually in a specialized dermatology centre, a burns unit or an intensive care unit. In some centres, liaison has been established between dermatology teams and intensive care units.

The patient must be nursed in a side room to limit the risk of infection, with a constant temperature of 30–32°C being maintained. This will reduce calorie loss through the skin and the resultant shivering and stress. If the patient has a high fever any attempt to decrease their central temperature by cooling the environment will result in added energy expenditure and this will prove another threat to their survival. However, lowering the central temperature with antipyretics will help reduce heat loss from the skin and improve the cardiac index.

The fragile state of the skin means that the patient will need to be nursed on a bed which reduces the amount of pressure on every area of the body. In a unit which is likely to admit such patients, it is well worth researching the bed situation, so when needed, the best possible bed can be obtained. Air-fluidized beds are good at pressure reduction but may not give full pressure relief when the patient is sitting up. Also, it is difficult for a patient to get on and off an air-fluidized bed and this may hamper attempts to keep the patient mobile. It should also be noted that some very oily preparations cannot be used on an air-fluidized bed. Some of the newer air beds can give very low pressures, even when the patient is sitting up. Sections of these beds can be deflated or inflated independently to help the patient get in and out of bed. It is also ideal to have a bed which can be both temperature regulated and have a facility for weighing the patient.

The patient's limbs should be carefully positioned in the bed. It is essential to ensure that skin lesions do not heal with contractures. Passive exercise may be carried out on some patients to keep joints and muscles from becoming stiff. It is often useful to call in the physiotherapist for advice.

Topical therapy

The skin needs to be kept clean and well lubricated. When at all possible, the best way of cleaning is with an antiseptic and emollient bath. This may be a long and traumatic procedure for both the patient and the nurse and care must be taken not to let the patient get too cold. The bath should be kept at 35–38°C. When it is not possible for the patient to get into the bath, antiseptic solutions and emollients can be used for washing the patient in bed.

The skin needs to be kept well lubricated at all times to prevent sticking and rubbing and to maintain comfort. Bland emollients, such as 50% liquid paraffin in 50% white soft paraffin or aqueous cream, should be used. This can be carefully applied to the skin; warming the creams by placing the container in a bowl of warm water prior to application can help the cream to go on more easily and be less painful. Aqueous cream can also be applied to foam sheets, such as Lyofoam or Gautex sheets, for the patient to lie on. Dressings may or may not be used. Some patients will find that plenty of emollients act as a cover to their lesions whereas others may be more comfortable with certain areas covered with dressings. When dressings are used, plenty

of emollients should be applied first to prevent sticking and the dressing should be secured with a light bandage; tape must never be stuck to the patient's skin. Areas need to be cleaned and dressings changed regularly to prevent infection.

Topical steroids may be used in some patients, especially those with autoimmune blistering disorders. Topical antibiotics are indicated in others, either on large or small areas or around catheters or lines.

Mouth care

This is extremely important especially as many patients have a lot of oral lesions. Antiseptic mouthwashes can be used every hour. Analgesic mouth washes may be useful before eating. When the patient is too sick to perform their own mouth washes, the nurse will need to carry out mouth-care procedures for the patient.

A clear airway must obviously always be maintained. When the patient has a lot of oral lesions, great care needs to be taken to ensure that lesions or peeling skin do not obstruct the airway.

Eye care

Patients with extensive lesions on or around the eyes may need daily examination by an ophthalmologist. Eyes need to be cleaned and antiseptic or antibiotic eyedrops applied every 1–2 hours and synechiae must be disrupted. Ointments are useful prior to the patient going to sleep to keep the eyes from drying.

Care of catheters and lines

Anything which provides another portal of entry for infection should be avoided but at times catheters and intravenous lines are necessary. Great attention must be paid to the care of these and local infection control policies adhered to strictly. Central lines should be avoided and peripheral lines should be sited in non-lesional areas when possible. Catheters should be changed and cultured regularly and bacterial sampling performed at least every 2 days.

Fluid replacement and electrolyte balance

The patient may have unconsciously limited oral intake for several days prior to clinical presentation, due to a sore throat and generally feeling unwell. This is an important point because the patient may already be dehydrated before the onset of the extensive fluid loss associated with diseases such as TEN.

Intravenous fluid replacement must be initiated as soon as possible. During the first few days, IV fluids will be required with the type and amount of fluid administered being adjusted daily. Intravenous fluids should be gradually replaced by oral or nasogastric administration. Exclusive nasogastric or oral fluid replacement is rarely possible before the second week from commencement of therapy. Fluids given will include normal saline, albumin and potassium. Regular blood analysis of urea, electrolytes, albumin and blood glucose will dictate which fluids are prescribed.

Nutrition

Nasogastric feeding must also be initiated as soon as possible for nutritional support, to minimize protein losses and promote healing. Even if patients are able to eat orally, it may still be necessary to give tube-feeding supplements overnight. In all cases enteral feeding is preferable to parenteral therapy considering the risk of venous line contamination. It is essential to involve the dietician for advice on the nutritional regime. The diet should be high in protein and calories, to counteract losses and aid healing.

Patients may have poor gastric emptying which gives rise to the risk of regurgitation and inhalation. It is necessary to check residual gastric volume periodically by aspiration and if more than 50 ml is present in the stomach, feeding should be stopped (Roujeau & Revuz 1990).

Pain relief

Patients with extensive skin lesions experience a lot of pain which may be very hard to control. Not only is there pain from the extensive skin lesions but those with mucosal lesions will also suffer with pain from mouth, throat and eye lesions. Advice should be sought from the pain relief team where available. Often, morphine-based drugs are needed to keep the patient as free from pain as possible. The patient will be in most pain when activities and procedures are being carried out, such as bathing or applying the treatment. In very severe cases an anaesthetist may consider giving IV midazolam, to enable dressings to be carried out. Pain relief must be given regularly and especially to co-incide with activities.

Monitoring systemic treatment

Most patients will need antibiotics at some stage of their disease but it is recommended that these are given as soon as signs of sepsis are noticed,

---

Box 8.3 Observations on patients with acute skin disorders (adapted from Roujeau & Revuz 1990)

Frequency	Observation
Every hour	Respiration rate
	Blood pressure
	Heart rate
	Urinary volume
	Glycosuria
	Urinary osmolality
Every 3–4 hours	Temperature/shivering
	Consciousness
	Gastric emptying
Once or twice daily	Extension of skin lesions
	Body weight
	Calculation of fluid losses
	Arterial blood gases
	Chest X-ray
	Blood examinations
	Blood cell counts
	Urea, nitrogen, creatinine
	Glucose
	Electrolytes
	Albumin
	Phosphorus
	Enzymes
	Urinary examinations
	Urea, nitrogen, creatinine
	Glucose
	Electrolytes
Every other day	Bacteriology of skin lesions

rather than prophylactically. This is so that specific organisms can be targeted rather than broad-spectrum antibiotics given for long periods, giving rise to the risk of resistance to antibiotics.

Patients with extensive skin diseases have a combination of factors which make them prone to thromboembolisms. Pulmonary embolism has been known as a cause of death in patients with extensive skin disease. Therefore, most patients are put onto anticoagulant therapy during the course of their treatment.

Oral steroids tend not to be used now to treat SJS and TEN but will be used in very high doses, up to 320 mg/day, in patients with autoimmune blistering disorders (Savin 1987). Side effects will be present with doses this high and treatment to counteract them, such as insulin for raised blood sugar, will need to be initiated. It should also be remembered that high-dose oral steroids can temporarily change a person's personality; for example, they can become manic or depressed.

In generalized pustular psoriasis, cytotoxic drugs such as methotrexate will be given and the reaction to doses and level of clearing with each dose must be carefully observed so that future doses can be prescribed precisely.

Psychological support

Critically ill patients with extensive cutaneous lesions will need psychological support. SJS and TEN are conditions which have sudden onset and the patient and family have to cope with the speed at which the patient becomes so acutely ill.

The autoimmune blistering disorders, especially pemphigus, can take a long time to get under control. During this time the patient will suffer from large open wounds and pain as well as from the effects of high doses of steroids.

Generalized pustular psoriasis and erythrodermic psoriasis can take weeks to stabilize, during which time the patient is extremely ill and may suffer a succession of improvements and deterioration of the disease.

An added problem with being so acutely ill with skin disorders is that they are very visible, both to the patient and to relatives.

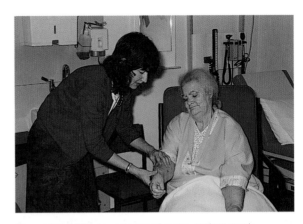

Figure 8.8   The importance of nurse–patient touch.

Counselling at this acute stage is best carried out by the nurse during the 24-hour care that the patient will need. It will not be formal counselling but will arise from the caring and understanding of the nurse looking after the patient and the building of a therapeutic relationship (Fig. 8.8).

The relatives must not be forgotten. They will find it extremely distressing to see a loved one in such an obviously ill state. It is helpful to discuss aspects of the patient's care with them. There are often some things they can do to assist with care and this may alleviate the feeling of 'helplessness' which is common.

It must also be remembered that staff caring for these patients will need support too. When the patient is critically ill they will often need a nurse present at all times. When a procedure is difficult and painful it will be psychologically distressing for both the patient and the nurse. As these patients tend to be in hospital for several weeks, if not longer, nurses get to know the patients very well and whilst this can have an extremely positive effect on the patient and the nurse, it can also be psychologically exhausting.

CONCLUSION

Life-threatening dermatology conditions are rare but when they do occur, intensive medical and nursing care is needed.

It is essential that such patients are cared for in a specialized area used to dealing with these conditions. Much of the treatment is nursing care, as the patient has to be supported and infection minimized to allow survival whilst reepithelialization occurs.

REFERENCES

Bastuji-Garin S, Rzany B, Stern R S et al 1993 Clinical classification of cases of toxic epidermal necrolysis and erythema multiforme. Archives of Dermatology 179: 92–96

Blank I H 1987 The skin as an organ of protection. In: Fitzpatrick T B, Eisen A Z, Wolff K, Fredberg I M, Austien K F (eds) Dermatology in general medicine, 3rd edn. MacGraw Hill, New York, pp 337–342

Born T E, Zawada, E T 1989 Toxic epidermal necrolysis: a medical student's perspective. South Dakota Journal of Medicine 42(II): 15–19

Bystryn J C 1984 Adjuvant therapy of pemphigus. Archives of Dermatology 170: 941–951

Fitzpatrick T B, Johnson R A, Wolff K, Polano M K, Suurmond D 1997 Colour atlas and synopsis of clinical dermatology. Common and serious diseases: erythroderma, 3rd edn. McGraw-Hill, New York

Gamelli R L 1988 Nutritional problems of the acute and chronic burn patient. Relevance to epidermolysis bullosa. Archives of Dermatology 124: 756–759

Irvine C 1991 'Skin failure': a real entity: discussion paper. Journal of the Royal Society of Medicine 84: 412–413

Murphy J T, Purdre G F, Hunt J L 1997 Toxic epidermal necrolysis. Journal of Burns Care and Rehabititation 18: 417–420

Ohkacuara A, Yasuda H, Kobayashi H et al 1996 Generalized pustular psoriasis in Japan: two distinct groups formed by differences in symptoms and genetic background. Acta Dermato-Venereologica 76(1): 68–71

Pasulka P S, Wachtel T L 1987 Nutritional considerations for the burned patient. Surgical Clinics of North America 67(1): 109–131

Roujeau J C 1994 The spectrum of Stevens–Johnson syndrome and toxic epidermal necrolysis: a clinical classification. Journal of Investigative Dermatology 102: S28–S30

Roujeau J C, Revuz J 1990 Intensive care in dermatology. In: Champion R H, Pye R J (eds) Recent advances in dermatology, no. 8. Churchill Livingstone, Edinburgh, pp 85–99

Revuz J, Penso D, Roujeau J C et al 1987 Toxic epidermal necrolysis: clinical findings and prognosis factors in 87 patients. Archives of Dermatology 123: 1160–1165

Savin J A 1987 Death in bullous pemphigoid. Clinics in Dermatology 5: 52–59

Strong D 1998 Dermatological emergencies. In: Till M J (ed) Dermatological nursing essentials: a core curriculum. Pitman, New Jersey, pp 319–332

Wojnarowska F 1998 Subepidermal immunobullous disease. In: Chapman R H, Burton J L, Burns D A, Breathnach S M (eds) Textbook of dermatology, vol. 3, 6th edn. Blackwell Science, Oxford, pp 1865–1892

Wolkenstein P, Revuz J 1995 Drug-induced severe skin reactions. Incidence, management and prevention. Drug Safety 13(1): 56–68

PATIENT SUPPORT GROUP

Pemphigus Vulgaris Network
Flat C, 26 St Germans Rd
London SE23 1RJ

9

Psoriasis

Julie Van Onselen

INTRODUCTION

Psoriasis is a chronic, inflammatory and non-infectious skin condition which recurs throughout life, affecting up to 3% of the UK population (Camp 1998). In practical terms, this means that in an average-sized practice of 9000 patients, an estimated 250–300 are likely to suffer from psoriasis.

Psoriasis is characterized by well-demarcated red plaques which are thick, scaly, uncomfortable, often itchy and unsightly. Psoriasis affects males and females equally, although female onset is often earlier. Psoriasis affects children, adults and older people and may occur at any age. There are several forms of psoriasis and areas can occur anywhere on the body, with severity ranging from small patches on the elbows and knees to total body. Scalp psoriasis affects approximately 50% of all psoriatics (Helm & Camisa 1998).

Psoriasis is often underestimated as a cause of physical suffering and great psychological distress. Psoriasis can have a profound impact on quality of life for the sufferer and their family. Finlay & Coles (1995) explored the effect of severe psoriasis on the quality of life of 369 patients. One aspect of the study involved a comparison with three chronic 'life-threatening conditions': diabetes, asthma and bronchitis. The results showed that having psoriasis was worse than having any of the three comparative diseases.

RECOGNITION AND TYPES OF PSORIASIS

Psoriasis is a chronic skin condition characterized by inflamed and scaly skin, commonly in a plaque form. The size of the plaques can range from a few millimetres to several centimetres in diameter; whole areas of the body can be covered with one plaque, e.g. the back. Psoriasis may affect any part of the skin surface. It is not infectious but relapses and remits through the patient's life. Psoriasis is unsightly; the skin integrity is compromised and psoriatic areas may be uncomfortable, itchy and sore.

There are several different forms of psoriasis: chronic plaque, scalp, guttate, flexural, localized (palmoplantar), generalized pustular and erythrodermic (see Figs 9.1–9.7, respectively). These are all outlined in Table 9.1. Additional features of psoriasis are outlined in Box 9.1.

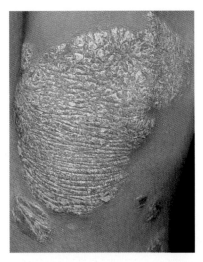

Figure 9.1
Chronic plaque psoriasis (reproduced with the permission of St John's Institute of Dermatology).

Box 9.1 Other features of psoriasis

- *Face* – facial plaques are rare. Common involvement includes the forehead, hairline, external auditory canal or small scaly patches generally on the face, especially the upper eyelids
- *Flexures (body folds)* – associated with all types of psoriasis, commonly affecting the groins, natal cleft, antecubital and popliteal fossae
- *Genital areas* – 2–5% of male patients have psoriasis on their penis. Genital psoriasis is less common in females and affects the perivulval skin with minimal scaling
- *Psoriatic arthropathy* – arthritis occurring in approximately 7% of all psoriasis sufferers. Often small joints are affected but larger joints with varying degrees of physical disability occur
- *Nails* – 25–50% of all psoriasis sufferers, commoner in older patients. Psoriatic nail changes include pitting, salmon patches, onycholysis or subungual hyperkeratosis
- *Sites of trauma* – the Köebner phenomenon is the tendency for psoriatic lesions to develop at the site of trauma (usually 10–14 days after the trauma)

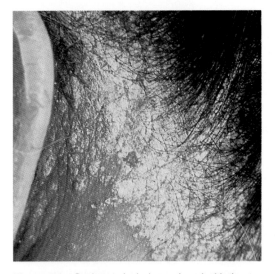

Figure 9.2 Scalp psoriasis (reproduced with the permission of Dr Tony Burns, Consultant Dermatologist, Leicester Royal Infirmary).

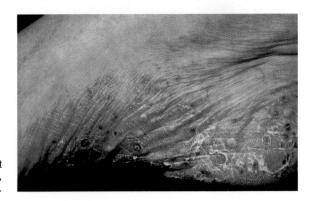

Figure 9.3 Localized pustular psoriasis on a foot (reproduced with the permission of Dr Tony Burns, Consultant Dermatologist, Leicester Royal Infirmary).

Table 9.1 Types of psoriasis

	Appearance and sites	Onset, course and other features
Chronic plaque psoriasis	Well-demarcated, raised pink plaques with dry silvery white scales (type 2)	Affects 90% of all patients with psoriasis
	Elbows, knees, lower back, common sites Rare in children, especially under-5s Peak prevalence (type 1) in 25–34 year age group with second smaller peak (type 2) in 55–74 year age group	Mid-teens to early 20s peak Nail involvement, pitting and onycholysis common
Scalp psoriasis	Mild – scalp will be dry and flaky Psoriasis can occur on the scalp only Moderate/severe – scalp will also be red and inflamed with well-demarcated plaques Any hair loss/thinning is temporary	50% of all patients additionally have scalp psoriasis
Guttate psoriasis	Small, extensive round red papules Frequently preceded by a streptococcal throat infection 'like raindrops' appear commonly on trunk or develop into chronic plaque form	Most common in children and teenagers Can clear in 2–3 months, or be recurrent
Flexural	Well-demarcated red smooth plaques Often confused with fungal infections with little scale. Affects submammary, and intertrigo axillary and anogenital skinfolds	More common in obese and elderly patients, especially women
Localized pustular	Palms and soles are inflamed and scaly with yellow sterile pustules Pustules dry to form brown patches	More common in middle-aged females. Associated with smoking
Generalized pustular	Acute form of psoriasis – dermatological emergency Fluid and electrolyte imbalance Confluent sterile pustules High outputs/cardiac decompensation on a background of generalized erythema Intensive nursing care	Develops rapidly, all ages Withdrawal of systemic steroids
Erythrodermic	Entire skin surface is inflamed (erythematous) As above	As above

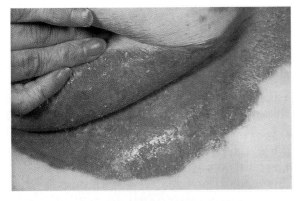

Figure 9.4 Flexural psoriasis (reproduced with the permission of Dr Tony Burns, Consultant Dermatologist, Leicester Royal Infirmary).

WHAT HAPPENS IN THE SKIN? THE PATHOPHYSIOLOGY OF PSORIASIS

The skin is composed of many layers contained in the epidermis and dermis. In normal skin the cells reproduce and move from the dermis to the epidermis to be shed. This process in normal skin takes approximately 28 days and is known as proliferation.

In psoriasis the new skin cells (keratinocytes) reproduce too quickly and move up to the skin surface whilst the unmatured surface cells are still present (Fig. 9.8). The turnover time is reduced to 4 days and the proliferation of the epidermal cells is increased 30-fold, which results in

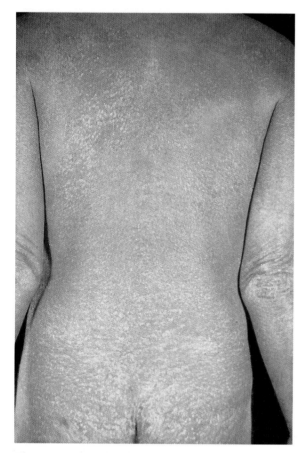

Figure 9.5 Erythrodermic psoriasis (reproduced with the permission of Dr Tony Burns, Consultant Dermatologist, Leicester Royal Infirmary).

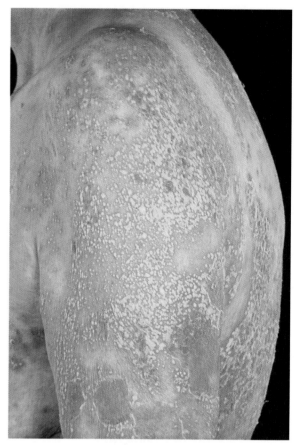

Figure 9.6 Generalized pustular psoriasis (reproduced with the permission of Dr Tony Burns, Consultant Dermatologist, Leicester Royal Infirmary).

the loose silver scaling. Psoriasis also produces a thickened epidermis with an associated increased blood flow to the skin. The capillaries become dilated and surrounded by an infiltrate composed of white blood cells due to the activation of the immune system. This increased blood supply affects temperature control and causes raised erythemic areas (Camisa 1994).

The uninvolved skin around the plaques appears normal but is often generally dry. This skin often remains dormant but can be activated intermittently. There is an underlying abnormality with the entire skin of a psoriasis sufferer. Therefore plaques can form anywhere in the body and an individual may experience several different patterns and sites of psoriasis in a lifetime.

WHAT CAUSES PSORIASIS?

The exact causes and the genetics of psoriasis are not known. Psoriasis is likely to be inherited as the condition is familial; one-third of psoriasis patients have a relative who suffers (Ahnini 1999). Psoriasis may be in a person's genetic make-up and is often triggered by certain factors. These include:

- *infection* – streptococcal upper respiratory tract infections in guttate psoriasis
- *some medications* – e.g. antimalarials, lithium, propranolol and other beta blockers, quinidine, oral steroids, indomethacin and tetracyclines
- *alcohol and smoking* – there is a reported association between developing and

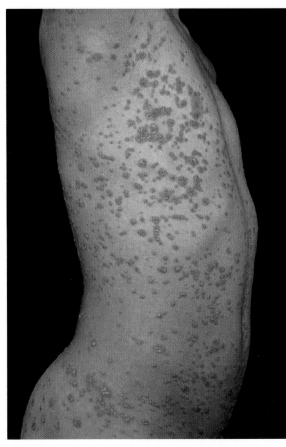

Figure 9.7 Guttate psoriasis (reproduced with the permission of St John's Institute of Dermatology).

aggravating psoriasis and high intakes of alcohol and cigarette smoke (Naldi et al 1992)

- *climatic changes* – sunlight is generally helpful but in 10% of patients is a trigger factor. Autumn and winter often aggravate psoriasis
- *skin trauma* – psoriasis can appear at the site of skin trauma after 7–14 days (known as the Köebner phenomenon)
- *stress* – stressful life events often precipitate an episode of psoriasis.

PSORIATIC ARTHROPATHY

In the past 30 years psoriatic arthropathy has been recognized as a separate entity from rheumatoid arthritis. The incidence of arthropathy in psoriasis sufferers has been estimated at between 5% and 7%. The most common presentation of arthropathy is asymmetrical oligoarthropathy, affecting the interphalangeal joints (distal or proximal) (Fig. 9.9). A minority of patients with psoriatic arthropathy will suffer with more mutilating and severe forms of arthritis extensively affecting all joints.

In the mildest forms, psoriatic arthritis should be treated as any other form of arthritis, with aspirin or non-steroidal antiinflammatory drugs. Other forms of treatment can involve using heat pads, warm soaks and exercise programmes. Treatment for severe psoriatic arthropathy will involve referral to a rheumatologist for arthritis

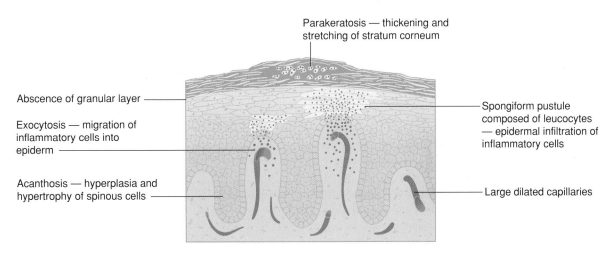

Figure 9.8 Normal and psoriatic skin.

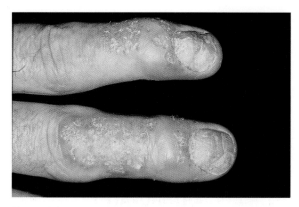

Figure 9.9 Psoriatic arthropathy (reproduced with the permission of Dr Tony Burns, Consultant Dermatologist, Leicester Royal Infirmary).

treatments such as antiarthritis medication, local injections of steroids, gold injections, physiotherapy and reconstructive surgery. Methotrexate is an effective treatment for patients with severe psoriatic arthritis.

PSYCHOSOCIAL IMPLICATIONS OF PSORIASIS

Psoriasis has many physical effects but the psychological and social impact can have devastating effects on the sufferer's self-esteem and self-perception. Psoriasis, like other skin conditions, can often not be hidden. Gollnick (1998) describes the far-ranging psychological and social effects of psoriasis. These include experiences of being an outsider in a family, experiencing less social interaction and understanding from friends, effects on personal and sexual relationships and being excluded from some professions. The psoriasis sufferer may experience stigmatization, resignation and helplessness and dysmorphobia (distorted body image).

The type and extent of psoriasis do not necessarily equate to patient distress (Penzer 1996). A patient with a minimal amount of psoriasis could suffer psychologically and socially as much as someone who has over 50% of their body affected. This is particularly evident when the patient has facial, palmar or genital psoriasis. A survey of the social and psychological effects of psoriasis showed that 72% of patients avoided swimming,

40% avoided all sport, 34% avoided the hairdresser, 64% said their choice of clothes was restricted and 50% said that psoriasis inhibited their sexual relationships (Ramsay & O'Reagan 1988).

Nurses need to understand and be aware of the psychological effects of psoriasis. The nursing assessment should always include the patient's perception of their psoriasis and it is important to ask the patient what their psoriasis stops them doing and how their psoriasis has made them feel in the past. Remember that a small area can cause the patient great distress, especially on a visible area such as the face. Genital psoriasis is another example of a special site which, even at the most minimal, can cause great distress to patients. Patients can be very fearful of sexually transmitted disease and will feel very embarrassed and often their relationships can be affected.

Stress is often perceived to be a causative factor in psoriasis. Physical and psychological stress can trigger psoriasis. A research study (Al'abadie et al 1994) has shown that psoriasis patients do not experience more stressful life events than other patient groups but they perceive the events to be more stressful. Treatment itself can often be stressful, as it can be time consuming, inconvenient and messy.

The risk of psoriasis is higher in smokers (more than 15 cigarettes a day) compared with non-smokers. Alcohol consumption (more than three drinks a day) is also linked to a higher risk of developing psoriasis (Naldi et al 1992).

Case study 9.1 Patient's view

They're used to skin things – they don't say disgusting or something just because you've got it. The main problem is being out and about, because the skin problem is the sort of thing that people would not think you would have to go into hospital for, because it doesn't kill you or anything. People don't realize just how important it is to have clear skin and it does make a difference, not just socially but mentally. You know you can't go swimming or say you feel comfortable with friends. I mean, the summer is the worst obviously because you can't wear the clothes you would like to wear. But it's not just that it's uncomfortable, so that it cracks and that sort of thing. A lot of people get it too.

Patient on a dermatology ward (Ersser 1996)

MANAGING AND TREATING PSORIASIS

The nurse can offer support and advice on the treatments and practicalities of topical application and skin care. An integral part of nursing assessment in dermatology is using touch to feel the patient's skin condition. Touching the psoriasis can provide many psychological benefits for the patient. Patients with psoriasis can experience isolation through lack of touch from people close to them, which in turn can be emotionally disabling. Psychosocial support is paramount in providing education and advice on treatments.

Psoriasis is treated topically in the majority of patients and systemically (phototherapy and oral medication) for the minority. Most patients being treated with topical therapy will be managed by primary care and most patients treated systemically will be managed by secondary care. All psoriasis treatments take weeks rather than days to clear the condition. Patients and their families require much support and motivation which can be provided by nursing care. Lack of success with topical treatments is likely to be due to insufficient practical demonstration and advice. Useful questions to ask patients during assessment are shown in Box 9.2.

Box 9.2   Questions to ask patients concerning practicalities of topical treatments (Van Onselen 1998)

1. Ask patient to demonstrate the technique they use to apply treatments. Is the technique correct and do they use enough? Can they reach all areas affected?
2. Does the patient have adequate supplies of treatments? Where does the patient keep their treatments? Moisturizers can be carried around in a small pot for reapplication during the day.
3. Treatment application needs to become a routine part of everyday life and minimize disruption to the patient's lifestyle. So does the patient have a routine for applying treatment? At the same time each day?
4. If the patient has a partner, can they help with treatment applications, especially to difficult areas (e.g. scalp treatments)?
5. When the patient is away from home, do they still treat their psoriasis?
6. What does their psoriasis stop the patient from doing and are they motivated to self manage their skin condition?

Case study 9.2   Attending a nurse-led primary care dermatology clinic

First visit
The main problem with psoriasis is that you don't die *from* it but you are sure to die *with* it. When I was in my 30s I used to pray that my psoriasis would become malignant. I felt so desperate and really thought this was the only way I would get some help.

Last visit
Put me down as your success story! I have just returned from one of the best holidays in years because my psoriasis is minimal. I feel I owe you a great thank you. I have had psoriasis for 45 years and this is the best yet and I honestly believe at least half the question was time. No medical practitioner has ever had the time to discuss treatments, show pamphlets and ask for feelings and emotions. They always have a crowded surgery of more serious complaints. I'm not moaning, it is just the way things are. Quote me, use what I say, it has worked and my skin has been super this summer.

TOPICAL THERAPIES

Emollient therapy

Emollients (bath oils, soap substitutes and moisturizers) provide a surface lipid film on the epidermis which diminishes water loss and stops the skin from drying. The aim of using emollients in psoriasis care is to improve the general skin condition by moisturizing, lubricating, soothing and removing scale from the areas of psoriasis, which assists in preparing the plaque for active topical therapies (Finlay 1997). Patients should moisturize their entire skin (including their psoriasis plaques) at least once a day and also prior to applying active treatments. Apply the moisturizer in long downward strokes following the line of the hair to avoid folliculitis. Moisturizers must be allowed to soak into the skin before topical therapies are applied (Dawkes 1997a).

Vitamin D analogues

Vitamin D analogues are highly effective topical treatments for psoriasis. There are two vitamin D analogues available: calcipotriol and tacalcitol. Vitamin D analogues act by promoting normal skin turnover by being antiproliferative, promoting differentiation of keratins and by immunological action (Berth-Jones 1998). They are not steroids and are therefore safer for long-term continuous use. Vitamin D analogues are non-staining and cosmetically acceptable.

Vitamin D analogues will improve psoriasis after 2 weeks and clearance can be achieved within 12 weeks. The cream or ointment is applied to the psoriasis plaque in a smear and rubbed in gently (optimally twice or once daily up to 100 g/week in a thick smear for calcipotriol and once daily in a thin smear for tacalcitol up to 10 g/day for a 12-month maximum course). Calcipotriol only is licensed for children over the age of 6. Calcipotriol scalp solution is applied daily to the areas of psoriasis, parting the hair systematically around the scalp and gently rubbing it in (one to two drops will cover an area the size of a postage stamp).

Rarely, vitamin D analogues can produce an irritant reaction with some redness, soreness and pruritus. Often, this redness will be a normal reaction as the scaling lessens and the plaque appears more red. Mild irritation should therefore not be a reason for stopping treatment. The psoriasis plaques will clear from the inside to leave a ring and then gradually fade. A systemic review of comparative efficacy and tolerability of calcipotriol shows it is superior to most other treatments and effective (Ashcroft et al 2000).

Dithranol

Dithranol was first used as a treatment for psoriasis in 1877. It effectively clears psoriasis by inhibiting mitosis and slowing down the excessive rate of keratinocyte division. In hospital treatment, daily dithranol application is combined with tar baths and UVB (ultraviolet light therapy) which is known as the Ingram regimen.

Dithranol is available as commercially produced preparations for short-contact treatments, most effective on distinct areas of chronic plaque psoriasis. It is unsuitable for patients with extensive chronic plaque psoriasis and guttate psoriasis. Flexural psoriasis can be difficult to treat due to smudging skin, resulting in burning and soreness. The hairline can be treated with low percentages of dithranol but it will stain the hair. The higher the concentration of dithranol, the more effective the treatment. The unwanted effects of skin irritancy and staining can be offputting for patients.

The technique of applying dithranol is extremely precise and this does need to be taught, supervised and monitored carefully. Short-contact dithranol is rubbed in precisely onto the psoriasis plaque only for 30 minutes once daily, until absorbed (Fig. 9.11). Start with the lowest strength and gradually increase strengths over several weeks. The dithranol must then be carefully washed off with lukewarm water. The treated areas of psoriasis will flatten and become stained purple/brown, which gradually fades after treatment.

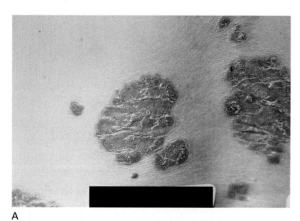

A

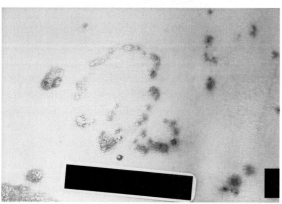

B

Figure 9.10 Psoriasis plaque treated with Dovonex. **A:** Week 4. **B:** Week 12 (reproduced with permission of LEO Pharmaceuticals).

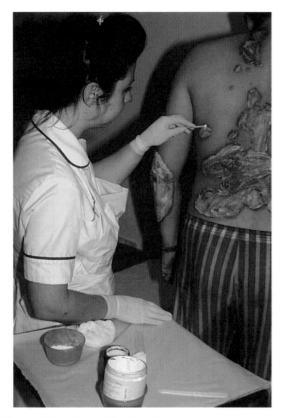

Figure 9.11 Dithranol treatment.

Coal tar

Coal tar, used since the 19th century, is a chemical complex made up of thousands of compounds, distilled, purified and dispersed in a suitable vehicle (creams, lotions, gels, scalp and bath preparations). In 1925 a combination of using tar and UVB to treat psoriasis, called the Goekerman regime, was devised, which is still widely used for hospital care, especially day-care treatments. Coal tar helps clear psoriasis by an antimitotic effect but its exact action is still unknown. There have been recent concerns about the carcinogenicity of coal tar. The European Commission has suggested limiting concentrations of benzolapyrene, so it is likely that in the future coal tar preparations will not be used so widely (Schooten et al 1995).

Coal tar preparations can be applied moderately by wiping onto the entire plaque once or twice daily (Fig. 9.12). Coal tar is messy and smelly so old clothes and night clothes need to be worn but purified tar preparations are less staining. The evidence on the efficacy of coal tar is limited but shows the maximum benefit is achieved at 5% of tar (Williams et al 1992). Coal tar can irritate the skin, especially if applied to skin which is then exposed to the sun. Sterile folliculitis can develop in areas of the skin covered in hair.

Coal tar scalp preparations with keratolytics are extremely effective at removing thick scale. The hair needs to be parted and the scalp ointment rubbed very generously into every area of psoriasis or scaling. The ointment is best left on the scalp overnight, with a shower cap and old pillows used to keep the ointment on the scalp and protect bedding. This descaling process may need to continue for several nights (Dawkes 1997b). Coal tar shampoos are used the next day to wash out the ointment and scales.

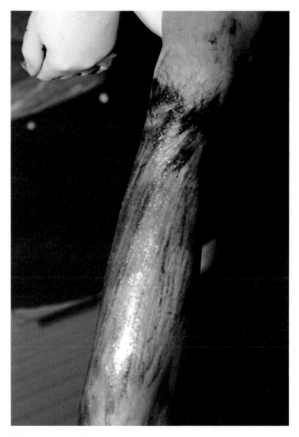

Figure 9.12 Coal tar treatment.

Topical retinoids (vitamin A derivatives)

Tazarotene gel, the first topical retinoid developed for psoriasis, was introduced in 1997 for the treatment of mild to moderate psoriasis. The exact mechanism of action is unclear but is believed to work by normalizing epidermal differentiation, thus reducing hyperproliferation and the inflammatory skin cells (McClelland 1997).

Tazarotene is a gel formulation which is odour free, non-staining and can be used for the body only. The UK licence for tazarotene indicates usage for stable plaque psoriasis covering less than 10% of the body surface area (area equivalent to one arm) in patients over the age of 18 years. Tazarotene is applied precisely to the psoriasis plaque, once daily for up to 12 weeks. It is contraindicated in pregnancy and lactation and adequate contraception must be ensured for all patients of child bearing age. Other side effects include irritation to non-psoriatic skin.

Topical steroids

Mild and moderate topical steroids are often used to treat special body sites (e.g. the face, scalp and genitals) and for flexural psoriasis. Mild and moderately potent steroids can be used in moderation for limited areas, e.g. mild steroids for the hairline and face and moderately potent steroids combined with antifungals for flexural areas. Potent and very potent steroids should only be used on the advice of a dermatologist. Guidelines on the use of topical steroids in psoriasis are provided by the British Association of Dermatologists (Gawkrodger 1997) and outlined in Box 9.3.

Topical steroids may be as effective at clearing psoriasis as other topical treatments but the side effects and disadvantages far outweigh any need to use long-term topical steroid therapy. Corticosteroids suppress the inflammatory component of psoriasis but do not treat the proliferation. When potent and very potent topical corticosteroids are discontinued, the patient may experience a rebound phenomenon when the condition recurs, which can precipitate severe

---

Box 9.3 BAD guidelines for use of topical corticosteroids in the treatment of psoriasis (Gawkrodger 1997)

- No topical corticosteroid should be used regularly for more than 4 weeks without critical review.
- Potent corticosteroids should not be used regularly for more than 7 days.
- No unsupervised repeat prescriptions should be made: patients should be reviewed every 3 months.
- No more than 100 g of a moderately potent or higher preparation should be applied per month.
- Attempts should be made to rotate topical corticosteroids with alternative non-corticosteroid products.
- Use of very potent or potent preparations should be under dermatological supervision.
- The fingertip measurement is helpful, so patients know how much ointment or cream to apply.

---

pustular psoriasis. Other local side effects from topical steroids may occur with long-term use, including skin thinning (atrophy) and broken small capillaries (telangiectasia), which are reversible, or permanent unsightly stretch marks (striae) on the treated area.

SCALP TREATMENTS

Scalp psoriasis often appears in conjunction with plaques on the body and affects 50% of all patients with psoriasis. The presentation of scalp psoriasis often differs between patients. Some patients may have discrete, well-demarcated plaques on their scalp similar to the plaques on their body. Alternatively, scalp psoriasis can occur as diffuse scaling throughout the entire scalp. Patients with severe scalp psoriasis usually have thick plaques of keratin with the scaling extending along the hair shafts (Fry 1992).

Scalp psoriasis can be categorized into three groups:

1. *Mild* – dry flaking skin on areas of the scalp interspersed with normal skin. The hairline is unaffected and there is no hair loss.
2. *Moderate* – dry, flaking and scaling skin on the majority of the scalp with some normal skin. Psoriasis extends to the hairline with minimal hair loss.

3. *Severe* – the entire scalp is affected with minimal normal skin. The scalp is full of thick and lumpy scales. The hairline is affected with redness and scaling extending beyond the scalp margins. Temporary hair loss may occur (always reassure the patient that the hair will grow back).

There are many treatments for scalp psoriasis and it is important that patients and their relatives are taught to treat their scalps meticulously. Tar shampoos should be used for mild scalp psoriasis and a dry flaking scalp can also be improved by massaging emollients (oils/lotions) into the scalp. When thick scaling is present, the scalp will need to be descaled with emollients and keratolytics to remove the majority of scale (Fig. 9.13). Topical treatments in solution or lotion form can then be applied to treat the psoriasis.

The best method of descaling and treating scalp psoriasis is to descale the scalp overnight with generous applications of keratolytics and emollients, wash the hair in the morning with a tar-based shampoo and apply scalp solution or lotion during the day. The scaling may take up to a week of nightly applications to clear. The psoriasis may take weeks to clear.

Box 9.4   Treating scalp psoriasis successfully

- Assess the scalp
- Meticulous application of all scalp treatments
- Mild tar shampoos
- Descale first with coal tar/keratolytics overnight
- Topical steroids for inflamed scalps
- Topical vitamin D analogues – long term

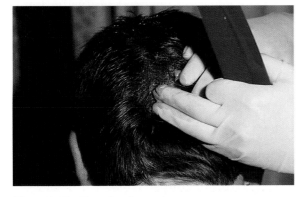

Figure 9.13   Descaling the scalp.

NAIL CHANGES AND TREATMENTS

There is no topical treatment that will help psoriatic nail changes. Keeping nails short will stop the onycholysis getting worst. Use good-quality nail clippers rather than nail scissors and soak fingertips in a bowl of warm water to soften the nails before manicure. Women can use nail varnish which will help camouflage the nail changes. Systemic treatments will help nail psoriasis but this is hard to justify unless psoriasis on the body is severe. Referral to a chiropodist will also be helpful, especially for patients who have problems cutting their thickened nails or who have subungual hyperkeratosis.

CHILDREN AND PSORIASIS

Psoriasis in children is rare under the age of 6 years, uncommon in childhood and likely to appear as a first episode in the teenage years (Hunter et al 1995). A National Child Development Survey showed the point prevalence of examined psoriasis was 0.5% at 11 years and 0.8% at 16 years (Williams & Strachan 1994). The onset of psoriasis under the age of 20 years has been shown to be 2% in infants, 8% in children and 25% in adolescents (Farber & Nall 1974). The mean age of onset in children is between 7 and 8 years and girls are more frequently affected than boys (Higgins & du Vivier 1996).

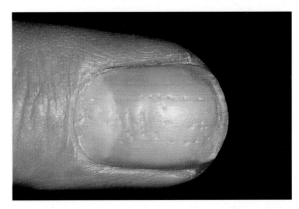

Figure 9.14   Nail psoriasis (reproduced with the permission of Dr Tony Burns, Consultant Dermatologist, Leicester Royal Infirmary).

Forms of psoriasis in children

Chronic plaque psoriasis and guttate psoriasis are the most common forms of psoriasis in children. Scalp psoriasis can be more severe in children. Flexural psoriasis is seen in infants as a napkin psoriasis. Psoriasis before the age of 2 years is generally in the napkin area. Napkin psoriasis can be difficult to differentiate from seborrhoeic dermatitis and napkin dermatitis but psoriform and silvery scales will be present. Localized pustular and erythrodermic forms are extremely rare and generalized pustular psoriasis is seldom seen.

Treatment in children

Table 9.2 outlines the treatment guidelines for children. Generally, with the exception of systemic drugs and extra caution with light therapy, similar treatments are used for children and adults. Children with psoriasis rarely require inpatient admission and day care or community care is the preferred option for the child with extensive psoriasis or the child who requires intensive topical and light therapies.

Table 9.2 Recommendations for topical psoriasis treatments in children

Treatment	Guidance
Emollients	As adult recommendations
Vitamin D analogues	Calcipotriol cream/ointment: child over 6 years, maximum 50 g/week; over 12 years, 75 g/week Tacalcitol – NOT recommended for children
Dithranol	As adult recommendations
Coal tar products	As adult recommendations Exception: Alphosyl HC – NOT recommended under 5 years
Topical retinoids	Tazarotene – NOT recommended under 18 years
Topical steroids	No specific guidelines known
Scalp treatments	Shampoos – as adult recommendations Cocois – NOT recommended under 6. Child 6–12, under medical supervision Calcipotriol scalp solution – NOT recommended for children

Family-centred nursing care for children with psoriasis

Children with psoriasis and their families will need help and understanding. The onset of psoriasis can be sudden and alarming. Psoriasis may run in the family but some parents will have no experience of, or knowledge, about psoriasis. Children and parents will require realistic information about treatment options, time involved and correct application techniques. The nursing care needs to be centred around the child and their family with minimal disruption to the child's life. The child will need to understand what is happening to their skin and the nurse needs to help the family get psoriasis into perspective. The child needs to understand that psoriasis is a nuisance and can be treated but may take some time to clear.

The child should continue as normal and attend school. Treatments can be fitted around the school day with applications at night, so there is no need for the child to go to school covered in messy treatments or wearing body suits. The child may need to use a moisturizer if their skin becomes uncomfortable during the day or after swimming. The child's teacher and school should be educated about psoriasis and the school nurse involved. The child may be subject to teasing from their peers; children can make cruel remarks, especially when someone has a visible problem.

When psoriasis first appears in the teenage years, it can be extremely difficult and upsetting for the teenager who is already coping with bodily changes and may be self-conscious. Teenagers will need time and privacy to learn about applying their own treatments. Some may

---

Case study 9.3 Parent's view

I was terribly upset when my daughter developed psoriasis ... I remember how awful it was when Dad had it ... but treatments are better now. There is no point in being cross with people who do a double take and stare at my daughter ... I asked my daughter's teacher to explain to the other children that it was not catching and it turned out she had it too. People just don't talk about it.

Psoriasis Association

want their parents' help but others may wish to be independent. The nurse needs to be very aware of this and tailor care towards the individual teenager's needs.

SYSTEMIC THERAPIES

Patients with severe psoriasis will usually require second-line/systemic therapies, often in combination with the above topical therapies. These patients will receive their treatments in a hospital dermatology department with shared care from the community for monitoring side effects and providing ongoing support.

Phototherapy

UVB

Ultraviolet radiation (UVB) is indicated for chronic plaque or guttate psoriasis in patients who fail to respond to topical treatment alone. The treatment is supervised and the patient exposes their whole body in the UVB cabinet, three times a week for 6–8 weeks. Narrow band UVB (311–313 nm) is becoming widely available and is indicated for moderate to severe psoriasis.

PUVA

Psoralen and UVA radiation (PUVA) is indicated for patients with moderate to severe chronic plaque psoriasis. Psoralen is a light-sensitive chemical that is taken orally 2 hours before light treatment or applied topically by soaking in a bath immediately before treatment. PUVA treatments are twice weekly for up to 8 weeks. Precautions include eye protection for 24 hours after taking oral psoralen.

Drug therapy

Adult patients with severe psoriasis and disabling psoriatic arthropathy can be treated with drug therapies. All the drug therapies will be commenced in secondary care and require monitoring for the many side effects. The drug therapies for psoriasis are shown in Table 9.3.

INCORPORATING PSORIASIS CARE INTO PRIMARY CARE NURSING

All primary care nurses can improve patient care through an awareness of psoriasis. The primary care nurse is well placed to set up a psoriasis care

Table 9.3 Summary of drug therapies for psoriasis

	Methotrexate	Acitretin	Cyclosporin
Action	Immunosuppressant	Retinoid	Immunosuppressant
Dose	Test dose 2.5 mg/week Start 10 mg/week Increase monthly by 2.5 mg/week to a maximum of 25 mg/week	Start 25–30 mg/day Increase to 70 mg/day Maintain at 25–50 mg/day Maximum treatment 6 months	1.5–2.5 mg/kg twice daily
Side effects	Bone marrow suppression Liver and kidney impairment GI symptoms Psychiatric disorders	Dryness of lips/mucous membranes, conjunctivitis, nose bleeds, skin peeling, sweating, muscle aches, hair thinning, nausea, vomiting and abdominal pain	Renal/hepatic dysfunction Hypertension GI disturbances Fatigue Muscle weakness/cramps
Precautions	Pregnancy Interactions with NSAIDs	Pregnancy X-ray thoracic spine	Long-term increased risk of lymphoma Avoid sunbathing, increased risk of skin cancer
Monitoring	Full blood count LFTs weekly initially then monthly Contraception advice	Contraception advice Monthly LFTs Fasting serum lipids, month 1, 3 and 6	Contraception advice Weekly blood pressure Monthly serum creatinine and LFTs

service for patients in the health centre, which could stand alone or be incorporated into a dermatology nursing clinic. The psoriasis care service can offer nursing support on treatments and lifestyle issues with assessment and review appointments.

The assessment visit needs to include an overview of the patient's history of psoriasis (including family history, hospital appointments and admissions). The whole body needs to be examined; when there are definite or isolated areas of psoriasis, do not forget to consider other areas such as nails, scalp and natal cleft and ask about joint stiffness. The nurse needs to ask about past and present treatments, including applications, techniques and amounts. Remember that different areas of the body often require different treatment. The patient's feelings and ability to cope with psoriasis must be included and there should be continual assessment of how their psoriasis affects them. The patient and nurse can work on a skin care plan and the patient can be monitored through regular review to optimize control and efficacy of treatment.

Patient's role

The patient has an important role to play in successful psoriasis care. Some patients may be very motivated and seek out help; these are usually people with extensive disease or those with mild disease who are very distressed. Other patients (estimated at 80%) may be less motivated and may have milder disease; they may have tried a treatment at one time and not liked it. Therefore, they have given up on treatment and need remotivation.

The patients need to be given information on the range of topical treatments available so they can make an informed choice as to which option they feel will suit them, their coping ability and their lifestyle the best.

The nurse needs to help the patient to:

- learn and become informed about their psoriasis and how they can manage their condition medically and cope socially
- participate in treatment by monitoring efficacy and impact on lifestyle between visits

- assimilate information so they understand their condition and treatment.

Box 9.5 Ten beneficial outcomes for a psoriasis care service

1. Patients will be supported and empowered to manage their own skin condition.
2. With nursing support, patients will learn to control their psoriasis.
3. Patient distress and return visits to the general practitioner will be reduced.
4. Quality of life will be improved and the support and understanding provided will help patients to lead a normal life.
5. Children will learn to cope with managing their psoriasis in the community setting and time away from school will be minimized.
6. The most effective treatment for the patient, considering extent/type of psoriasis and lifestyle, can be established and monitored.
7. Patients with severe psoriasis who are attending dermatology departments can have shared care, especially for the monitoring of systemic therapies.
8. Patients will be helped to apply their treatments correctly and effectively, thereby reducing wasted prescriptions. The treatment prescribed will be utilized appropriately and the total cost of prescribing will decrease.
9. Unnecessary hospital referrals will be reduced.
10. Necessary referrals to the dermatologist will ensure that topical treatments have been given adequate time and understanding and the patient will then receive a more useful referral.

PSORIASIS TREATMENT IN SECONDARY CARE

Caring for patients with psoriasis takes up approximately one-third of dermatology nursing time in secondary care. The majority of psoriasis patients referred to secondary care will be treated with intensive topical treatments, light therapy and monitoring systemic therapies. Dedicated dermatology beds remain essential for acutely ill patients with severe, erythrodermic and generalized pustular psoriasis.

TIPS FOR PATIENTS REGARDING LIFESTYLE ISSUES AND PSORIASIS

1. When people ask what is the matter with your skin, it is important to tell them that you have psoriasis which affects up to three

people in every 100 in the UK. It is a skin condition which runs in families, is not catching and is just a nuisance.

2. Be aware of addressing stress, by talking out feelings and expressing any upset or anger. This is important as how you feel in yourself can affect your general health and psoriasis.

3. Stop smoking; it is a known fact that smoking can make psoriasis worse.

4. Reduce alcohol intake and regard it only as a social pleasure, keeping to the general safe drinking levels (women 14 units/week and men 21 units/week).

5. Keep your home cool and central heating low; heat will dry the skin.

6. Dark clothing shows skin scales more; light-coloured tops will reduce the embarrassment of dandruff.

7. Beauty tips for ladies:
   - If your skin is sensitive use hypoallergenic make-up products
   - Avoid perfumed products (spray perfume on your clothes rather than your body)
   - Masking creams may be useful for covering small areas of psoriasis especially on the face or hairline
   - Hair removal: use cold rather than hot wax and avoid shaving
   - Regular manicures and pedicures will help with nail involvement; false nails and varnish can cover nails
   - Hair and scalp care: explain to your hairdresser that you have psoriasis; if they are not sympathetic, change your hairdresser
   - Have a hairstyle that avoids the need for grips or bands and pulls the hair
   - Heat will irritate the scalp and damage hair so avoid heated rollers and use a hairdryer at a distance
   - Avoid perms when the scalp is inflamed and ensure the perm is gentle
   - Don't use a medicated shampoo for months on end; occasionally change to a mild shampoo to allow the scalp to regain its normal balance.

8. Joint pain: regard this as part of your psoriasis and take extra care of your general health.

Help to minimize joint pain and damage by resting when joints are inflamed and using gentle daily exercises to keep them stretched and mobile.

9. Family support can make all the difference; talk to your family about the difficulties you face with your psoriasis and let them help you with treatments. Above all, try not to let your psoriasis interfere with family life.

10. Remember, you can control your psoriasis, especially if you tackle it at the earliest possible stage. Some of the recommendations for modifications in lifestyle will soon become the norm for you, but it is up to you to change habits.

TIPS FOR NURSES REGARDING TREATMENTS FOR PSORIASIS IN THE COMMUNITY

1. The majority of patients with psoriasis can be supported and treated in the community. The practice nurse has an essential role to play in the chronic disease management of psoriasis.

2. Psoriasis is a chronic skin condition so psoriasis sufferers and their families need ongoing advice and support, especially with their treatments.

3. Assessment of patients is essential to establish sites of psoriasis, previous treatment and application techniques and the patient's coping strategies.

4. Regular reviews of the patient are important in establishing individual treatment routines.

5. The key to helping patients with treatments is encouragement and motivation for their own self-care. Including families and partners is important, if the patient wishes.

6. Patient care needs to include the following:
   - Knowledge of the patient's understanding of psoriasis and dispelling myths
   - The importance of good general skin care, protecting and moisturizing the skin
   - Topical treatments available to the patient, how to apply and maximize the effectiveness of treatments
   - Treating the scalp, descaling and applying scalp treatments

- Coping with the psychological impact of psoriasis
- Support and practical advice on work, household activities and recreation.

7. Advice and support on treatments needs to be very practical. Adequate time needs to be allowed to demonstrate correct treatment application, then supervise the patient and/or relative and provide ongoing review of the treatment application. This may take several appointments but is time worth spending.

8. Remember if psoriasis is treated correctly, it will generally always improve and remission can last for years.

CONCLUSION

All nurses will meet patients suffering from psoriasis and can provide support and information on managing their skin. This chapter has given information and some practical advice on topical treatments and health education. In primary care, psoriasis care is an area in which PCGs could develop nurse-led services. In secondary care, the care of the skin is essential for all patients and nurses will care for patients with psoriasis in a variety of clinical areas. The patient may have had little advice on skin care in the past or may be an expert at managing their own condition.

Psoriasis is a very common skin condition and patients need nurses to provide them with understanding and practical advice.

REFERENCES

Al'abadie M, Kent G, Gawkrodger D 1994 The relationship between stress and the onset and exacerbation of psoriasis and other skin conditions. British Journal of Dermatology Nursing 130(2): 199–203

Ahnini R T 1999 Novel genetic association between the corneodesmosin (MHCS) gene and susceptibility to psoriasis. Human Molecular Genetics 8(6): 1135–1140

Ashcroft D M O, Li Wan Po A, Williams H C, Griffiths C E M 2000 Systemic review of comparative efficacy and tolerability of calcipotriol in treating chronic plaque psoriasis. British Medical Journal 320: 963–967

Berth-Jones J 1998 The emergence of vitamin D as a first line treatment for psoriasis. Journal of Dermatological Treatment 9(3): 13–18

Camisa C 1994 Psoriasis. Blackwell Science, Oxford, pp 7–24

Camp R D R 1998 Psoriasis. In: Champion R H, Burton J L, Ebling F J G (eds) Textbook of dermatology. Blackwell Science, Oxford, pp 1589–1650

Dawkes K 1997a How to apply emollients effectively. British Journal of Dermatology Nursing 1(1): 8–9

Dawkes K 1997b How to apply scalp treatments. British Journal of Dermatology Nursing 1(2): 8–9

Ersser S-E 1996 Ethnography and the development of patient-centred nursing. In: Fulford K W M, Ersser S, Hope T (eds) Essential practice in patient-centred care. Blackwell Science, Oxford, pp 53–68

Farber E M, Nall M L 1974 The natural history of 5,600 patients. Dermatologica 148: 1–18

Finlay A Y 1997 Emollients as an adjuvant therapy for psoriasis. Journal of Dermatological Treatment 8 (suppl 1): 25–27

Finlay A Y, Coles E C 1995 The effect of severe psoriasis on the quality of life of 369 patients. British Journal of Dermatology 132: 236–244

Fry L 1992 An atlas of psoriasis. Parthenon Publishing Group, Carnforth, Lancs

Gawkodger D J 1997 Current management of psoriasis. Journal of Dermatological Treatment 8: 27–55

Gollnick H P M 1998 The psoriatic patient and the use of topical antipsoriatics. Journal of Dermatological Treatment 9 (suppl 3): 7–11

Helm T N, Camisa C 1998 Scalp psoriasis. In: Camisa C (ed) Psoriasis handbook. Blackwell Science, Oxford

Higgins E M, du Vivier A 1996 Skin disease in children and adolescence. Blackwell Science, Oxford

Hunter J A A, Savin J A, Dahl M V 1995 Clinical dermatology. Blackwell Science, Oxford, p 51

McClelland P B 1997 New treatment options for psoriasis. Dermatology Nursing 9(5): 295–306

Naldi L, Parazzini F, Brevi A et al 1992 Family history, smoking habits, alcohol consumption and risk of psoriasis. British Journal of Dermatology 127: 212–217

Penzer R 1996 Psoriasis. Primary Health Care 6(5): 23–30

Ramsay B, O'Reagan M 1988 A survey of the social and psychological effects of psoriasis. British Journal of Dermatology 118: 195–201

Schooten F J, Moonen E J C, Rhijnsburger E 1995 Dermal uptake of polycyclic aromatic hydrocarbons after hairwash with coal tar shampoo. Lancet 344: 1505–1506

Van Onselen J 1998 Psoriasis care for primary care. Primary Health Care 8(8): 27–38

Williams H C, Strachan D P 1994 Psoriasis and eczema are not mutually exclusive diseases. Dermatology 189: 238–240

Williams R E A, Tilman D, White S I 1992 Re-examining crude coal tar treatment for psoriasis. British Journal of Dermatology 126: 608–610

FURTHER READING

Barker J N W N, Davison S, Poyner T F 1999 Pocket guide to psoriasis. Blackwell Science, Oxford

Camisa C 1998 Handbook of psoriasis. Blackwell Science, Oxford

Patient guides

Dave V K 1997 Skin care for psoriasis. Class Publishing, London

Gibbons S 1992 Beat psoriasis. Thorsons, London

Habets B 1993 The psoriasis handbook. Carnell, London

Lewis J 1996 The psoriasis handbook. Vermillion, London

Lowe N 1998 Psoriasis – a patient's guide. Martin Dunitz, London

Warin A 2000 Understanding psoriasis. British Medical Association, London

Wilson C 1989 Psoriasis – a practical guide to coping. Crowood Press, Marlborough

PATIENT SUPPORT GROUPS

The Psoriasis Association
7 Milton Street
Northampton NN2 7JG
Tel: 01604 711129
Fax: 01604 792894

Psoriatic Arthropathy Alliance
PO Box 111
St Albans
Hertfordshire AL2 3JQ
Tel/Fax: 01923 67837
Web site: www.paalliance.org

10

Eczema

Sandra Lawton

INTRODUCTION

The exact prevalence of eczema is unknown but it is thought to account for 20% of all patients seeking medical assistance with a skin condition (Hunter et al 1995). This chapter will define, describe and examine the classification of eczema. Each type will be covered in depth, identifying the prevalence, clinical features and the nursing and medical management of the disease. The impact on the patient, their quality of life and individual needs will be covered.

Nurses play an important role in the care of patients with eczema. Eczema is a miserable condition, which can have a major impact on the lives of not only patients but also their families. The aim of management is to provide good control and establish a routine that will improve the life of the patient. The nurse has a major role to play in this, providing support, education and the time for explanation and demonstration of treatments (Lawton 1996).

DEFINITION OF ECZEMA/DERMATITIS

The term eczema is derived from the Greek *ekzein*, meaning to boil over. Eczema and dermatitis are used synonymously and refer to a characteristic reaction pattern of the skin to a range of external and internal factors. The microscopic features of an eczematous reaction show inflammatory changes in the skin. Vascular dilatation leads to clinical erythema, whilst exudation of plasma and inflammatory cells from the vessels into the surrounding dermis produces swelling which is clinically manifest as papules or oedematous plaques. In some cases the exudation of fluid and cells extends into the epidermis to produce spongiosis and vesicle formation (Stevens et al 1989).

Classification of eczema

The current classification of eczema is inconsistent. Gawkrodger (1992) suggests that it is difficult to provide a suitable alternative as most eczema is of unknown aetiology. Different types of eczema may be recognized by morphology, site or cause and Gawkrodger divides the classification into endogenous (due to internal or constitutional factors) and exogenous (due to external agents in contact with the skin). In practice, however, classification is difficult as many patients may present with a combination of factors producing their eczema, e.g. a gravitational eczema with a superimposed contact allergic reaction. However, for the purpose of this chapter, the classification shown in Box 10.1 will be used.

Box 10.1 Classification of eczema		
Exogenous	*Endogenous*	*Unclassified*
● Contact irritant	● Atopic eczema	● Asteatotic
● Contact allergic	● Seborrhoeic	● Lichen
● Photosensitive	● Discoid	simplex
	● Gravitational	● Juvenile
	● Pompholyx	plantar
		dermatosis

Acute eczema (Fig. 10.1)

In an acute reaction, the skin clinically exhibits the cardinal signs of inflammation, calor (heat), rubor (erythema), tumour (swelling) and dolor (pain, often in the form of itch). Clinically, the appearance of the lesion is very mixed; there is usually a background erythema or a raised oedematous plaque, not sharply demarcated but merging with the surrounding skin. Vesicle formation is frequent in the early stages and may coalesce to form large bullae, which frequently

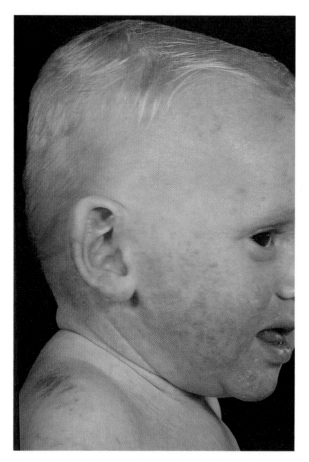

Figure 10.1 Acute eczema (reproduced with the permission of Professor H C Williams).

rupture with oozing of clear fluid and the formation of surface crust. Hence the term eczema or 'boiling' (Stevens et al 1989).

Subacute eczema

In subacute eczema there are histological features of both acute and chronic eczema. Stevens et al (1989) suggest that this may be more appropriately named 'chronic active' eczema. There are clinical changes with erythema but less vesicle formation. There is some thickening of the epidermis (acanthosis) due to inflammation, itching and scratching. Histologically, subacute eczema shows features of both acute eczema (spongiosis, vesiculation and exocytosis) and chronic eczema (acanthosis and papillomatosis).

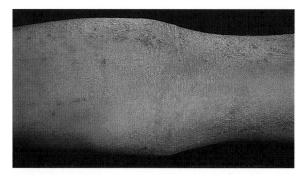

Figure 10.2 Chronic eczema (reproduced with the permission of Professor H C Williams).

Chronic eczema (Fig. 10.2)

In chronic eczema clinically the erythema varies. There is lichenification and scaling and sometimes increased pigmentation. Fissuring may be present but vesicles and large bullae will be absent. Chronic eczema represents the endstage of long-standing, incompletely resolved, acute or subacute eczema (Stevens et al 1989).

GENERAL PREVALENCE

The prevalence rates for eczema excluding atopic eczema and contact eczema (seborrhoeic eczema, discoid eczema, asteatotic eczema, pompholyx eczema, varicose eczema, photosensitive eczema and lichen simplex) are not available, but the NHANES (National Health and Nutrition Examination Survey (US)) study (Johnson 1978) suggested that around 1% of the population had clinically significant eczema that was not atopic or contact dermatitis. Seborrhoeic eczema was recorded separately in that study, and clinically significant disease was found to affect 2.8% of the population, mainly adults. Asteatotic eczema may be especially common in old age, affecting 29% of those in residential homes for the elderly (Williams 1997).

ENDOGENOUS ECZEMA

Atopic eczema

Prevalence

Atopic or childhood eczema is one of the most common and miserable skin diseases, currently affecting 20% of children by the age of 7 years in the UK (Williams 1994). With an onset in early years, this inflammatory skin condition is characterized by itching and eczema involving the face and skin creases. Although a tendency to dry skin and irritants may be lifelong, around 60–70% of these children will clear by their mid-teens. Prevalence estimates for adults suggest an overall frequency of atopic eczema of between 1.2% and 10%. There is also reasonable evidence to suggest that the prevalence of atopic eczema has increased substantially over the past 30 years, for reasons which are unclear, but it is likely that environmental factors associated with urbanization are important. Atopic eczema is also more common in wealthier families and Afro-Caribbean children.

Although there are no recent national prevalence studies of atopic eczema in the UK, data from a national birth cohort study point to considerable variation in disease prevalence and region (Williams 1997). There is, however, no doubt that atopic eczema has a major impact on the lives of the individual and their family.

Diagnosis

Atopic eczema is usually diagnosed on clinical grounds, basing it on the patient's history, family history and appearance of the skin rash.

Box 10.2 Diagnostic criteria for atopic eczema (McHenry et al 1995)

Must have
An itchy skin condition (or reported scratching or rubbing in a child)

Plus three or more of the following
- History of itchiness in skin creases such as folds of the elbows, behind the knees, fronts of ankles or around neck (or the cheeks in children under 4 years)
- History of asthma or hay fever (or a history of atopic disease in a first-degree relative in children under 4 years)
- General dry skin in the past year
- Visible flexural eczema (or eczema affecting the cheeks or forehead and outer limbs in children under 4 years)
- Onset in the first 2 years of life (not always diagnostic in children under 4 years)

Following a consensus of opinion formed at a joint workshop of the British Association of Dermatologists and the research unit of the Royal College of Physicians of London, diagnostic criteria for atopic eczema were suggested (Box 10.2).

Clinical patterns of atopic eczema (Fig. 10.3)

In babies and infants, atopic eczema tends to be vesicular and weepy. It often starts on the face with a non-specific distribution elsewhere, the nappy area often being spared. In older children, the eczema becomes lichenified, dry and excoriated, affecting mainly the elbow creases, backs of knees, wrists, ankles and ears (flexural). A stubborn 'reverse' pattern affecting the extensor aspects of the limbs is also recognized. Children often present with a 'discoid' pattern of atopic eczema which tends to be more stubborn to treat, becomes easily infected and requires stronger forms of treatment (Fig. 10.4). In adults, the pattern is similar to that of children but tends to be more chronic with lichenification and more widespread low-grade involvement of the trunk, face and hands.

The most common features of atopic eczema are the itching and scratching, often referred to as the 'itch–scratch cycle'. This is commonly cited as the most distressing aspect of atopic eczema, with loss of sleep and the impact it has on the child and the family being well recognized.

Bacterial infections are also common in patients with atopic eczema because the skin is often dry and damaged by scratching. Children with atopic eczema often present with secondary infections and flare-ups of their eczema because the characteristic dry skin and chronic scratching favour colonization by *Staphylococcus aureus* (Williams 1994).

Viral infections are less common but can occur. Most are caused by the herpes simplex virus: the patient may present with herpetic lesions (small vesicles, crusting, weeping or, more often, grouped 'punched out' erosions). The patient may also be systemically unwell with malaise and pyrexia. It is vital therefore to determine whether the infection is bacterial or viral. Swabs should be taken for culture and the appropriate

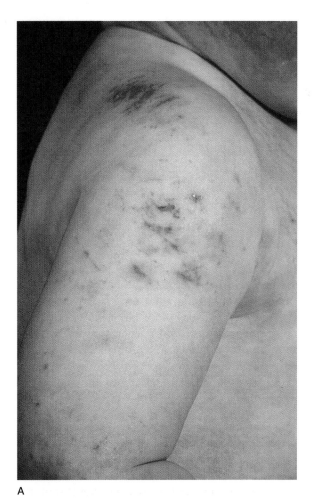

A

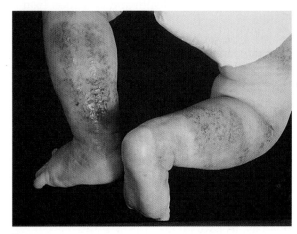

B

Figure 10.3   **A:** Atopic excoriations. **B:** Atopic infection (reproduced with the permission of Professor H C Williams).

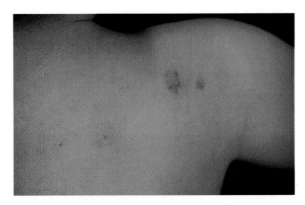

Figure 10.4   Discoid eczema in a child (reproduced with the permission of Professor H C Williams).

antibiotic/antiviral therapy given. For *S. aureus* flucloxacillin is usually the most appropriate antibiotic (erythromycin may also be given if there is a known penicillin allergy). For the herpes infection (eczema herpeticum), the antiviral treatment is aciclovir. Admission to hospital may be considered in cases of severe infection.

Molluscum contagiosum is a viral infection commonly found in children with atopic eczema. It presents with groups of pearly-pink umbilicated papules which are caused by a pox virus. Treatment is by cryotherapy or by expressing the contents. Children, however, do not tolerate either very well and if left alone, the condition will resolve (this can take several months).

Investigations

Skin prick tests and RAST (radioallergosorbent test) are unable to predict the outcome of avoiding appropriate antigens. These tests look at IgE concentration and identification of specific antibodies to common allergens such as house dust mite, pollens or foods. In the general population, approximately 15% of healthy people have raised IgE titres whilst 20% of patients with atopic eczema do not have raised IgE titres or a positive RAST test. They are therefore of little value in predicting disease or cause (McHenry et al 1995). Skin swabs may be taken only if there is clinical evidence of infection. Patch testing to detect contact allergy may be performed in patients whose condition has deteriorated but also in

those where sensitization to topical treatments, including topical steroids, may be suspected.

Assessment

Assessment of patients with eczema requires time for history taking, examination, explanation and treatment. A survey by the National Eczema Society showed that patients would not only like a diagnosis and treatment but also an explanation as to the nature of eczema and advice on how to use the treatments prescribed (Long et al 1993). History taking is important to gain an insight into the patient, their life with atopic eczema and their expectations. Box 10.3 gives an example of the assessment questions used within a specialized paediatric eczema clinic (Lynn et al 1997).

Box 10.3   Assessment questions for atopic eczema

1. Does anything make your child's eczema worse? Yes/No
   If yes, please specify.
2. Is your child on a special diet? Yes/No
   If yes, what foods are you avoiding?
3. Is your child's sleep disturbed because of his/her eczema? Yes/No
   If yes, is it: every night?   1–2 nights per week? 3–6 nights per week?
4. Does your child's eczema affect: school? Yes/No social life? Yes/No
   If yes, in what way?
5. What is the most distressing thing about your child's eczema?
6. Are all your child's immunizations up to date?
7. Is there a family history of: asthma? hay fever? eczema?
8. Does your child suffer from asthma? Yes/No
   If yes, what treatment is he/she on?
9. At the moment, what are you using to treat your child's skin?
10. What have you used in the past?
11. What do you hope to gain from attending the hospital?

A full skin examination should also be performed within the assessment, recording the extent and severity of the eczema and clinical pattern. Evidence of clinical infection should be noted and treated appropriately. The weight and height of children should be recorded on a growth chart for those with chronic severe eczema.

Quality of life

There is a real need for doctors and administrators to recognize that eczema is not necessarily a minor skin disorder but a major handicap with considerable personal, social and financial burdens on the family (Su et al 1997). Much work has been done lately to address these issues. Finlay & Khan (1994) developed a simple practical questionnaire to measure the impact of skin disease and its treatment on patients' lives. This is known as the Dermatology Life Quality Index (DLQI) and consists of 10 questions covering how the patient's skin disease has affected their life in the previous week. It covers symptoms of itching, soreness and pain, feelings about their skin condition, their ability to perform normal daily activities (leisure, work and school), personal relationships and treatment. The index has a simple scoring system that makes it easy to use. Each question has four possible answers: 'not at all' (0) 'a little' (1), 'a lot' (2) and 'very much' (3). The answers are then totalled to obtain a result (minimum of 0 and maximum of 30). The higher the score, the greater the impairment in quality of life.

The work of Finlay & Khan looked at adults; following this, a similar study was undertaken looking specifically at children. Lewis-Jones & Finlay (1995) undertook a study to create and initially validate a simple questionnaire to measure quality of life in children with skin disease – the Children's Dermatology Life Quality Index (CDLQI). The methods used in this study were based on those used in the creation of the DLQI for use with adults. These two measures have clearly documented that atopic eczema has a major impact on the lives of patients. Because of the lack of information concerning the effect on family function rather than on the individual, the authors of the two previous studies and their colleagues then looked at the family impact of childhood eczema (Lawson et al 1998). The questionnaire format was based on similar principles to the DLQI and CDLQI and highlighted what many of us working with eczema families consider are areas of concern and consideration when managing these children (Box 10.4).

Measuring the impact of skin disease on the quality of life directs us when making clinical decisions and planning clinical research. It improves our ability to audit services and to bid for further resources for dermatology patients.

Box 10.4 Family impact of atopic eczema (Lawson et al 1998)

Practical care issues	74% of parents described a general burden of extra care, i.e. household cleaning, washing, preparing food and shopping
Psychological pressures on the parents	71% described feelings of guilt, frustration, exhaustion, resentment and helplessness
Family lifestyle	66% said they did not lead a 'normal' family life
School	six out of 10 children had problems at school. All experienced teasing and bullying
Effects on child behaviour	54% of parents reported changes in behaviour such as being naughty, irritable, bad-tempered, easily bored and hurtful to other family members during flare-ups of eczema
Social life	34% of parents felt their social life was restricted due to tiredness. Finding suitable baby sitters was also a problem
Relationships	29% felt interpersonal relationships were affected by caring for a child with eczema. Tiredness from sleep loss caused friction
Sleep disturbance	63% of children had current sleep problems and most had had sleep disturbance at some time. The itching and scratching resulted in parental frustration and exhaustion in 64%. 63% of siblings were also losing sleep
Holidays	23% of families were restricted in their choice of holiday because of sleep problems, climate and the special needs of caring for a child with eczema
Financial aspects	Special diets, extra laundry, bathing and clothes add to the cost of family life
Practical support	17% reported receiving inadequate support from the teaching and medical professions

Management

Although a cure is unrealistic at present, 75% of children will clear by their early teens (McHenry et al 1995). It is therefore paramount that the patient and their family receive the advice, support and education they require to manage their eczema. Most patients should be able to achieve good control of their eczema if it is managed correctly. The nurse is in a privileged position to do this.

First-line treatment. To be managed effectively, a multidisciplinary approach is needed for the care of atopic eczema. The disabling effects and the psychosocial impact of atopic eczema are substantial. Support and education are essential to enable children and their families to manage the condition (Lynn et al 1997). Nurses are in a privileged position in both primary and secondary care to provide adequate time for explanation, discussion and education about the application of topical preparations and the amounts to use. Skin-care plans and information leaflets detailing various aspects of atopic eczema management can then further support this. They should be clear, factual, non-controversial and available in a variety of languages. The National Eczema Society produces a wide variety of information to meet this need.

● *Avoidance of provoking factors* – Irritants such as soaps and detergents, which remove the natural lipid from the skin surface, should be avoided. Eczema patients already have a dry skin so soap substitutes should be used to prevent further drying of the skin. Extremes of temperature, cold winds or a hot environment with low humidity will also exacerbate eczema, as will woollen clothing worn next to the skin. Cotton clothing is more comfortable. Keeping nails cut short will also prevent damage to the skin from scratching.

● *Bathing and emollients* – Bathing and the use of emollients is the mainstay of any skin-care regimen. Bathing is useful for cleansing the skin and removing old treatments and scale. It is also an excellent way of hydrating the skin. Overwashing can dry or irritate the skin. There are many emollients available and patients should be allowed to decide on the most suitable emollients and bathing regimen for them. Emollients come in a variety of forms and work by providing a surface lipid film which prevents water evaporation from the epidermis. They are most effective when applied after bathing, as this is when the water content of the skin is greatest. Emollients should then be reapplied regularly throughout the day to prevent drying of the skin and as prevention against external irritants, e.g. cold winds, water, soil, foods which young children may smear over their faces when eating such as yoghurts, fruits, etc. and the constant dribbling of young babies and infants. Generally the greasier the emollient the better but individual preference is important; patients may often wish to have different ones for day and night time use. Patients must be given adequate amounts of emollients with the average weekly amount for adults being 500 g and for children 250 g.

● *Infection* – Systemic antibiotics are important in treating overt secondary bacterial infections in patients with atopic eczema (McHenry et al 1995). Antibiotics of choice for isolated pathogens are:

● *Staphylococcus aureus*: flucloxacillin or erythromycin if there is allergy to penicillin
● *beta-haemolytic streptococci*: phenoxymethylpenicillin or erythromycin if penicillin allergy.

Use of topical antibiotics should be restricted to limited situations. They are generally not ideal for treating bacterial infections in patients with atopic eczema who often have widespread secondary infection. Treatment of staphylococcal carrier sites prophylactically (nose, axillae and perineum) with topical antibiotics may be appropriate in patients with recurrent infected eczema (McHenry et al 1995).

Eczema herpeticum caused by herpes simplex virus responds well to oral aciclovir which should be given early in the course of the disease. If patients are unwell it should be administered intravenously. Patients need advice about infection, when to recognize it and to seek medical advice.

● *Topical corticosteroids* – Topical corticosteroids are the mainstay of treatment for atopic eczema and can be used safely if certain precautions are taken. Use and abuse of topical steroids has caused considerable confusion and controversy and has resulted in the undertreatment of many patients with atopic eczema. Lack of adherence to treatment may often be traced back to the patients' or parents' fears of steroids. It is therefore important to explain the different potencies and the benefits and risks of topical corticosteroids. The basic principle is to use the least potent preparation required to keep the eczema under control and when possible, the corticosteroids should be stopped for short periods (McHenry et al 1995). As Watts (1997) states, a child will have more side effects from itching, scratching, sleepless nights, infection and missing school than from using correctly prescribed topical steroids.

• *Antihistamines* – Antihistamines are used for their sedative properties. They are useful short term in conjunction with topical treatments when there are relapses and severe pruritus. Long-term use is not recommended as tachyphylaxis may occur. They should be used an hour before bedtime for those patients who have trouble getting to sleep, who wake regularly during the night or who scratch whilst asleep. Daytime use should be avoided. Patients often find they have trouble waking for school or work. They are therefore of benefit only in the short term.

• *Psychology* – Patients often benefit from sharing knowledge and experiences so patient support groups can often be helpful. There are also cognitive behavioural techniques available to patients. A clinical psychologist may be able to suggest behaviour and habit reversal techniques, combining conventional topical treatment with a behaviour modification technique which aims to eliminate self-damaging behaviours characteristic of chronic eczema, e.g. repetitive scratching and rubbing (Bridgett et al 1996).

• *Ichthammol and tar* – The principal tars used for treatment of atopic eczema the UK are ichthammol and coal tar. They have an antipruritic effect and are useful in lichenified eczema. They can be applied using creams, ointments, and pastes, added to the bath and applied as paste bandages. They can be messy to use but do have a place in eczema management. They can also be used as an alternative to topical corticosteroids if parents/patients do not wish to use conventional treatment.

Bandaging. Bandages are an occlusive technique used in the management of eczema. Paste bandages are used for many types of eczema (see Boxes 10.5 and 10.6) and wet wraps are used more commonly for childhood atopic eczema.

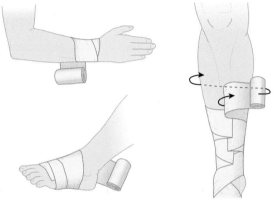

(a) Start at foot or wrist.

(b) Wrap around limb and fold back (pleating) upon itself and apply in the opposite direction, overlapping by half the width of the bandage.

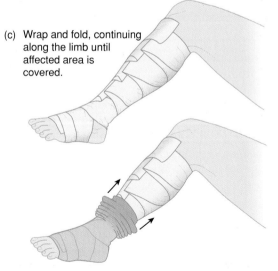

(c) Wrap and fold, continuing along the limb until affected area is covered.

(d) Cover bandage with tubular gauze or bandage (to prevent soiling of clothing/bed linen). Secure well with tape.

Figure 10.5   Application of medicated paste bandages.

Box 10.5 Paste bandages

Application	Advantages	Disadvantages
Choice depends on therapeutic action Over emollients/topical steroids Spiralling and folding to prevent tightening Secondary layer tubular bandage, crepe or compression bandage Can be left for 12–48 hrs	Refreshing and cooling Relieves irritated skin Useful for protection and difficult to unravel More useful for adults/older children Can be used on whole or parts of limbs	Messy and will stain clothing/bedding Secondary layer of bandage needed Therapeutic substances may irritate Possible to develop a contact dermatitis from constituents

Indications for bandages:

- useful for acute flares of eczema
- for excoriated and inflamed eczema on limbs
- to prevent scratching
- to protect skin
- for softening lichenified (thickened) skin.

Wet wrap dressings (Fig 10.6) are an occlusive technique used in the management of atopic eczema. Parents often find the itching and scratching the most frustrating and distressing symptom of eczema. This technique is frequently used to control the symptoms of the 'itch–scratch cycle' which in turn helps with the problem of sleep deprivation associated with it. Wet wraps can be used on any degree of eczema that has not responded to emollients and mild topical corticosteroids. They must not be used on weepy, infected eczema until the infection has been treated.

The wet wrap dressing is a warm, wet and occlusive treatment using an open-weave tubular dressing (Tubifast™) (Box 10.6) which is applied over prescribed topical preparations (emollients and mild topical corticosteroids). There are many modifications to the general approach of wet wrap dressings.

Their mechanism of action involves the following.

- *Evaporation* – the very gradual evaporation of water from the wet layer results in cooling of the skin, reducing the itching and discomfort.
- *Rehydration* – the skin is rehydrated using large amounts of emollients, which then last longer on the skin.

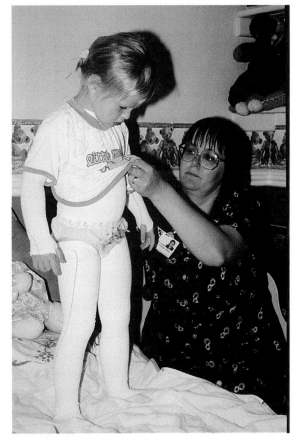

Figure 10.6   Wet wraps (reproduced with the permission of S Lawton).

- *Protection* – they provide some physical protection from scratching and allow the skin to heal.
- *Enhanced steroid penetration* – steroid absorption is enhanced so that they reach

both the superficial and deep inflammation of eczema. This in turn leads to better control and the need for less topical corticosteroids.

Items required for bandaging include:

- prescribed topical treatments – emollients and mild corticosteroids
- Tubifast™ bandages (Box 10.6)
- bowl
- scissors.

Box 10.6 Tubifast™ bandages

Brown line for larger children
Yellow line for the body
Green line for arms
Green line for legs (under 5 years)
Blue line for legs (over 5 years)
Red line for young babies' arms
Tubifast™ is available in 1 m, 3 m and 5 m packs on Drug Tariff

---

Before starting, the appropriate lengths of Tubifast™ bandages have to be prepared.

1. Measure the lengths of Tubifast™ required.
   - *For arms* – measure from top of the shoulders to the tips of the fingers and add approximately 2 inches. Cut four lengths (two for each arm) or double lengths if hands are to be wrapped.
   - *For legs* – measure from the thigh to the tips of the toes and add approximately 2 inches. Cut four lengths (two for each leg) or double lengths if feet are to be wrapped.
   - *For body* – measure from top of the neck to base of the bottom. Cut out two armholes. Cut two lengths.
   - *For ties* – cut 8 × 1 inch wide strips from the leftover bandages.
2. Bath as normal, with emollients rather than soap (emollients provide a surface lipid film which prevents evaporation from the epidermis). Pat dry.
3. Place two arm lengths, two leg lengths (or half of each double length) and one vest into a bowl of warm water.
4. Apply prescribed topical corticosteroids to eczematous areas and emollient liberally to remaining skin.

5. Squeeze out the wet Tubifast™ and apply, still wet and warm, to the body. Cover with the dry Tubifast™ as a second layer. Repeat this with each arm and leg. Holes may be made for the fingers and toes or the double length of bandage may be twisted at the toes or hand and pulled back up over the arm or leg.
6. Ties are then passed through holes in both layers of the bandage to secure the body suit in place. Usually two ties are required for each arm and leg.
7. Normal clothing or nightwear can then be worn over the bandages.

Wet wraps may be applied daily or at night only. They are used until the 'itch–scratch' cycle has been broken, the eczema is under control and the skin is well hydrated. They may be used with emollients only; this has been shown to be of benefit in preventing a flare-up of the eczema. If the bandages start to dry out, they may become hot and uncomfortable. It is important that they are kept moist and may be remoistened by taking down the outer dry layer and spraying the inner layer with water in a garden spray. Tubifast™ also can be washed and reused. It is important, however, to realize that wet wraps are not a cure for eczema but can be helpful in controlling its symptoms (Lawton 1999).

Most patients respond well to first-line management but for those who fail to respond, referral should be made to a specialist. McHenry et al (1995) indicated the following criteria for specialist referral.

- Diagnostic doubt.
- Failure to respond to maintenance treatment with mildly potent steroids in children or moderately potent steroids in adults.
- Second-line treatment required or commencement of dietary manipulation.
- When specialist opinion would be valuable in counselling patients and family.

Second-line treatment

House dust mite. Although the house dust mite may play an important role in atopic eczema, at present there are no effective ways of eradicating it completely and attempts to do so are not recommended. Research is still trying to determine to what extent reducing mite levels in the home can improve eczema. There are, however, some simple measures which can help.

- Remove feather pillows and quilts and replace with synthetic ones.
- Cover the mattress with a plastic cover. This can be wiped down with a damp cloth.
- Use cotton sheets, pillow cases and quilt covers. Turn down the sheets every day to let the mattress air. Change bedlinen weekly (or more often if desired). Wash at 50°C or above. Don't forget the curtains, which preferably should be cotton so that they may be washed frequently.
- Vinyl flooring, plain floorboards or cork tiles are easier to clean and can be wiped with a damp cloth. Most houses have carpets in the bedrooms. If it is not practical or too costly to remove them, they must be thoroughly vacuumed (daily if possible), along with the headboard, mattress, base or divan. Remember to keep the child away from the area when cleaning.
- Damp dusting keeps the levels of house dust mite down and must include all surfaces which attract dust.
- All children have a favourite toy or comforter, which they take to bed and love. Wash them frequently in the washing machine at 50°C. Do not have too many soft toys gathering dust. If unable to wash the toy, put it in a plastic bag and place it in the freezer overnight.
- If the child shares a room these principles apply to all soft furnishings. If bunk beds are used the child with eczema should use the top bunk.
- House dust mites like warm, damp conditions. Keep the room cool and well ventilated and minimize soft furnishings.

Dietary restrictions. The role of foods in initiating or perpetuating atopic eczema has been extensively investigated. Dietary manipulations are generally indicated only when the patient's history strongly suggests a specific food allergy or when widespread eczema fails to respond to first-line treatment. In general, dietary restriction is of little or no benefit in adults or older children with atopic eczema. In infants, a 4–6-week trial of egg and milk exclusion with the introduction of hydrolysate infant formula may be recommended. This will be followed by a supervised rechallenge. A dietician must be involved to ensure an adequate diet for the growing child. No dietary measures should be taken on an ad hoc basis.

Immediate type I hypersensitivity reaction can also occur following contact or ingestion of some foods. This reaction is not unique to atopic patients but patients must avoid the substances they know cause the problems. Common foods which can give this reaction are nuts, shellfish and eggs. Reactions range from a contact urticaria to anaphylaxis. Treatment will usually require antihistamines or adrenaline injections for severe reactions.

Phototherapy and photochemotherapy. Psoralen plus UVA (PUVA) and to a lesser extent UVB have been helpful in some patients with atopic eczema. There are, however, some concerns about the long-term effects of skin ageing and malignancies.

Third-line treatment

- *Oral steroids* are occasionally required for patients with a severe exacerbation of their eczema. They should not be used routinely and should be avoided during adolescence when there is a growth spurt (potential growth retardation).
- *Evening primrose oil* – evidence on the therapeutic value of this oil remains inconclusive. If used, adequate doses should be given: 160–320 mg daily in children aged 1–12 years and 320–480 mg daily in adults for 3 months. If no benefit is noted after 3 months it is unlikely to be helpful (McHenry et al 1995).
- *Other drugs* – azathioprine, ciclosporin, Chinese herbs and interferon have been reported to be effective in atopic eczema, but are only used by specialists for those with severe eczema. Hepatotoxicity has been reported following Chinese herbs, so liver function tests should be performed regularly. Homeopathic and other complementary remedies have little scientific evidence to support their use at present.

Seborrhoeic eczema

The cause of seborrhoeic eczema is now thought to be associated with skin colonization by pityrosporum yeasts in adults and is not associated with seborrhoea. This term is very confusing and is used for two very distinct patterns of eczema seen in adults and neonates. The patient usually presents with erythema and characteristic greasy scaling on the central face, eyebrows and scalp, around the ears, central chest and back.

Adults – seborrhoeic eczema (Fig. 10.7)

In adults the pattern is very similar with scalp and facial involvement. The scalp shows excessive white scaling (dandruff) associated with itching and variable skin erythema; the face, the ears, the cheeks, the sides of the nose and forehead are the common sites. Less commonly, the rash occurs on the trunk and intertrigenous regions (particularly in overweight patients)

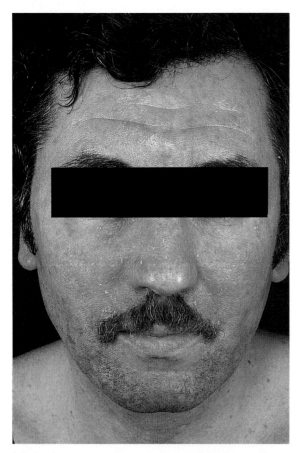

Figure 10.7 Seborrhoeic eczema (reproduced with the permission of Dr J S English and Professor H C Williams).

such as the submammary folds and perineum (Stevens et al 1989).

Neonates – cradle cap

In infants, the first manifestation of the disease is the presence on the scalp of waxy yellow scales, often thick and confluent, and difficult to remove from the scalp and hair. This inflammation then spreads down onto the face, particularly around the eyebrows and ears. An identical rash may also originate in the nappy area and extend up to the trunk and into the axillae.

Treatment and management (adults)

If treatment is to be successful the patient needs to understand the principles of treatment and how to apply the treatment effectively. The array of various preparations can be daunting for the patient; they need practical demonstrations and support. As seborrhoeic eczema often involves the scalp, the choice of vehicle and application of treatment are important. A shampoo is the easiest to use and most acceptable for the patient. Shampoos, however, only come into contact with the scalp for a limited time so should only be used for mild cases. Lotions are also used to treat scalp disease but are not very effective at removing scale. Creams and ointments are messy and difficult to use but are the most effective when treating scale. They are best applied in a systematic, methodical manner by parting the hair and then leaving on overnight to achieve maximum benefit. All the preparations mentioned above are used to carry an active treatment agent, depending on the severity of the disease. The principles of care for scalp seborrhoeic eczema are:

- *mild cases* – shampoo (usually with antipityrosporum activity, e.g. ketoconazole, selenium sulphide)
- *moderate cases* – steroid or combination of steroid/keratolytic agents
- *severe cases* – if scaling is present, cream or ointment containing salicylic acid is required.

A proprietary product called Cocois™ (coconut oil, sulphur, salicylic acid and coal tar) is widely used to treat a variety of scaly scalp conditions.

When both scale and inflammation are present, a keratolytic preparation can be used in conjunction with topical corticosteroids. Once the condition is controlled the regimen may be adjusted to a maintenance treatment which can then be adjusted for exacerbation and flares.

Antiyeast agents. Several of these agents are used to treat adult seborrhoeic eczema. Their therapeutic effect is partly responsible for the belief that the yeast commensal pityrosporum is involved in the pathogenesis of seborrhoeic eczema.

- Sulphur: a traditional remedy that is still widely used.
- Zinc pyrithione: this is the active base of several medicated shampoos.
- Selenium sulphide: present in some shampoos.
- Ketoconazole: several studies have shown that Nizoral™ shampoo is an effective treatment for seborrhoeic eczema. It is available over the counter and on prescription. A twice-weekly application for 2–4 weeks is recommended.

Coal tar. Coal tar has a mild antiproliferative effect. There are numerous preparations containing coal tar and they are produced in a variety of vehicles. They do, however, stain bedding and clothing.

Salicylic acid. Salicylic acid is a keratolytic agent used for removing skin scale.

Corticosteroids. Corticosteroid applications come in a variety of formulations and combinations. They should be used for short intensive bursts and then stopped to avoid side effects.

Emollients. For seborrhoeic eczema involving flexures, a skin-care regimen will always involve the use of emollients and the therapeutic treatment required to treat symptoms of the disease. For intertrigenous areas a combination treatment, e.g. Canesten HC or Daktacort (mild corticosteroid/antifungal cream), or antifungal cream alone, e.g. ketaconazole, may be used. Care must be taken in the use of potent topical corticosteroids in flexures, as absorption will be increased.

Discoid eczema

The cause of discoid eczema (see Fig. 10.4) is unknown but it is commonly seen in middle-aged and elderly men. The patient usually presents with several rounded 2–5 cm areas of raised red skin bearing tiny vesicles and papules. The edges of the lesions are sharply defined and the scaling, if present, is evenly spread across the lesion. In elderly men the lesions are more common on the trunk and extensor surfaces of limbs. In women, although less common, the lesions will be seen on the dorsal surfaces of the hands and fingers. The lesions are extremely itchy so they are then scratched and the vesicles deroofed. The vesicular fluid then oozes onto the surface, producing crusting. This scratching often leads to secondary bacterial infection with staphylococci (Stevens et al 1989). Patients with atopic eczema often present with a 'discoid pattern'.

Treatment and management

Emollients and topical corticosteroids may be used in conjunction with occlusive techniques such as paste bandages or wet wraps in children. This type of eczema does, however, often require a stronger topical corticosteroid.

Pompholyx (Fig. 10.8)

Pompholyx ('a bubble') is the term given to eczema that typically occurs on the palms, soles and sides of fingers and toes. The cause is usually unknown and it may occur at any age, often in warm weather and in the young adult. The patient presents with a sudden onset of crops of clear vesicles, which appear deep seated and 'sago-like'. Severe itching may precede this. There is no redness but the patient may experience a sensation of heat. The vesicles may become confluent and present as large bullae (Rook et al 1986). When these blisters resolve there is severe peeling and cracking of the skin, which is very painful and liable to secondary infection. Attacks may occur at intervals of weeks, months or years with the cause often unclear.

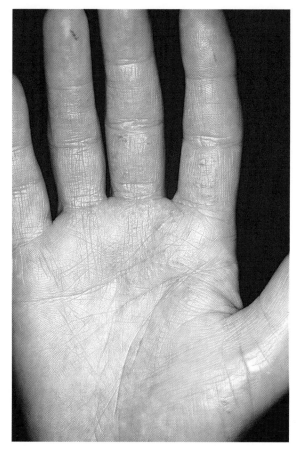

Figure 10.8 Pompholyx (reproduced with the permission of Dr J S English).

Treatment and management

In the early stages of the disease the application of emollients and corticosteroids will be sufficient. If the disease has progressed to large bullae:

- aspirate the blister
- potassium permanganate soaks are useful for wet and weepy eczema. They are very effective for drying up these areas but should only be used for a few days at a time as they may irritate the skin. They also stain skin, baths and linen brown so care should be taken when using potassium permanganate
- apply topical corticosteroids under plastic occlusion (Clingfilm or plastic gloves with cotton gloves or socks over the top)

- systemic corticosteroids may be used if the disease is severe
- antibiotics can be taken for secondary infection
- antihistamines may be used if there is sleep loss and itching
- patch testing may be performed at a later date to exclude contact allergy
- always look for severe toe–web fungal infection as this can trigger pompholyx on the hands or feet.

Gravitational eczema (see Chapter 7)

EXOGENOUS ECZEMA

Photodermatitis (Fig. 10.9)

Drugs (topical and systemic) or chemicals on the skin can interact with ultraviolet light to cause a

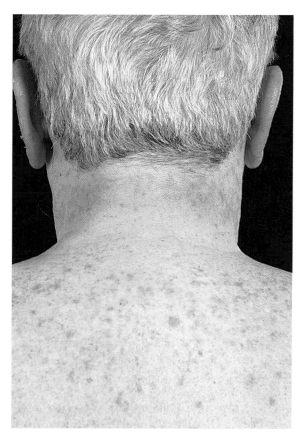

Figure 10.9 Photodermatitis (reproduced with the permission of Dr J S English).

photosensitive eczema. The areas exposed to the UV rays become inflamed and eczematous. The reaction will occur on exposed areas such as the hands, the V of the neck, the nose, the chin, the ears, and upper forehead. Areas which tend to be spared are the upper lip under the nose, the eyelids and submental region.

Several exposures to ultraviolet will be required before an eruption occurs (Hunter et al 1995). The patient presents with an itchy eruption of lesions – red patches, plaques, vesicles and bullae. In a chronic reaction, blistering will be less common but in an acute flare, such as that seen with phytophoto reactions, there will often be large bullae present.

Treatment and management

- Remove the trigger.
- Avoid further exposure to UV light.
- Wear appropriate clothing.
- Wear a total sunblock.
- Topical corticosteroids.
- If severe systemic corticosteroids.

Contact dermatitis

Prevalence

In the UK, the term eczema usually implies an endogenous cause whilst dermatitis is often associated with a contact factor such as exposure to irritants or specific allergens. The prevalence of contact dermatitis and others (not atopic eczema) is around 9%. Overall estimates of the prevalence and incidence of contact dermatitis in the general population are scarce.

Contact dermatitis is especially common in certain occupational groups (car, leather, metal, food, chemical and rubber industries) and those frequently exposed to irritants (hairdressers, cleaners, nurses and nursing mothers). It has been estimated that eczema or contact dermatitis accounts for 85–98% of occupational skin disease. Hand eczema can be crippling, leading to permanent disability and potential loss of earnings (Williams 1997).

Contact irritant dermatitis (Fig. 10.10)

Contact irritant dermatitis is much more common than allergic contact dermatitis. Contact irritant may result from an acute toxic insult to the skin, as with exposure to acids, or be due to cumulative damage from more marginal irritants, both physical and chemical, i.e. water, abrasives, acids and alkalis, solvents and detergents.

The skin provides the first and most important line of defence against exogenous agents. However, many substances can penetrate readily in and through the epidermis even when it is intact. If the stratum corneum is damaged then there will be an increase of percutaneous absorption and transepidermal water loss. If the irritants are applied for sufficient time (months or years) and in sufficient concentrations, dermatitis will occur. The repair capacity of the skin may be exhausted or penetration of chemicals may incite an inflammatory response in the skin, usually the hands.

Individuals with a history of atopic eczema and those with very fair skin are more susceptible to irritants, as are those working with irritants, e.g. hairdressers and nurses. Protection therefore plays an important part in the prevention of contact irritant dermatitis. The diagnosis and management are, however, not always clearcut. Patients often present with a combination of both irritant and allergic contact dermatitis. The pattern of reaction does not always indicate the cause, so patch testing should be performed to identify allergies.

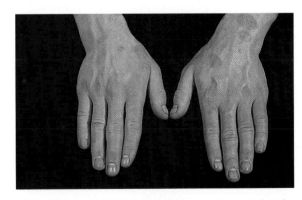

Figure 10.10 Contact irritant dermatitis to oils (reproduced with the permission of Dr J S English).

Treatment and management.

Skin care. Regular skin-care regimen using emollients and topical corticosteroids for exacerbations.

Avoid exposure to irritants. Cold weather, soaps, detergents, polishes, solvents, and any cleaning agents.

Note: The following guidelines are borrowed from Queens Medical Centre Hand Care Leaflet, with permission.

Handwashing. Always wash hands in lukewarm water. Do not use soap; instead, use a moisturizer as a soap substitute. Pat hands dry with a soft towel, taking extra care between the fingers. Finish off with another application of moisturizer.

Moisturizer. Always carry a small pot of moisturizer. Use it for washing hands and at frequent intervals throughout the day.

Gloves. Wear cotton gloves to protect hands. Avoid woollen gloves as they may irritate the skin. Whenever possible, wear plastic gloves for wet work and when in contact with any irritating substances. Gloves should be worn if in contact with fruit or vegetable juices whilst preparing food, e.g. citrus fruit, potatoes and tomatoes. Plastic gloves are preferable to rubber gloves, as they are less likely to cause allergies.

Limit the time gloves are worn to a maximum of 20 minutes at any one time. If water enters the glove it should be removed immediately, turned inside out, rinsed and left to dry.

Cotton gloves worn inside plastic gloves prevent excess perspiration. Several pairs will be required to ensure a clean dry set is always available.

Cotton gloves should be worn for dry, dusty or dirty work.

Jewellery. Remove rings during housework and don't wash hands with rings on. Keep rings clean by brushing with a soft brush.

Contact allergic dermatitis (Fig. 10.11)

Contact allergic dermatitis is a type IV (cell-mediated or delayed) hypersensitivity. This means that the first contact with a substance causes no immediate problems. Over a period of time, the allergen entering the skin sets up an immune response, with further subsequent exposures resulting in an inflammatory eczematous reaction. Common sensitizers are shown in Box 10.7.

Box 10.7 Common sensitizers (reproduced with permission from Gawkrodger 1992)	
Allergen	*Source*
Chromate	Cement, tanned leather, primer paint, anticorrosives
Cobalt	Pigment, paint, ink, metal alloys
Colophony	Glue, plasticizer, adhesive tape, varnish, polish
Epoxy resins	Adhesives, plastics, mouldings
Fragrance	Cosmetics, creams, soaps, detergents
Nickel	Jewellery, zips, fasteners, scissors, instruments
Paraphenylene diamine	Dye (clothing, hair), shoes, colour developer
Plants	*Primula obconica*, chrysanthemums, garlic, poison ivy/oak (USA)
Preservatives	Cosmetics, creams and oils
Rubber chemicals	Tyres, boots, shoes, belts, condoms, gloves

The management of contact dermatitis is not always easy because many factors influence the disease process. The principal objective is to identify the offending irritant or allergen by patch testing.

Patch testing

Patch testing is a very specialized procedure for the determination of specific chemicals or materials suspected of causing allergic contact dermatitis. Patch testing is indicated in all cases of suspected allergic contact dermatitis when the cause is unknown or uncertain.

During patch testing, low concentrations of potential allergens are applied to healthy skin. The allergens are applied under occlusion for 48 hours to allow penetration of the allergen. The testing should not be performed when the eczema is acute or widespread, as the entire skin may be irritable at this stage and there may be false-positive reactions, resulting in 'angry back'

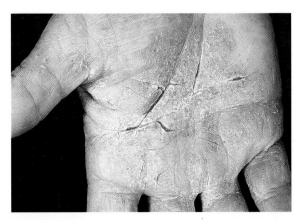

Figure 10.11 Contact allergic dermatitis to IPPD (reproduced with the permission of Dr J S English).

Box 10.8. Patient history – contact dermatitis

General
How long has the condition been present?
Where did the eczema first start?
What areas are affected now?
Does the condition improve when away from work?

Occupation
What is your occupation?
Previous occupations?
What objects, materials, substances are used regularly at work?
What special or protective clothing is worn at work?

Hobbies and leisure time
What are your hobbies?
What materials and substances are used for those hobbies?
Is there any contact with animals or pets?
In the garden are there any plants or flowers which make the eczema worse?
Does the eczema improve or get worse in sunlight?

Clothing, skin care, jewellery
What type of clothing fabrics are usually worn?
What everyday products, e.g. shampoo, are used?
What skin-care products have and are being used?
What types of make-up, perfumes and after-shave are worn?
What types of watches and jewellery are worn?
Gloves and type worn?

Medication
What medicines are taken regularly?
What topical medicaments are used?

syndrome. Patients should not be patch tested whilst taking high-dose oral corticosteroids and must stop antihistamine therapy prior to patch testing and whilst the patches are in situ. Patients should not sunbathe or use sunbeds before or during the procedure. The history is very important, as the patient's story will give a good indication of allergen exposure and possible cause (Box 10.8). Patch testing involves much detective work if an accurate cause is to be found.

The procedure. Patch tests are grouped into 'batteries'. The standard battery is known as ESB (European Standard Battery) which contains the current most common allergens. Additional batteries containing chemicals relevant to the individual's disease or employment may be required (e.g. medicaments, hairdressing).

1. Patch tests are prepared. Small amounts of test substances are applied to the small aluminum discs on adhesive tape (Finn chambers) used for patch testing (Fig. 10.12). The exact range of test substances is selected depending on the clinical problem, site of the dermatitis, patient's occupation and other factors all identified from the patient's history.

2. Patch tests are applied. The ESB is applied to every patient, with the identified additional allergens as required. Precise documentation and identification of allergens are required. The patches are applied to the upper back, left for 48 hours and then removed. The sites of applica-

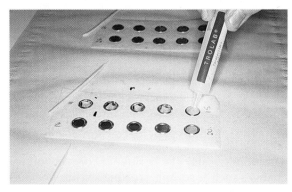

Figure 10.12 Patch testing (reproduced with the permission of Dr J S English and Professor H C Williams).

tion are marked on the back to identify them and they are read again after a further 48 hours. Accuracy and precision are vital.

3. Patch tests are read. Forty-eight hours after application, the patches are removed and the initial reading is taken. After a further 48 hours the final reading is taken. A positive allergic response is manifested by a localized eczematous reaction, scored according to the following:

+/−   doubtful: faint erythema

+   weak: erythema, maybe papules

++   strong: vesicles, infiltration

+++   extreme: bullous

IR   irritant (of various types, but often showing a glazed circumscribed area, frequently with increased skin markings)

Following patch testing the patient requires advice and support to understand the relevance of the results and how to avoid their particular allergens. Information sheets are given to the patient, their carers and GP so that they are all aware of what should be avoided. They may also require advice about their hand care and use of protective clothing, emollients and other topical applications.

UNCLASSIFIED ECZEMA

Lichen simplex (Fig. 10.13)

Lichen simplex is an area of lichenified eczema caused by repeated rubbing or scratching. This may start with any itchy skin lesion, which becomes constantly rubbed or scratched due to habit or stress. It is more common in women and rarely seen in children.

The patient will present with either single or multiple sites; which include the nape of the neck and sides, the lower legs and ankles, the scalp, the upper thighs, the vulva, pubis or scrotum and the extensor forearms (Rook et al 1986). There may also be evidence of secondary changes such as scaling, crusting, excoriation and fissuring.

Treatment and management

The aim of treatment is to prevent further damage from scratching and reduce the inflammation. Coal tar and Ichthammol paste bandages

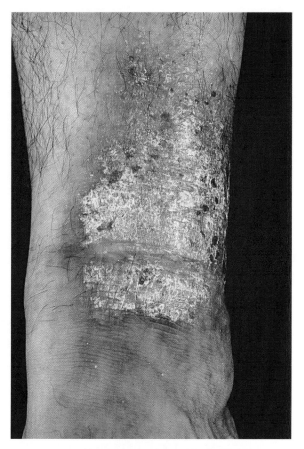

Figure 10.13   Lichen simplex (reproduced with the permission of Professor H C Williams).

can help with the irritation, inflammation and lichenification. They are used in conjunction with topical corticosteroids and may be left in place for up to a week. For smaller, more localized areas, topical corticosteroids under a hydrocolloid dressing may be used.

Juvenile plantar dermatosis
(See Chapter 7)

Asteatotic eczema (See Chapter 7)

CONCLUSION

As stressed, the management of patients with an eczematous reaction requires a sympathetic approach to care. The nurse is able to provide the support, education and advice required by this group of patients and their families. Many of the principles apply to all types of eczema, the key being the initial assessment of the patient and their disease. Eczema is an itchy, miserable condition; the nurse is able to help in a very practical way to improve the quality of life for the eczema patient.

Signpost Box

page 154, 159, 160	Icth–scratch cycle	→ Chapter 2
page 154, 155	Bacterial and viral infections	→ Chapter 13
page 155	Cryotherapy	→ Chapter 5
page 155	Nursing assessment	→ Chapter 2
page 157	Emollients	→ Chapter 3.1
page 158, 163	Topical treatments	→ Chapter 3.1
page 159	Antihistamines	→ Chapter 3.2
page 161	Type I hypersensitivity	→ Chapter 1
page 161	Phototherapy	→ Chapter 4
page 162	Cradle cap	→ Chapter 7
page 166	Type IV hypersensitivity	→ Chapter 1

REFERENCES

Bridgett C, Noren P, Staughton R 1996 Atopic skin disease: a manual for practitioners. Wrightson Biomedical Publishing, Petersfield

Finlay A Y, Khan G K 1994 Dermatology Life Quality Index (DLQI) – a simple practical measure for routine clinical use. Clinical and Experimental Dermatology 19: 210–216

Gawkrodger D J 1992 Dermatology: an illustrated colour text. Churchill Livingstone, Edinburgh

Hunter J A A, Savin J A, Dahl M V 1995 Clinical dermatology, 2nd edn. Blackwell, Oxford

Johnson M L T 1978 Skin conditions and related need for medical care among persons 1–74 years, USA 1971–1974. Vital and Health Statistics series 11, no. 212. DHEW publication no. 79–1660, US Department of Health, Education and Welfare, National Centre for Health Statistics, pp 1–72

Lawson V, Lewis-Jones M S, Finlay A Y, Reid P, Owens R G 1998 The family impact of childhood atopic dermatitis: the Dermatitis Family Impact Questionnaire. British Journal of Dermatology 138: 107–113

Lawton S 1996 Living with eczema: the dermatology patient. British Journal of Nursing 5(10): 600–609

Lawton S 1999 How to ... wet wrap. British Journal of Dermatology Nursing 3(1): 8–9

Lewis-Jones M S, Finlay A Y 1995 The Children's Dermatology Life Quality Index (CDLQI): initial validation and practical use. British Journal of Dermatology 132: 942–949

Long C C, Funnell C M, Collard R, Finlay A Y 1993 What do members of the National Eczema Society really want? Clinical and Experimental Dermatology 18: 516–522

Lynn S E, Lawton S, Newham S, Cox M, Williams H C, Emerson R 1997 Managing atopic eczema: the needs of children. Professional Nurse 12(9): 622–625

McHenry P M, Williams H C, Bingham E A 1995 Management of atopic eczema. British Medical Journal 310: 843–847

Rook A, Wilkinson D S, Ebling F J G, Champion R H, Burton J L 1986 Textbook of dermatology. Blackwell, Oxford

Stevens A, Wheater P R, Lowe J S 1989 Clinical dermatopathology: a text and colour atlas. Churchill Livingstone, Edinburgh

Su J C, Kemp A S, Varigos G A, Nolan T M 1997 Atopic eczema: its impact on the family and financial cost. Archives of Disease in Childhood 76: 159–162

Watts J 1997 Eczema and the family. Community Nurse September: 35–37

Williams H C 1994 Epidemiology of atopic eczema. Current Medical Literature (Allergy) 2: 3–7

Williams H C 1997 Dermatology. In: Stevens A, Raferty J (eds) Health care needs assessment (series 2). Radcliffe Medical Press, Oxford

PATIENT SUPPORT GROUP

National Eczema Society
163 Eversholt Street
London NW1 1BU
Tel: 020 7388 4097

11

Acne and rosacea

Mandy Boston   Dawn Preston

INTRODUCTION

Acne vulgaris and rosacea are two reasonably distinct conditions with a very different aetiology. Acne vulgaris is a very common inflammatory skin disorder affecting the face, chest and back and is most frequently seen in adolescents. It is estimated that at any one time there are 1.7 million people in the United Kingdom either receiving or requiring treatment for acne (Chu et al 1997). Virtually all teenagers (85%) experience some degree of acne in its various forms.

Rosacea is essentially an inflammatory cutaneous disorder affecting an older age group than acne vulgaris (between 30 and 60 years of age). It is rare in adolescence.

Some patients find the effects of acne or rosacea socially and psychologically devastating.

ACNE VULGARIS

What is it?

Acne vulgaris is one of the commonest skin disorders affecting young teenagers. It is due to inflammation arising around the pilosebaceous follicles on the face, neck, shoulders and upper back. Acne is characterized by seborrhoea (increased skin greasiness), non-inflamed lesions such as blackheads (open comedones), whiteheads (closed comedones) and inflamed lesions such as papules, pustules and nodules. The precise cause is unknown but is associated with an increased sebum production, retention of hyper-proliferating ductal keratinocytes, ductal colonization with *Propionibacterium acnes* (*P. acnes*) and subsequent peri-follicular inflammation.

Incidence, age and onset

Acne usually starts to develop between the ages of 11 and 14 and reaches its peak between 17 and 21 years. Peak severity occurs earlier in females than males due to the earlier onset of puberty. Acne will remain at the level of severity for 2–3 years, gradually improving and disappearing by the age of 25 years in most cases. However, 5% of females and 1% of males between the ages of 25 and 40 years still experience clinical acne (Cunliffe 1991).

Aetiology

There are three main interrelated factors which influence the development of acne.

1. An increase in the production/excretion of sebum from the pilosebaceous glands which are under the influence of circulating androgens. Patients with acne have a consistently high sebum excretion rate which is controlled by the androgens from adrenal glands and the gonads. The elevated sebum excretion rate is likely to be due to the increased sensitivity of the sebaceous glands to androgens although a small number of females have hyperandrogenetic syndromes such as polycystic ovarian syndrome (Fig. 11.1).

2. The follicles become enlarged due to an increase in the horny layer (accumulation of dead keratinocytes) partially blocking the duct and so form comedones (blackheads and whiteheads), which also contain sebum and bacteria. Microcomedones are a precursor of clinically obvious comedones (Fig. 11.2).

3. *P. acnes* is a normal skin bacteria which colonizes the pilosebaceous duct, in particular comedones. Changes in the micro-environment of the comedone favours the proliferation of *P. acnes* and the production of soluble factors which diffuse into the dermis invoking an inflammatory response (Fig. 11.3).

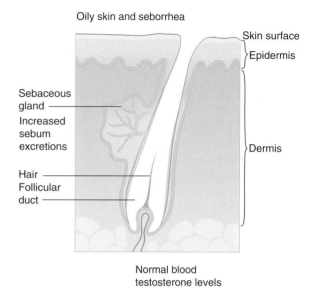

Oily skin and seborrhea

Skin surface

Epidermis

Sebaceous gland

Increased sebum excretions

Dermis

Hair

Follicular duct

Normal blood testosterone levels

Figure 11.1 Increase in the sebum excretion rate.

Clinical presentation

The clinical appearance of acne can be quite diverse. The characteristic lesions seen in acne are described in Box 11.1.

Box 11.1 Characteristic lesions involved in acne

Non-inflamed lesions

Open comedones (blackheads): black in colour, contain sebum and melanin, rarely become inflamed

Closed comedones (whiteheads): non-inflamed, frequently become inflamed (Fig. 11.4)

Inflamed lesions

Papules: small, inflamed, red lesions (Fig. 11.5)

Pustules: contain pus, resolve in 5 days (longer if they are deeper) (Fig. 11.5)

Nodules: deeper lesions which are often painful, may take several months to resolve and scarring may occur (Fig. 11.6)

Scars

Atrophic: loss of tissue (Fig. 11.9)

Hypertrophic/Keloids: representation increased, fibrous tissue (Figs 11.7, 11.8)

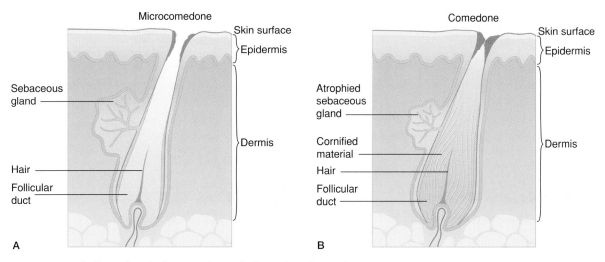

Figure 11.2   A: Formation of microcomedones. **B:** Formation of comedones.

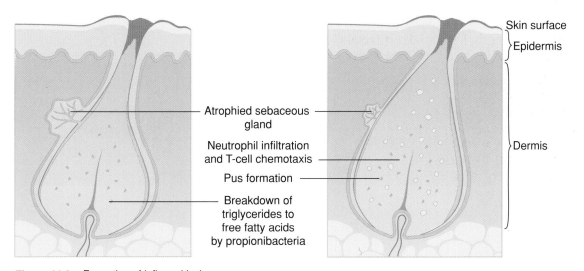

Figure 11.3   Formation of inflamed lesions.

Scars

Scarring will occur commonly in those patients with severe inflammatory acne and those who are left untreated. Scars may be either atrophic (depressed) or hypertrophic/keloid (raised) (Figs 11.7, 11.8). The most common sorts of scarring are atrophic macules (Fig. 11.9) and 'ice pick scars' which can be treated with collagen injections, excision or dermabrasion. Hypertrophic and keloid scars occur less frequently and can be treated with variable response with potent topical steroids, intralesional triamcinolone or cryotherapy. More recently, treatment with laser therapy has been used for various forms of acne scarring, but unfortunately only a few centres offer laser treatment on the NHS.

Classification

Acne can be divided into mild, moderate and severe. Other factors may influence the severity, e.g. persistent disease, poor response to therapy,

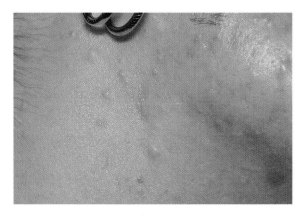

Figure 11.4   Comedones (whiteheads).

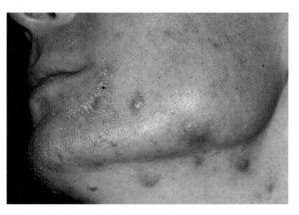

Figure 11.5   Papules and pustules.

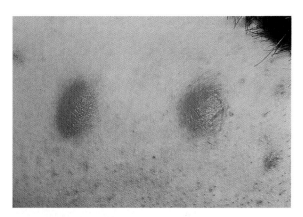

Figure 11.6   Nodules.

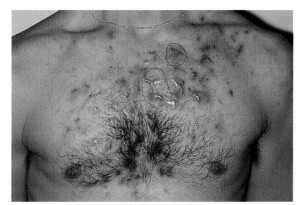

Figure 11.7   Hypertrophic scar.

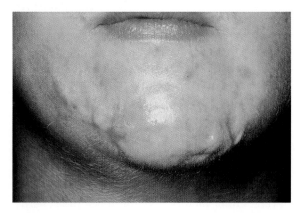

Figure 11.8   Keloid scar.

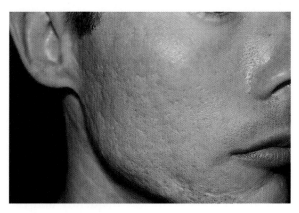

Figure 11.9   Atrophic macular scar.

scarring and increased patient anxiety will make the acne more severe.

Erythema and excoriation may occur in conjunction with the above lesions. Acne can occasionally be itchy and excoriated lesions may be present.

Sites

The face, back and/or chest are the most common sites as there are many sebaceous glands in these areas (Box 11.3). Patients may have acne on one

---

Box 11.2 Classification of acne

- *Mild acne*: this consists of inflammatory lesions, e.g. small papules, pustules and non-inflamed lesions, comedones
- *Moderate acne*: the inflamed lesions are more extensive and deep-seated, i.e. papules, pustules and nodules. In addition to the inflamed and non-inflamed lesions, scarring may occur (Fig. 11.10A)
- *Severe acne*: is many pustules, papules and nodules with significant scarring, often affecting more than one site (Fig. 11.10B)

Box 11.3 Percentage incidence of sites affected (Cunliffe 1989)

Face	99%
Back	90%
Chest	78%
All three sites	75%

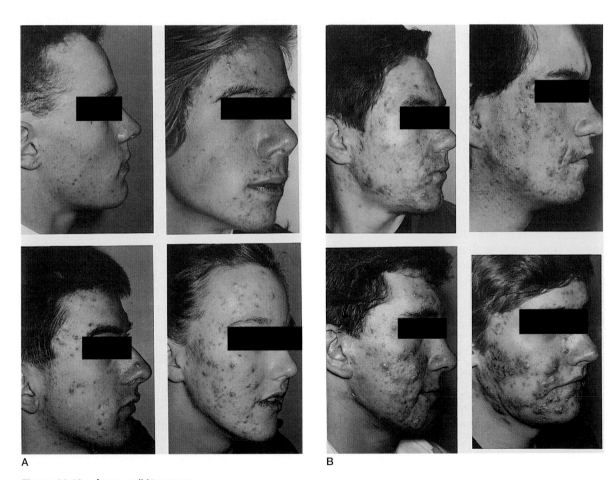

A

B

Figure 11.10 Acne – mild to severe.

or more sites. It is important for the nurse to be aware that whilst the face may be clear, the patient may have acne on the trunk.

Treatment

By the time the patient seeks medical help, they will probably already have tried many over-the-counter products. Any treatment must aim to prevent new lesions occurring, prevent scarring and minimize the psychological trauma that may result from acne.

Choosing a treatment that is convenient to use, has few obvious side effects and shows early improvement will increase patient compliance. It is important that patients understand that their treatment may continue for many years and that compliance is essential (Chu 1998). Ninety percent of patients will show 50% improvement once they have received 3 months of treatment.

Topical treatment

Benzoyl peroxide. Available in cream, gel or lotion form in concentrations from 2.5% to 10%. It has both antimicrobial and anticomedonal properties and is effective for both inflamed and non-inflamed lesions. It is applied once or twice a day. Patients must be advised that mild redness and peeling are normal initially and that the preparation may cause bleaching of clothes.

Retinoic acid or derivatives. Topical retinoids loosen and decrease the retention of cornified material in the follicular canal and so help prevent the formation of non-inflamed (come-donal) lesions. They are thought to reduce the thickness of the stratum corneum, so allowing other topical medications to penetrate more easily. Currently tretinoin, isotretinoin and adapalene are all available. Patients using these may experience mild skin irritation, particularly on exposure to the sun.

Topical antibiotics. These are useful for patients with mild or moderate acne who are unresponsive to benzoyl peroxide. Clindamycin and erythromycin are considered to be equally effective. For some patients, a regimen of topical antibiotics alternated with either benzoyl peroxide or a retinoid may be more successful. Benzoyl peroxide reduces the emergence of *P. acnes* resistance. Patients need to be aware that they must be applied twice daily and that mild irritation is to be expected.

Azelaic acid. This acts as an antibacterial and anticomedonal agent. It is applied twice daily and, as with most topical treatments, it can cause mild scaling and erythema which may be minimized by reducing the number of daily applications.

Combined topical preparations. Novel topical therapies combining treatments, e.g. erythromycin with zinc, benzoyl peroxide or isotretinoin, are also available.

Systemic treatment

Oral antibiotics remain the standard treatment for acne. Antibiotics cause suppression of *P. acnes* and reduce the free fatty acid content of the surface lipids. They act as both an antibacterial and anti-inflammatory agent. The antibiotic of choice is oxytetracycline (500 mg bd), although non-compliance can occur as the capsules need to be taken 30–40 minutes prior to food and dairy products should be avoided. Other commonly used antibiotics include erythromycin, minocycline, doxycycline and trimethoprim.

Some antibiotics have been shown to produce resistant *P. acnes*. Resistance may correlate with poor clinical response to treatment. At present, minocycline produces fewer resistance problems than the other commonly used antibiotics. However, it is the most expensive. It has few side

Table 11.1 Treatment for acne in relation to severity

Classification	Treatment
Mild inflammation	Topical benzoyl peroxide bd Topical antibiotics bd Combined topical preparations bd Azelaic acid bd
Moderate	Appropriate topical therapy Oral antibiotics Dianette® (females)
Severe	High-dose antibiotics Oral isotretinoin

effects and as it is taken once daily, it aids patient compliance.

It is important that any treatment is continued for at least 3 months before assessing its success. Patients must be made aware that response to treatment is slow and good compliance is essential. Combining topical benzoyl peroxide with antibiotics will reduce the incidence of *P. acnes* resistance.

Antiandrogen hormone therapy. Commonly used for females with moderate acne, particularly if oral contraception or period regulation is also required, antiandrogens work by reducing sebum production. The preparation of choice is Dianette® (cyproterone acetate 2 mg and ethinyloestradiol 35 µg).

13-Cis-retinoic acid (isotretinoin). Oral isotretinoin dramatically inhibits sebum production, comedone formation and reduces the number of *P. acnes* and the inflammatory response. This is the only therapy which will suppress the four main factors which influence the development of acne. It can only be prescribed by hospital dermatologists and requires close monitoring during therapy (Layton et al 1993).

The standard dose of oral isotretinoin is 0.5–1 mg/per kg per day for a period of 4 months. However, if these doses are not tolerated, lower doses can be used over a longer period. The cumulative dose, i.e. 120 mg/per kg, relates to better long-term remission. Virtually all patients will show 100% clearance at the end of a 4–5-month course and in 70% there will be no recurrence (Cunliffe 1991). Retreatment can be given if necessary. Isotretinoin is teratogenic therefore patients must be advised to avoid pregnancy. A negative pregnancy test must be provided pretreatment and adequate contraception must be ensured throughout the course and for 6 weeks post therapy.

The common side effects of dry lips, dry skin and nasal crusting will usually occur during the treatment. These can be combatted by regular use of emollients and lipsalve.

Oral isotretinoin is an expensive therapeutic option although when compared with the expense of long-term rotational antibiotics, its cost features favourably as does its excellent results.

Other treatments

Comedone removal. Blackheads can be removed using an extractor and big whiteheads (macrocomedones) can be treated with cautery after the application of local anaesthetic cream.

Ultraviolet light. Some patients find that sunlight improves their acne; there is recent scientific evidence to support this.

UVB has a short-term antiinflammatory effect but the immediate improvement is not sustained and long-term adverse effects of ultraviolet light outweigh any short-term benefit.

Less common variants of acne

Acne conglobate. An aggressive form of acne with large nodules, abscesses and commonly nodules which fuse together to form sinuses.

Acne fulminans. A severe form of acne, most common in younger males. It is often accompanied by the patient feeling systemically unwell with fever, joint pain and general malaise. It is aggressive and causes scarring.

Pyoderma faciale. This is uncommon but mainly affects women aged 20–40 years. Pustules and nodules erupt suddenly, usually on the face. Scarring can occur if not treated promptly.

Gram-negative folliculitis. Usually a sudden development of many pustules, which looks like an acne flare. It is a complication of long-term antibiotic therapy. Treatment is either oral trimethoprim or oral isotretinoin.

Infantile acne. Presents within 3 months of birth with localized lesions, mostly on the cheeks. The acne may reoccur at puberty.

Acne excoriée. Predominantly occurs in females where there are few or no lesions. Patients 'pick' or 'fiddle' with the lesions and topical treatment can exacerbate the problem. Patients must be advised not to touch the spots and if the condition is severe, psychotherapeutic intervention may help.

Patient education and advice

Acne is sometimes incorrectly viewed as a natural part of growing up. However, patients with acne often feel unattractive, have low self-esteem and rarely, psychological problems have led to suicide (Cotterill & Cunliffe 1997). One study has demonstrated the significantly higher unemployment rates in individuals with acne (Cunliffe 1986). It is vital that no patient is ever left believing that they do not require treatment because it is a condition that they will grow out of. Dismissive attitudes from friends or health-care professionals may explain why many patients with acne do not seek medical attention (Dudley & Poyner 1998).

It is important that adequate time is available when treating patients with acne. The therapeutic outcome is influenced by empathic history taking and a caring attitude will promote trust and compliance, which is essential for patients with acne (Plewig & Kligman 1993). 'One of the first and best interventions the nurse can do is to allow patients to express their feelings' (Poorman & Webb 1992). The work of Poorman & Webb demonstrates how to use such an approach with a patient with acne.

All health-care professionals treating a patient with acne must ensure that they accurately determine the effect acne is having on their patient's life. The physical severity of the disease and psychological effects on the patient's life do not necessarily correlate, hence it is important to consider the psychosocial disability in all patients regardless of the severity of the disease (Chu et al 1997). The most effective method of determining the extent of psychological problems arising as a result of acne is to use a questionnaire as part of the initial holistic assessment. Layton et al (1997) evaluated the Assessment of the Psychological and Social Effects of Acne (APSEA) Questionnaire in order to determine the benefit of using such a questionnaire as a clinical tool (Fig. 11.11). Patients who are experiencing significant psychological problems should be commenced on an early effective therapy and occasionally some patients may require referral for psychological support.

Nurses working in either primary or secondary care settings may meet patients who are attending an appointment for reasons other than their acne. For this reason it is important that all nurses have a basic understanding of the psychological distress that acne can cause and an overview of the many treatments that are available. In any health-related consultation, the nurse can then ensure that the patient is aware of how to access effective treatment and can discuss general health advice in relation to acne. The nurse must emphasize the importance of complying with treatment and ensure that the patient understands that it may take 6–12 weeks to show definite improvement. Patients with acne should be advised to use mild soap and water for washing and to use cosmetic lotions or sun lotions rather than ointments which have a tendency to be greasy. Whilst using any topical treatment, moisturizers will help combat associated dryness. It is worth reminding those with acne not to pick or squeeze spots as this lengthens healing time. Female patients should be made aware that an approaching menstrual cycle can worsen acne.

As with many conditions, stress can worsen acne and advice should be offered on stress management strategies.

Box 11.4 Acne myths	
Myths	*Reality*
Acne is caused by poor diet	There is no evidence to support this; acne is not made worse by eating chocolate or sweet food
Acne is caused by poor hygiene	There is no evidence to support support this; frequent washing does not improve acne
Acne is infectious	Acne is not contagious, so is not passed from one person to another
Acne is worsened by lack of exercise	There is nothing to support this
Greasy hair can cause spots	There is no evidence to support this

ROSACEA

What is it?

Rosacea is a relatively common, highly visible, chronic, non-infectious, inflammatory skin disorder mainly affecting the central third of the face, particularly the convexities, i.e. the nose and cheeks. It can, however, extend to the scalp, forehead and eyelids (blepharitis). Only rarely does it affect the trunk and scarring is exceptional.

THE LEEDS TEACHING HOSPITALS

APSEA Form

WQN 116

Patient's name ....
Patient's Address ....
Date of Birth .... Hospital No ....
Consultant.. Ward ....

Overall clinical grade of acne. Mild ☐ Moderate☐ Severe☐

APSEA score *(value)* ☐

APSEA score *(significance)*   Insig. ☐ Low ☐ Medium ☐
High ☐ Very high ☐

Numbers 1–6, tick the most appropriate answer to each question

IN THE PAST WEEK

1.   Worrying thoughts go through my mind
☐   a great deal of the time
☐   a lot of the time
☐   from time to time, not often
☐   only occasionally

2.   I can sit at ease and feel relaxed
☐   not at all
☐   not often
☐   usually
☐   definitely

3.   I feel restless, as if I have to be on the move
☐   very much indeed
☐   quite a lot
☐   not very much
☐   not at all

AT THE MOMENT

4.   I like what I look like in photographs
☐   not at all
☐   sometimes
☐   very often
☐   nearly all the time

5.   I wish I looked better
☐   not at all
☐   sometimes
☐   very often
☐   nearly all the time

6.   On the whole I am satisfied with myself
☐   strongly disagree
☐   disagree
☐   agree
☐   strongly agree

Questions 7–15, read the following carefully and put a line at the point that most accurately represents how you feel because of your acne

7.   Do you enjoy the things you used to?
Never 0 _____ 10 All the time

8.   Are you more or less irritable than usual?
Never 0 _____ 10 All the time

9.   Do you feel that you are useful and needed?
Never 0 _____ 10 All the time

How has your skin condition limited the following activities or made them more difficult or awkward, or less enjoyable since you have had acne?

10.   Going shopping
Not at all 0 _____ 10 All the time

11.   Going out socially to meet friends from outside the home
Not at all 0 _____ 10 All the time

12.   Going away for the weekends, holidays and outings
Not at all 0 _____ 10 All the time

13.   Eating out
Not at all 0 _____ 10 All the time

14.   Using public changing rooms/swimming pools
Not at all 0   10 All the time

15.   Do you think your appearance will interfere with your chances of future employment ?
Strongly disagree 0 _____ 10 strongly agree

'Designed and Printed by The Leeds Teaching Hospitals NHS Trust Print Unit (November 1998)

Figure 11.11   Assessment of the Psychological and Social Effects of Acne (reproduced with permission from The Leeds Teaching Hospitals Trust).

The physical signs relating to rosacea include:

- flushing (Fig. 11.12)
- persistent symmetrical erythema
- telangiectases (small dilated vessels in the skin which are permanently visible caused by a reduction in the mechanical integrity of the upper dermal connective tissue)
- episodes of inflammation which can include papules, pustules and nodules
- connective tissue dysplasia.

Patients with rosacea, unlike those with acne vulgaris, do not have comedones. In a minority of cases, rosacea can also be associated with ocular complaints including conjunctivitis, blepharitis, keratitis and iritis. Complications which are associated with rosacea occur more frequently with a prolonged or protracted course. The frequency of acute attacks tends to decrease with time.

The course of this disease is often persistent and chronic, with periods of remission punctuated by acute exacerbations of inflammatory lesions and swellings. Rosacea may cause unsightly persistent erythema on the cheeks and nose which may become more violaceous with time. Additionally, the skin over the nose may thicken and become coarse, irregular and very oily. This condition is known as rhinophyma (pronounced enlargement of the nose) (Fig. 11.13) and may be the only sign of rosacea. Rhinophyma occurs most commonly in males in their late 50s or over. The ratio of male to female is 10:1. As rosacea progresses, lymphatic failure results in a sustained inflammatory response in the cutaneous tissues. The accumulating plasma proteins may play a role in the fibroplasia that underlies the development of rhinophyma.

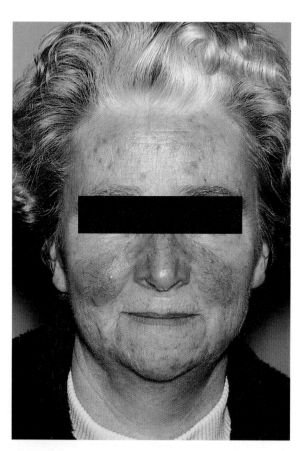

Figure 11.12 Flushing in rosacea.

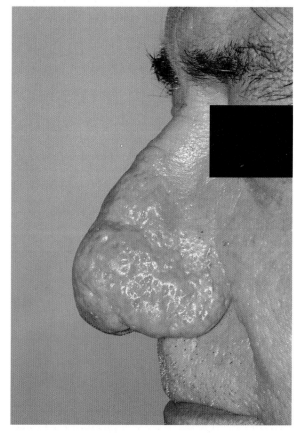

Figure 11.13 Rhinophyma.

Incidence, age and onset

Rosacea affects women more commonly than men. The average age for onset of rosacea is between 30 and 50 years, although it can occur at any age. Fair-skinned people, particularly those of Celtic origin and those who blush easily, are the most likely to be affected. The incidence of rosacea varies, according to different studies, from 2% to 10% The most common form of rosacea, occurring in four out of five cases, is the erythemotelangiectatic form. One in five cases presents with inflamed lesions in the papulopustular form.

Aetiology

The aetiology of rosacea is unknown. There is no laboratory test to confirm the diagnosis but there are a number of current theories.

Rosacea is considered to be the curse of the Celts, seen most commonly in fair-haired, freckled, pale-skinned individuals, suggesting that skin type and actinic damage may play some part. It is controversial whether the demodex mite is implicated in the aetiology. Some studies have shown increased numbers of demodex mites in inflammatory rosacea. Other studies have suggested the demodex mite might provoke a full-blown reaction.

There are a number of aggravating factors in the deterioration of rosacea.

Environmental

Ultraviolet light causes deterioration in 70% of patients. Sun exposure, strong winds and extremes of temperature should be avoided.

Diet

Hot drinks cause exacerbation of rosacea and the vasodilatation may last for 40 minutes following a hot drink (see also Box 11.5).

Systemic and topical medications

Drugs that produce dilatation of venules can produce rosacea-like symptoms. It is well recognized that topical corticosteroids can produce a rebound effect in patients with rosacea, i.e. they appear to improve the problem initially but discontinuing the treatment leads to relapse of the problem, thus topical steroids should **not** be used in rosacea. Topical applications containing hydroalcoholic or sorbic acid vehicles, e.g. sun screens, cosmetics and hair sprays, may also aggravate acne rosacea.

Box 11.5 Foods that may aggravate rosacea

- Spicy food, e.g. pickled, marinated, fermented, smoked, soy sauce, vinegar
- Tea, coffee
- Chocolate
- All wines and liquors
- All cheeses except cottage cheese
- Yoghurt, soured cream
- Citrus fruits, bananas, red plums, raisins, figs
- Tomatoes, avocados, aubergine, spinach
- Liver and some types of meat

Psychopathology

There is no doubt that stress causes exacerbation of rosacea although it is perhaps not regarded as a primary aetiological factor. This is more evident in rosacea fulminans.

When considering the pathophysiological sequence in rosacea it appears that there is a susceptible group of individuals. Ultraviolet light and environmental factors can produce dermal damage which can lead to small blood vessel dilatation. This makes the small vessel incompetent and results in increased fluid and leakage of molecules from the vessels, producing both inflammation and oedema. The inflammatory component results in papules and pustules. Susceptible individuals flush; this leads to increased blood flow which in turn leads to further small blood vessel dilatation.

Clinical presentation

Rosacea can be divided into different clinical forms.

I   Can present with persistent erythema which continues until treated. This is associated with telangiectasia and often with actinic damage (e.g. response to sunlight)

II Erythema as above and associated with papules and pustules

III As above with nodules, plaque-like inflammation which can disturb the facial contours

IV As above with connective tissue changes producing hyperplasia and clinically presenting as phymas (swellings)

Differential diagnosis

The following conditions may commonly be confused with acne rosacea (Garver & Wilkin 1992).

- Seborrhoeic dermatitis may coexist with rosacea but the distribution is dissimilar.
- A perioral dermatitis rebound after discontinuing topical corticosteroids may mimic rosacea.
- Acne vulgaris lacks the vascular component of rosacea; comedones do occur in rosacea.
- Discoid lupus erythematosus presents quite well-developed plaques which show pigmentary changes, atrophy and scarring, unlike rosacea.

Variants/complications of rosacea

Persistent oedema.   The site of the oedema is the central portion of the face, cheeks and eyelids.

Ophthalmic rosacea.   This is more common than recognized. Clinical presentations include blepharoconjunctivitis, keratitis, sicca syndrome and lupus granulomatous rosacea. The site of ophthalmic rosacea is the lower eyelids and it presents as brown/red papules and diascopy/lupoid infiltration.

Rosacea fulminans.   This is synonymous with pyoderma faciale. It occurs rarely, mostly in females aged over 25. The site is predominantly on the face.

Phymas.   These occur in 1% with a male-to-female ratio of 10:1. Phymas usually occur on the nose, less so on the chin, forehead, earlobes and eyelids.

Treatment

Garver & Wilkin (1992) advise that initially patients minimize or stop their exposure to heat, cold, sunlight, vasodilator drugs, hot drinks,

Table 11.2   Treatment for rosacea in relation to severity

Telangiectatic rosacea	Inflammatory rosacea	
Consider cosmetic camouflage	Mild	Topical metronidazole bd Sunblock
Laser therapy	Moderate	As mild Oral antibiotics (oxytetracycline 1 g daily or erythromycin 1 g daily)
	Severe	As moderate Minocycline 100 mg daily Consider oral isotretinoin if not responding

alcohol, spicy foods and chocolate. Ice chips held in the mouth have been found to be helpful in preventing flushing stimulated by a hot environment or menopausal causes for up to 30 minutes. Treatments are either topical, systemic or surgical. There is limited evidence to suggest that combined limited therapy for acne rosacea produces more rapid results and better efficacy. Since the rate of progression of rosacea varies amongst individuals, dermatologists usually tailor a combination of therapies to suit each patient (Table 11.2).

Rosacea is often a progressive disease characterized by periodic exacerbations and remissions and long-term therapy may be required.

Topical treatment

Antibiotics are commonly used. Metronidazole is better applied in a cream than a gel. Other topical antibiotics available include erythromycin, clindamycin and tetracycline but are used infrequently. Azelaic acid can also be used. Sun screens are important as 70% of patients will show deterioration on exposure to sunlight. Cosmetic camouflage could also be considered.

Systemic treatment

Although rosacea is not caused by bacterial infection, it responds well to antibiotics probably due to their antiinflammatory effects. Corticosteroids will potentiate the permanent telangiectasia and therefore are not used. Oxytetracycline, minocycline, doxycycline and metronidazole have all been used. Beta blockers may help reduce anxiety and emotional flushing.

Severe inflammatory rosacea which is resistant to antibiotics can be treated with oral isotretinoin. Relapsing and poorly responding cases and those with persistent oedema, inflammatory rosacea or phymas may require continuous or intermittent treatment with oral isotretinoin.

Surgical treatment

Advice should be given that once the inflammatory response is settled, patients may be left with telangiectasia. Patients must be warned about this as they may have unrealistic expectations of their disease outcome. The pulsed tunable dye laser can help the telangiectasia. Phymas may be reduced by dermabrasion, although CO_2 laser is now more frequently used.

Ocular lesions will usually require referral to an ophthalmologist.

Patient education

The distressing physical effects of rosacea can often exacerbate the condition and the healthcare professional must be aware that the patient will need more support during times of relapse (Sober 1992). Time spent developing a rapport with the patient and learning about their lifestyle is essential. It aids compliance and helps the patient to understand the disease. Chalmers (1997) advises that patients should be taught how to recognize substances that trigger flushing in order to avoid them. Garver & Wilkin (1992) recommend many methods for reducing or eliminating potential triggers (Box 11.6).

Patients with rosacea very quickly lose their self-esteem as they try to manage their conspicuous and often embarrassing facial symptoms. If rosacea is treated at the earliest opportunity and the prescribed treatment carefully followed then it is likely to be more successfully controlled. It is important that myths are dispelled at the earliest possible stage, e.g. that rosacea sufferers misuse alcohol. Alcohol is known to produce flushing and so exacerbates the problem in some sufferers.

It is very important that patients with rosacea are aware that it is a chronic condition but emphasize that although there is no permanent cure, the

---

> **Box 11.6** Patient advice
>
> - Avoid: pulling or rubbing the skin; using abrasive cloths, harsh soaps or astringent applications.
> - Use a gentle cleanser or soft natural sponge.
> - Tepid water should be used.
> - Remove make-up carefully and following cleansing, the face should be patted dry.
> - After washing, allow face to dry for 30 minutes prior to applying topical medications.
> - Make-up should be water based and fragrance free; avoid powder.
> - Prefoundation base in shades of sheer green or camouflage make-up can reduce redness.
> - Use a non-irritant sunblock.
> - Avoid foods or drinks known to aggravate the condition, e.g. alcohol, tea, spicy foods.

---

physical and psychological impact can be greatly reduced with the appropriate treatment and support.

CONCLUSION

Although there is no connection between acne vulgaris and acne rosacea, patients suffering from either diagnosis will require regular reassurance, encouragement, early advice and appropriate medication. 'An individual's sense of physical attractiveness is in part defined by the quality of the skin' (Poorman & Webb 1992). Today's media and fashion magazines portray and reinforce the need for perfect unblemished complexions and those failing to meet these standards can experience overwhelming feelings of embarrassment and shame which can ultimately manifest as anxiety, lack of confidence and depression. Early referral to a specialist for treatment avoids risk of scarring, both physically and psychologically.

Due to the range of treatments available these potentially debilitating diseases can be treated effectively and nurses are ideally placed to facilitate both early medical intervention and appropriate psychological and social support.

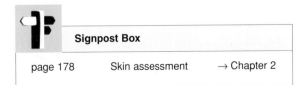

	Signpost Box	
page 178	Skin assessment	→ Chapter 2

REFERENCES

Chalmers D A 1997 Rosacea: recognition and management for the primary care provider. Nurse Practitioner 22(10): 18–30

Chu T 1998 Value for money from acne treatment. Prescriber (acne management suppl). A & M Publishing, Surrey, pp 10–11

Chu T, Cunliffe W J, Layton A, Mitchell T 1997 Pocket guide: acne. Medical Imprint, London

Cotterill J A, Cunliffe W J 1997 Suicide in dermatological patients. British Journal of Dermatology 137(2): 246–250

Cunliffe W J 1986 Acne and unemployment. British Journal of Dermatology 115: 386

Cunliffe W J 1989 Acne. Martin Dunitz, London

Cunliffe W J 1991 A brief guide to the treatment and management of acne. Schering Healthcare, Berlin

Cunliffe W J 1994 New approaches to acne treatment. Martin Dunitz, London

Cunliffe W J, Gray J A, Macdonald Hull S, Hughes B R, Calvert R T 1991 Cost effectiveness of isotretinoin. Journal of Dermatological Treatment 1: 285–288

Dudley A, Poyner T 1998 Fear and loathing among acne sufferers. Prescriber (acne management suppl). A & M Publishing, Surrey, pp 3–7

Garver J H, Wilkin J K 1992 Flushing and rosacea: overview and nursing interventions. Dermatology Nursing 4(4): 271–277

Layton A M, Stainforth J M, Cunliffe W J 1993 Ten years experience of oral isotretinoin for the treatment of acne vulgaris. Journal of Dermatology Treatment 4 (suppl 2): S2–S5

Layton A M, Seukaran D, Cunliffe W J 1997 Scarred for life. Dermatology 195 (suppl): 15–21

Plewig G, Kligman A M 1993 Acne and rosacea. Springer-Verlag, Berlin

Poorman S G, Webb C A 1992 Sexuality and self-concept: issues in skin disease. Dermatology Nursing 4(4): 279–284

Sober A J 1992 Management of rosacea. Dermatology Nursing 4(6): 454–456

FURTHER READING

Acne Distance Learning Programme for Nurses – available from the Acne Support Group (see below)

Boston M 1997 Acne: avoiding permanent damage. Community Nurse 3(4): 15–16

Cunningham M 1999 Diagnosis of rosacea. British Journal of Dermatology Nursing 3(3): 10–12

Preston D, Nicholson N 1999 More than just skin deep. Nursing Times Sept, 15 (skin care suppl): 7–8

PATIENT SUPPORT GROUP

Acne Support Group
First Floor, Howard House
The Runway, South Ruislip
Middlesex HA4 6SE
Tel: 020 8561 6868
http://www.m2w3.com/acne
http://www.stopspots.org

12

Skin cancer

Gillian Morrison

INTRODUCTION

Skin cancer is a phenomenon of the 20th century. Excessive exposure to ultraviolet radiation (UVR) is linked to both non-melanoma type skin cancer and malignant melanoma (Mackie 1989a). Prior to the 1920s modesty and fashion ensured that almost all sections of society kept their skin covered and took a pride in a pale complexion, even when living abroad. A tanned skin was synonymous with manual work and poverty. In the late 1920s Coco Chanel brought about a change in fashion and a sun tan became a symbol of health, youth and glamour. A sun tan proved you could afford to holiday abroad and had time for leisure activities. It rapidly became a status symbol and is still a desired fashion accessory today. However, this change in society's behaviour has had far-reaching effects and the incidence of skin cancer has now reached almost epidemic proportions, in many parts of the world being the commonest form of cancer (Cancer Research Campaign 1991).

The Government's *Health of the nation* White Paper highlighted the need to halt 'the year-on-year increase in the incidence of skin cancer by the year 2005' (DoH 1992). This will only be achieved by primary prevention working towards an increased awareness of skin cancer and its association with sun exposure and an ultimate change in fashion regarding sun-tanned skin.

To understand skin cancer, it is important to understand a little about ultraviolet radiation. That skin cancer and UVR are closely linked is something that people find hard to understand. The energy from sunlight is essential for life on earth; in ancient times, the sun was worshipped as a god and on a personal level people feel better and happier when the sun is shining. Yet there is a dark side to this life-giving sun in that it has the capacity to damage the human skin with, in some instances, deadly results.

Ultraviolet light is divided into three ranges according to their wavelengths (measured in nanometres): UVA, UVB and UVC.

Box 12.1	Ultraviolet radiation
UVA	Wavelength 315–400 nm. Main source of UVR. Does not burn the skin's surface but causes deeper damage within the dermis.
UVB	Wavelength 280–315 nm. Smaller proportion of UVR. Causes damage to the epidermis ranging from erythema to blistering burns.
UVC	Wavelength 200–280 nm. Short wavelengths removed by ozone layer.

UV radiation is more intense the nearer a country is to the equator as the sun's rays strike more directly. The sun's rays also strike more directly when the sun is highest in the sky, around midday. The sun's rays are also more intense at high altitudes and can be reflected, for example by snow or sand, causing greater intensity.

The ozone layer is a condensed form of oxygen which forms a protective layer between the atmosphere and the earth. UVA and UVB rays pass through, but UVC is blocked by the ozone layer. Any damage to the ozone layer by manmade gases such as CFCs (chlorofluorocarbons) and halon gases will allow these extremely damaging UVC rays to penetrate to earth where they can cause immense damage to all forms of animal, marine and plant life, as well as to the human skin.

The nursing of patients with both melanoma and non-melanoma skin cancer is based on three main points: recognition, treatment and prevention.

- *Recognition* – based on knowledge of the clinical features of skin cancer, an understanding of its causes and an awareness of those most at risk and how they are most likely to present.
- *Treatment* – includes both physical treatment of the tumour and psychological care following diagnosis.
- *Prevention* – in the form of education to recognize skin cancer and primary prevention to reduce sun exposure and prevent sunburn.

BASAL CELL CARCINOMA

This is sometimes called a rodent ulcer as, if left untreated, it will break down to form an ulcer which will relentlessly erode all localized tissue, including cartilage and bone.

Basal cell carcinomas (BCC) are the commonest form of skin cancer. They are traditionally seen in the older age group, although it is now becoming more common to see patients presenting with basal cell carcinomas in their 30s and 40s.

Although the tumours can cause substantial damage in a localized area, to all intents and purposes they almost never metastasize (Mackie 1989a).

Histology

Histology shows the presence of basophilic cells which have invaded the dermis and formed clumps of mitotic activity, leading to degenerative change (Fig. 12.1).

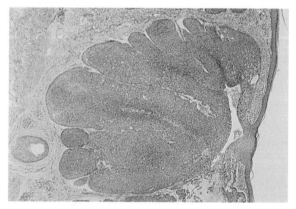

Figure 12.1 Basal cell carcinoma – histology (reproduced with permission from Dr M Walsh, Consultant Dermatopathologist, Royal Group of Hospitals, Belfast).

Recognition

Nurses can play a particularly valuable role by detecting basal cell carcinomas. These tumours particularly affect the elderly, many of whom may, due to a diminished mental capacity or failing eyesight, fail to recognize the significance of these lesions.

Clinical features

Basal cell carcinomas are visible to the naked eye through observation of the skin (Fig. 12.2). There are four main types of BCCs, all of which have slightly different features (Table 12.1).

Areas of pigment may be found in all types of BCC.

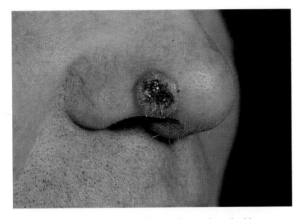

Figure 12.2 Basal cell carcinoma (reproduced with permission from Dr J R Corbett, Consultant Dermatologist, Department of Dermatology, Royal Group of Hospitals, Belfast).

Table 12.1 Classification and clinical features of BCC

Classification	Clinical features
Nodular BCC	Skin-coloured glistening papule. Telangiectasia. Rolled pearly edge. Sometimes central necrosis
Cystic BCC	Similar to nodular, but more telangiectasia and more tense
Morphoeic BCC	White/yellow morphoeic plaques resembling enlarging scar. Ulceration and crusting common
Superficial BCC	Superficial expanding plaques with rim-like edge

Aetiology

The most common cause is cumulative damage from sun exposure over many years (Mackie 1989a).

Any form of chronic scarring, including X-irradiation, may predispose to basal cell carcinoma.

Multiple BCCs occur in a variety of inherited syndromes such as naevoid basal cell syndrome or xeroderma pigmentosum. These conditions are, however, relatively rare.

At-risk groups

- Individuals with a fair skin which burns easily, particularly the Celtic type of fair hair and skin and blue eyes.
- The closer the individual's proximity to the equator, the higher the incidence of basal cell carcinoma.
- Outdoor workers, such as farmers, builders, etc. who have had a high degree of sun exposure.
- Individuals who enjoy outdoor hobbies such as gardening, sailing and golf.

Presentation

Typically, the patient will be middle aged to elderly with a lesion on the face which has grown slowly, possibly over 2–3 years. The lesion may have appeared to heal and then reappeared, thus duping the patient into thinking it was clearing. BCCs occur mainly on the sun-exposed sites, most commonly on the face around the nose, inner canthus or temple. However, it is also common on the tips of ears and on bald heads, backs of hands and chests which have had long-term sun exposure (Fig. 12.3).

The importance of early recognition of basal cell carcinomas cannot be overemphasized since a small lesion requires less extensive surgery and therefore causes less scarring, trauma and worry, particularly to elderly patients. If in any doubt about the likelihood of a lesion being a BCC, a good rule of thumb is to seek medical advice about all lesions which are not healing and may be enlarging.

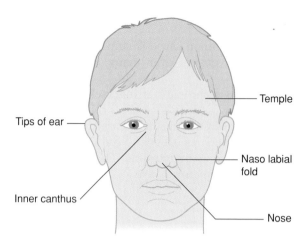

Figure 12.3 Sites for basal cell carcinoma.

Treatment

Initially, the diagnosis is confirmed by a punch biopsy. This is followed by a wide surgical excision of the tumour.

For aggressive or recurrent tumours and those with difficult-to-define edges, Mohs' micrographic surgery is the most effective treatment (see Chapter 5).

Following surgery, patients have regular follow-up appointments to check for any recurrence or for any new lesions and to receive health education regarding sun care.

Radiotherapy is only used where surgical treatment is contraindicated, mainly in very elderly patients.

Nursing care

The nursing treatment of patients with BCC is on two levels: the practical care of patients undergoing dermatological surgery and the psychological care of patients who have been given a diagnosis of cancer. The pre- and postoperative nursing care of dermatological patients is extremely important.

Patients' reactions to a diagnosis of BCC are very varied. At the time of diagnosis, very often the only word the patient hears is 'cancer' and it is important that the nurse at this visit and subsequent visits reinforces to the patient that this particular type of cancer will not metastasize. It may be some time before the patient is completely reassured. If the patient gives permission, it is often helpful, especially if the patient is elderly, to bring the relatives into this discussion.

Scarring, particularly for younger women if the face is involved, may cause a deep psychological problem. It is important to explore the patient's reaction to their scar. In some instances, cosmetic camouflage may be a help. However, some patients may even require counselling or psychiatric help.

Prevention and education

Education about good sun-care habits is the main method of preventing BCC. Amongst elderly patients, much of the sun damage will probably already have occurred. However, 'there is a strong possibility that if further photo-damage is prevented, then repair takes place in both the dermis and epidermis' (Marks 1992). Despite a lack of strong evidence to support this, it would be unwise to expose the skin to even further solar damage.

Sun-care education should be aimed at all who work outdoors and enjoy outdoor hobbies, in particular those with a fair skin which burns easily. When dealing with more elderly patients, however, it is important to address the advice more particularly towards them (see Box 12.2).

Many elderly people may never have used a sun screen or been abroad. Many elderly men in particular find applying creams 'fussy' and few realize the importance of protecting their skin on overcast days, cloud giving little protection from UVR. In many instances, it is sensible to include the family or carers in the sun-care advice as their understanding of the need for a sun-care regimen may help with compliance.

It is important to check any drugs being taken by elderly patients as certain medications used in the treatment of blood pressure, heart disease, fluid retention, etc. can cause photosensitivity. The label on the drug should have a printed warning and if it has, the patient should be advised to contact their doctor in the light of their diagnosis of basal cell carcinoma.

Patients with basal cell carcinomas and, when appropriate, their carers should be advised about the importance of early detection of further tumours or recurrence at the site of the old tumour. Recurrence rate following removal of a BCC is approximately 5% at 5 years (Gawkrodger 1992).

Key points	
Recognition	Be suspicious of any slow-growing lesion which fails to heal.
Treatment	Excision of lesion effects a cure.
Prevention	Good sun-care habits.

SOUAMOUS CELL CARCINOMA

Squamous cell carcinoma is an invasive carcinoma which, if left untreated, may metastasize. It arises on already damaged skin or mucous membrane, the most common cause of damage being ultraviolet radiation (Champion et al 1992). It is unusual in those under 55 and is more common in men than in women. However, this statistic may change with the increasing number of women who spend leisure and working time outside (Gawkrodger 1992).

Histology

Histology shows malignant keratinocytes which have a capacity to form keratin which invades the dermis (Fig. 12.4).

Recognition

Early recognition of squamous cell carcinomas is vital as they are faster growing and more aggressive than basal cell carcinomas (Champion et al 1992). Once again, the elderly are particularly vulnerable and nurses should be alert to the clinical features of squamous cell carcinomas (Table 12.2).

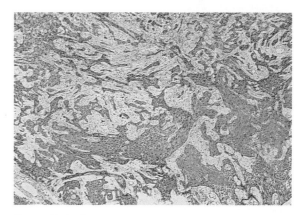

Figure 12.4 Squamous cell carcinoma – histology (reproduced with permission from Dr M Walsh, Consultant Dermatopathologist, Royal Group of Hospitals, Belfast).

Table 12.2 Classification and clinical features of squamous cell carcinoma

Classification	Clinical features
Sun-exposed skin which shows signs of skin damage	A small pimple which may have arisen on the site of a keratosis. Unlikely to metastasize
Nodular type – usually on sun-exposed skin (Fig. 12.5)	Hard nodule on indurated skin which increases in size quite rapidly and may develop into an ulcer. More aggressive, more likely to metastasize
Ulcerating forms of squamous cell carcinoma	Nodular area on the edge of an ulcer or an area of an ulcer or scar behaving differently from the rest of the ulcer or scar edge. More likely to metastasize

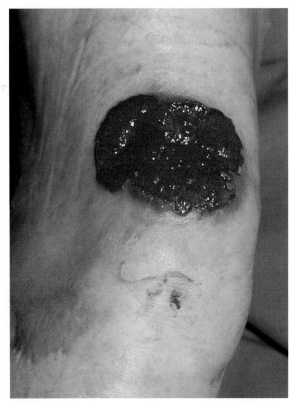

Figure 12.5 Squamous cell carcinoma (reproduced with permission from Dr J R Corbett, Consultant Dermatologist, Department of Dermatology, Royal Group of Hospitals, Belfast).

The clinical features of squamous cell carcinomas are mainly dependent on cause and site.

Aetiology and at-risk groups

Long-term sun exposure is the main cause of squamous cell carcinoma. It is therefore more prevalent in the elderly and particularly in those with fair skin and fair hair. A history of sun exposure in a foreign country close to the equator increases the risk factor.

Other causes include skin damage due to:

- chronic destructive skin disorders, such as lupus erythematosus or lupus vulgaris
- chronic scarring, for example from burns
- chronic ulcers
- genetic disorders, e.g. xeroderma pigmentosum

- immunosuppressed patients, e.g. following renal transplant
- photochemotherapy.

Presentation

Typically, the patient will be over 50 with a tumour on a sun-exposed site such as the face, neck, forearm or hand. The patient will give a history of a fast-growing lesion on an area of skin which will often show signs of sun damage and keratosis. Alternatively, the patient will present with a scar or ulcer which fails to heal normally.

Treatment

Patients with squamous cell carcinomas should be treated promptly to reduce the danger of metastases. An initial biopsy is taken to confirm the diagnosis followed by a wide excision of the tumour.

Radiotherapy may be used for the elderly and frail but is not usually the first line of treatment as it may cause further damage to the skin, thus encouraging new tumours (Mackie 1989a).

Patients are examined for lymph node metastasis at the time of diagnosis and at all follow-up visits.

The pre- and postoperative nursing treatment of patients with squamous cell carcinoma is similar to that of patients with basal cell carcinoma. The psychological care, however, is more complex. It is not possible to give the patient complete reassurance that the tumour will not metastasize. However, it is essential to reassure the patient with an early lesion that this is unlikely, that they will be followed up carefully and that the original tumour has been removed.

Prevention and education

Patient education should mainly be directed towards preventing further sun damage to the skin. The advice given should be similar to that for patients with basal cell carcinomas (see Box 12.2).

Patients should also be advised to look out for further lesions and to be aware of the significance of any enlarged lymph nodes.

As many of these patients will be elderly, it is often advisable to make carers and attending nursing staff aware of the possibility of further primary tumours, the risk of secondaries and the need to act quickly in referring patients for medical advice.

Key points	
Recognition	May grow rapidly to form a fleshy nodule which may ulcerate.
Treatment	Wide excision and careful follow-up to observe for metastases.
Prevention	Sun care and skin observation.

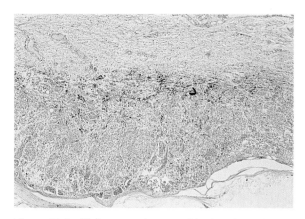

Figure 12.6 Malignant melanoma – histology (reproduced with permission from Dr M Walsh, Consultant Dermatopathologist, Royal Group of Hospitals, Belfast).

MALIGNANT MELANOMA

Cutaneous malignant melanoma is a form of skin cancer which affects the pigment-producing cells, the melanocytes. It arises in the epidermis and appears on the skin as a new or changing mole. It is a rare type of skin cancer, accounting for 11% of all skin cancers (Cancer Research Campaign 1991). However, it is also the most dangerous of the skin cancers, as it has the capacity to metastasize via the lymphatic and circulatory systems. To date, there is no proven curative treatment for advanced melanoma. Tumours are radiotherapy resistant but advances are being made in systemic therapy (Grob et al 1998).

Figures show that the number of patients with melanoma is increasing each year (Pedlow et al 1997). Worldwide melanoma rates show an increase of between 2% and 5% annually in white people (Marks 1992). Melanomas tend to occur in the relatively younger age group, being the most common cancer in women between 25 and 29 and second only to breast cancer in the 30–35 age group (Marks 1992).

Histology

Malignant cells (melanocytes) first appear in the epidermis which, if undetected, then proceed to invade the dermis and deeper tissues (Fig. 12.6).

Pathology

Accurate histopathology is of the utmost importance to assess the depth of the tumour and therefore the prognosis. Tumour thickness is measured as the Breslow depth (Breslow 1970). The measurement is taken through the vertical distance of the thickest part of the tumour, from the granular layer in the epidermis to the deepest melanoma cell (Fig. 12.7).

Breslow depth is the most important factor in determining the management and prognosis of the patient. Figure 12.8 shows the expected 5-year survival rate in relation to tumour depth. However, other histological factors do play a part in determining the prognosis. The Clark level of assessment relates to the invasion of tumour cells at the different levels within the dermis, both vertically and radially. The rate of mitotic activity also provides information.

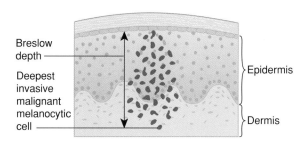

Figure 12.7 Measurement of Breslow depth.

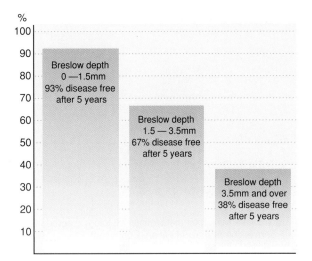

%

Figure 12.8 Breslow depth prognostic indicators for 5-year survival rate.

Anatomic site and sex may also have some bearing on prognosis. Studies have shown that patients with melanomas on limbs do better than those with melanomas on the head, neck or trunk (Johnson et al 1995). Women have a better survival rate than men but melanomas in women are often sited on the limbs, especially the leg, and are frequently thinner (Johnson et al 1995).

Recognition

The patient's nurse, whether in the community or hospital setting, may be the first person to notice a suspicious mole. Nurses see patients undressed and should make it part of their practice to comment on moles and enquire about any changes. Also, nurses are often approached by members of the public who are concerned about moles but are unsure as to whether they need to 'bother' a doctor. It is vital that nurses in these instances give the correct advice; as can be seen from Figure 12.8, the thinner the tumour, the better the prognosis.

Early detection and treatment is the most important factor in reducing mortality rates in patients with malignant melanoma (Johnson et al 1995). It is therefore of the utmost importance that all members of the medical profession and the general public are aware of the warning signs of melanoma.

Warning signs of melanoma

As an aid to detection of malignant melanoma, a seven-point checklist has been drawn up (Mackie 1989b) (Box 12.3). Nurses should refer patients with pigmented lesions who have any of these signs or symptoms to their general practitioner or hospital doctor.

Box 12.3 Checklist of symptoms or signs for suspected melanoma (adapted from Mackie 1989b)	
Change in size: either a mole has got larger or a new mole has appeared (all new moles should have been acquired by the age of 40)	Inflammation of mole or surrounding skin; rare in benign moles
	Crusting or bleeding; not seen in normal naevi unless traumatized
Change in shape: the development of an irregular border in a symmetrical, round or oval mole or a newly developed, irregular-shaped mole	Change in sensation: pain, tenderness or itch. The most common early symptom of malignant melanoma is itch in a mole (Johnson et al 1995)
Change in colour: variation of brown or black pigment in old or newly acquired mole (may be speckled)	Diameter larger than 7 mm. Most benign naevi are smaller than this

Classification and clinical features

Malignant melanomas fall into four main groups. Each has slightly different features but all have some of the signs and symptoms from Mackie's seven-point checklist.

Superficial spreading melanoma. The most common type of malignant melanoma. It develops over several months, initially spreading horizontally. The most common sites are the calf in women and the trunk in men. If left undetected, it will invade into the dermis, the surface will become more nodular and may crust and bleed. A superficial spreading malignant melanoma may appear as an irregular-shaped, variably coloured, pigmented area usually larger than 1 cm (Fig. 12.9).

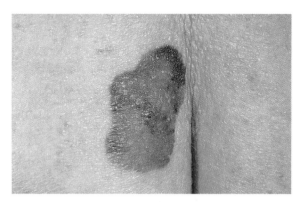

Figure 12.9   Superficial spreading melanoma (reproduced with permission from Dr O M Dolan, Consultant Dermatologist, Department of Dermatology, Royal Group of Hospitals, Belfast).

Nodular malignant melanoma.   As the name implies, this appears as a pigmented nodule which may be black or brown and is more likely to bleed than to crust or ooze. Nodular melanomas often grow quite rapidly and invade deeply to become an aggressive tumour (Fig. 12.10).

Acral melanoma and subungual melanomas. Acral melanomas occur on the palms of the hands or soles of the feet, subungual under the nail. These tumours are easily missed as they appear as flecks of painless pigment under the nail and may not be noticed on the feet. Therefore, they often present late and have a poor prognosis.

Lentigo maligna melanoma.   This is seen in elderly patients on sun-exposed skin, usually the face. The surrounding skin is usually photodamaged and the patient gives a history of long-term sun exposure. The initial lentigo maligna is an area of stained pigmented skin which is flat and grows gradually outwards. If left untreated, over a period of years, it will invade downwards and at this stage will present as a malignant nodule within the stained area.

Aetiology

Overexposure to UVR is the main cause of most skin cancer including malignant melanoma (Cancer Research Campaign 1995). However, in the case of malignant melanoma (apart from lentigo maligna melanoma), it is thought to be the relationship between short, intermittent, intense sun exposure and sunburn rather than long-term regular sun exposure that causes the damage (Mackie 1983). Therefore, it is not necessarily the outdoor worker who develops melanoma but may be the office worker who spends holidays abroad in intense burning sunshine. It is thought that a single episode of severe sunburn, especially in childhood, is enough to trigger off a melanoma in later life (Austoker 1994).

Although the relationship between intense sun exposure, melanoma and age is complex, there is evidence to support this theory. Studies have shown that Europeans migrating to Australia and New Zealand before the age of 5 have a higher incidence of melanoma than those who arrive after the age of 15 (Mackie 1989b).

The incidence of malignant melanoma in white people is also closely linked to their skin type. White-skinned races have little protective melanin in their skin compared with black or brown-skinned races. Individuals are classified by their skin's reaction to sun exposure and an ability to tan.

Table 12.3   Skin types and effects of sun exposure

Type	Skin reaction
I	White skin, always burns, never tans
II	Usually burns, sometimes tans
III	Sometimes burns, always tans
IV	Never burns, always tans
V	Moderately and heavily pigmented
V	Black African skin

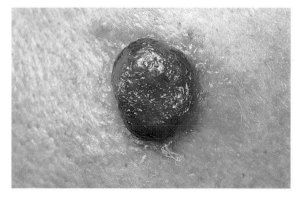

Figure 12.10   Nodular malignant melanoma (reproduced with permission of LEO Pharmaceuticals).

Individuals with skin types I or II have a greater risk of sunburn and therefore of developing melanoma.

At-risk groups

There are a number of factors which affect an individual's potential for developing melanoma. A personal risk factor chart was drawn up (Mackie 1989b). This defines the strongest personal risk factors as being:

- those with family history of malignant melanoma
- individuals with a larger than average number of small, benign, pigmented naevi which are above 2 mm in diameter
- those with skin types I or II and a tendency to freckling
- those with atypical or dysplastic naevi
- a history of severe sunburn
- those who already have a malignant melanoma.

Some individuals may have a combination of more than one of these risk factors.

None of these risk factors is under personal control, apart from sunburn, but they should be taken into account when advising patients about prevention and detection of melanoma.

Presentation

The patient with a melanoma presents with a newly acquired or changed mole which has at least one feature of the seven-point checklist (Box 12.3).

A history of the lesion will reveal how long the patient has had the mole and in what way it has changed. Examination of the skin will reveal skin type and whether the patient has other benign or atypical naevi. A general history will reveal any family history of melanoma and episodes of sun exposure and sun damage. However, not all melanomas present on areas of skin that have been sunburnt or even had particular sun exposure.

Melanoma is more commonly seen in women than in men. The leg is the most common site in women with 47% of all melanomas in women

being sited on the lower leg (Mackie 1989b). For men, the commonest site is the back followed by the head and neck (Fig. 12.11). In patients with lentigo maligna melanoma, the commonest site is the face.

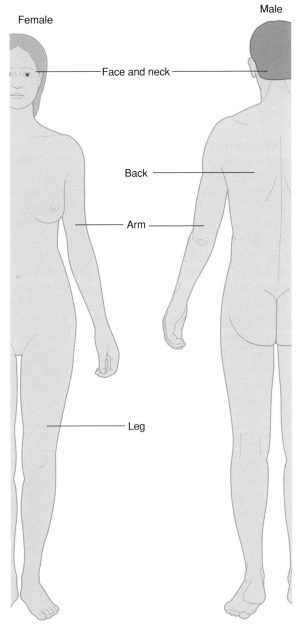

Figure 12.11 Most common sites for malignant melanoma.

Treatment

Any suspected pigmented lesion should be referred to a dermatologist without delay. In most instances, there is no waiting list for a lesion deemed urgent by a general practitioner.

Complete excision of any pigmented lesion which is causing concern is the appropriate treatment. The excised lesion is sent to histopathology for analysis. Biopsying part of a lesion for diagnostic purposes is inappropriate as it will destroy accurate evidence of tumour depth if the lesion turns out to be a melanoma. Tumour (Breslow) depth is the single most important factor in determining treatment and prognosis of the melanoma patient.

If the excised lesion proves to be a malignant melanoma, the second stage of the treatment is a wider excision of the normal skin around the melanoma scar with at least a 1 cm margin in order to reduce the risk of recurrence. It is important that the excision is also of adequate depth, usually to subcutaneous fat.

At the time of diagnosis, the patient should undergo a complete physical check. All other naevi should be checked and any that appear unusual should be measured and photographed. A history should be taken of the patient's general health and factors which would increase the likelihood of further melanoma should be discussed with the patient. Lymph nodes should be palpated, particularly those local to the scar, and a chest X-ray may be obtained. Initially, the patient will be reviewed every 3–4 months for the first 2 years, then 6 monthly and eventually yearly for an indefinite duration. A full physical examination should be carried out at each visit.

If at any stage lymph nodes are detected, a fine needle biopsy should be performed to check for malignant cells. If these are positive, a lymph node dissection is required. The melanocytes can spread via the lymphatic system to any organ, the most common secondaries being sited in the lung, liver, brain, bone and gastrointestinal tract. Cure once metastasis has occurred is rare (Johnson et al 1995). The decision on whether to attempt treatment or not should be based on the age and condition of the patient and if any palliative relief can be expected. Nursing care at this stage is mainly based on palliative care alone.

New therapies

A new technique has been developed which can help in identifying lymph node involvement. At the time of excision of the tumour, blue dye is injected which is taken up by the lymphatic system. An incision is then made over the expected lymphatic drainage pathway and the first lymph node identified by the dye, the sentinel node, is removed and sent for a frozen section biopsy. If positive, the need for lymph node resection is immediately identified.

Other forms of therapy being studied are gene therapy and tumour vaccines but as yet these are not standard therapy. Adoptive immunotherapy is also being explored, which involves the transfer of activated immune cells into the cancer-bearing host to try to reduce the tumour (Johnson et al 1995).

A trial of the administration of high doses of interferon to advanced melanoma patients has shown some improvement in relapse and mortality (Kirkwood et al 1996). Low-dose interferon has also been shown to be beneficial to patients with primary melanoma thicker than 1.5 mm without clinically detectable node metastases (Grob et al 1998).

Radiotherapy has proved to be of little benefit to patients except in the case of lentigo maligna melanoma. Studies of different chemotherapy regimens for thicker tumours are under constant review and some successes are now being reported.

Psychological care

Everybody reacts differently to a diagnosis of cancer, each individual's emotions being unique to themselves. It is normal to go through several stages of adjustment and the patient who initially appears to be accepting and understanding the diagnosis and prognosis may have more difficulty coming to terms with the situation than first expected.

The social implications of a diagnosis of malignant melanoma should not be ignored as not only do they have an effect on the patient's lifestyle but also a psychological effect by acting as a constant reminder of the diagnosis of cancer. Social issues include difficulty in obtaining a mortgage or life insurance, curtailment of holidays abroad, sports activities and concerns for children due to the hereditary aspect of melanoma.

Patients often find it difficult to come to terms with the lack of physical treatment available for melanoma. For many, a surgical excision performed under local anaesthetic appears inadequate and they may find it hard to understand that little other treatment is necessary in the case of thin tumours and is of limited use with aggressive tumours.

It is important to strike the right balance between advising patients about the necessary precautions that need to be taken and encouraging them to resume a full and active life. This is particularly important for patients with thin lesions who fail to understand the extremely good prognosis they should expect (see Fig. 12.8). Psychological shock impairs the ability to absorb and retain information so time should be set aside at each visit to discuss all aspects of living with a melanoma and patients encouraged to discuss their concerns and fears.

For some patients, joining a support group can provide help and information. Written information and leaflets, such as 'Living with melanoma' (Fig. 12.12) written by Pauline Perkins on behalf of the Wessex Cancer Trust, give a positive message of the outcome of early melanoma and incorporate information about melanoma, its treatment and follow-up advice.

Another leaflet which provides information on the signs and symptoms of melanoma is the Cancer Research Campaign's *Be a mole watcher for life*.

Patient advice and education

It is very often the nursing staff who undertake this important aspect of the patient's treatment. At the time of diagnosis, the patient will be in a state of shock and will be unable to take in very much of the advice being given. It is therefore important to reemphasize points with an appropriate leaflet or handout about mole watching and sun care (see Box 12.4).

Following diagnosis, the patient will have many questions. It is reassuring to have the name of the nurse and the clinic phone numbers for any queries or support between visits.

At each follow-up visit, the advice should be reasserted, particularly to ensure that the patient is aware of the signs and symptoms of early melanoma because 8–10% of patients do develop a second primary tumour (Mackie 1989b). As follow-up visits become more widely spaced, it is essential that the patient takes responsibility for their own mole watching.

Box 12.4   Mole watching

One easy rule to teach patients is the ABCD danger signs to look for in moles.

- *Asymmetry*   One half of the mole unlike the other
- *Border irregular*   Looks like a map
- *Colour variety*   From one area of mole to another, i.e. brown/black
- *Diameter*   Larger than 6 mm

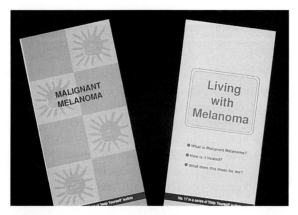

Figure 12.12   Information leaflets (reproduced with the permission of the Wessex Cancer Trust).

Examining the skin

Advice should be given on the importance of regularly examining the skin for changes in moles or new moles. This can either be by self-

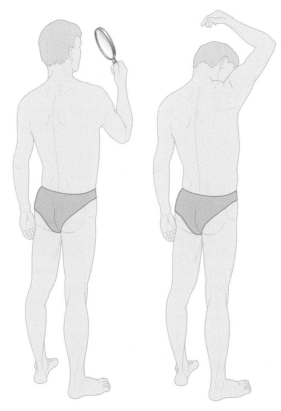

Figure 12.13   Self-examination.

examination using a mirror (Fig. 12.13) or by the use of photographs or a partner's cooperation in examining the skin for changes.

Pregnancy

There is no statistical evidence that pregnancy influences the recurrence of melanoma, but it is usual to advise patients to wait for 2 years following diagnosis before becoming pregnant.

Family

It is important that patients realize that their immediate family has a higher risk of melanoma and should be advised about examining their skin and seeking referral about any suspicious lesion.

Sun-care protection

To reduce the risk of further melanomas.

Risk reduction

Nurses are in an ideal position to provide primary preventative education. The aim should be to effect a change in sun-related behaviour in order to reduce sun exposure and prevent sunburn, especially in children and adolescents. For those who spend a lot of time outside, the aim should be never to have reddened or sunburned skin.

The message should convey a positive approach so that individuals can enjoy outdoor activities without increasing the risk of skin cancer or melanoma. It is also important to work towards changing attitudes which perceive a suntan as healthy and attractive.

Australia is one of the leading pioneers of sun care in the world. Their Slip, Slap, Slop slogan – slip on a shirt, slap on a hat and slop on a sun screen – is extremely simple yet effective, giving a light-hearted approach to a serious message. Another such example is Fried Bloke Break (Sanofi 'Be Aware, Take Care' Campaign) (Fig. 12.14).

How to protect the skin from sun exposure

Covering up

Covering up with clothing is the easiest, cheapest and most effective way of protecting the skin. Loose-fitting clothes keep you cool and comfortable.

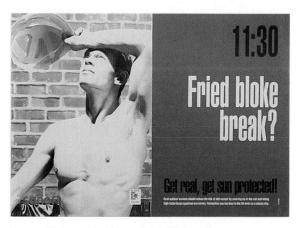

Figure 12.14   Fried Bloke Break (© Sanofi).

Cloth should be tightly woven; when held up to the light, it should not penetrate. Dark colours offer more protection than light colours.

A hat will provide good protection; a hat with a brim size of 4 cm will reduce ultraviolet rays by 50% (Fig. 12.15).

Shade and sun

Seek shade whenever possible; this can be under umbrellas, trees or buildings. Clouds do not provide adequate shade as one-third of the sun's rays can penetrate cloud.

Reflection from water, snow and sand increases UVR and the risk of sunburn.

The nearer to the equator, the stronger the sun's rays. This also applies to higher altitudes.

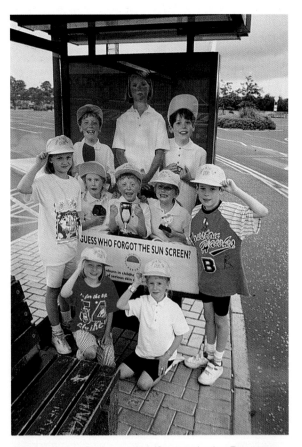

Figure 12.15 Sun protection (Communication Resource and Information Service, Eastern Health and Social Services Board, Belfast).

Don't be fooled by cool breezes, the ultraviolet rays are still as strong.

Avoid the sun between 11.00 am and 3.00 pm. Ultraviolet rays are strongest when the sun is highest in the sky. Sunburn in the UK has the same damaging effect as sunburn abroad. A study carried out on 100 melanoma patients in Scotland revealed one-third of them had never left the UK (Mackie 1989b).

Sunbeds

Sunbeds should be avoided. Patients should be warned that sunbeds and sun lamps can cause premature ageing, cataracts, sunburn and skin rashes and they appear to be a risk factor for skin cancer (Walter et al 1990). Patients sometimes suggest using a sunbed to give some protection to the skin prior to a sunshine holiday. However, 'tans' produced by UVA radiation from sunbeds do not result in the thickening of the skin which follows UVB exposure and therefore will give little protection against sunburn.

Sun screens

Sun screens contain filters which absorb UVB and most absorb a certain amount of UVA or act as a physical barrier that reflects and scatters ultraviolet rays.

Sun protection factors (SPF)

The SPF number on a sun screen gives an indication as to the amount of time that can be spent in the sun without becoming red or burnt compared with the amount of time spent with no sun screen on. Thus, a person who would normally go red and burn after 20 minutes of sunlight could in theory spend 15 times as long in the sun if wearing a factor 15 sun screen. However, this should be treated with caution as SPF figures are based on testing under laboratory conditions which does not take account of normal movement and rubbing which reduces the amount of sun screen. Figures are also based on applications of cream of 2 mg/cm^2, a great deal thicker than is normally cosmetically acceptable (Ley 1997).

Table 12.4   Percentage reduction in UVB by SPF number

SPF number	Reduction in UVB (%)
4	75
8	88
16	94
32	97

A factor 15 is generally agreed as being adequate protection. Above factor 15, there is relatively no greater improvement in the overall reduction in radiation (Ley 1997) (Table 12.4).

Sun screens should block both UVA and UVB rays. UVB rays cause the reddening and burning of the skin whilst UVA rays penetrate more deeply, causing chronic photodamage and ageing. Skin protected by only a UVB sun screen could in theory remain in the sun longer without burning; thus, the skin would absorb more UVA rays.

Choosing a sun screen

Choice of sun screen is dependent on the individual's lifestyle, taking into account time spent outdoors, sporting activities, age group and cosmetic requirements.

It is the vehicle or base of the sun screen that determines both its effectiveness and its cosmetic appeal and it is the cosmetic appeal which determines patient compliance (Box 12.5).

Application

Patients should be advised to apply sun screens liberally and evenly to all exposed skin.

Box 12.5   Vehicles of sun screens

Lotions	Spread easily, not greasy
Creams	May be applied more thickly
Gels	Less greasy but easily rubbed off
Sticks	Useful for lips and nose
Aerosols	Convenient, particularly for scalps, but may not give even enough coverage for whole body
Cosmetics	Many cosmetics incorporate a sun screen, useful to ensure year-round protection

Sun screen should be applied 20 minutes before going out to allow sufficient time for it to 'set' on the skin. It should be reapplied regularly, at least every 2 hours and after exercise and swimming.

Special instructions

Children.   Infants under 6 months should not be exposed to the sun as their skin has insufficient melanin protection. Protective clothing should be used (choose a close weave) and a sun hat. Always seek shade. Canopies on prams should be used but remember, they do not give total protection as rays can penetrate the sides.

By the age of 18, a child will have had the majority of their lifetime sun exposure.

Sun protection cannot be overemphasized. Studies have shown that children of parents who follow a good sun-care regime are more likely to comply with this regime as adolescents (Ley 1997).

Teenagers with acne.   They may complain about putting extra grease on their skin so should be advised to use an alcohol-based preparation or gel.

Sensitivity.   Patients may develop an allergy to sun screens. Photo patch testing may need to be carried out to isolate the allergen and a suitable product found that does not contain the particular allergen.

Vitamin D.   Patients using total skin protection may enquire about a lack of vitamin D. A study in Australia has shown no significant lack of vitamin D metabolism with patients using sun protection (Ley 1997). However, elderly patients who are more susceptible to fractures might be advised to take a vitamin D supplement.

Key points	
Recognition	Awareness of the significance of newly acquired moles or changes in existing moles.
Treatment	Early detection leads to removal of a thin lesion, effecting a cure.
Prevention	Protection of skin from sunburn. Seek advice about any changes in a mole.

CUTANEOUS T-CELL LYMPHOMAS

A rare group of malignant T-cell infiltrates which arise in the skin, namely mycosis fungoides and Sézary syndrome.

Mycosis fungoides

A slowly evolving lymphoma characterized by the presence of T-helper lymphocytes mainly in the epidermis and peripheral dermis (Diamandidou et al 1996).

The disease is more common in the older age group and twice as common in men (Diamandidou et al 1996, Demierre et al 1997). The disease usually evolves through three distinct phases.

Premycotic plaque phase

- May last for many years
- Small, round or oval erythrodermic scaly plaques
- Main symptom pruritius
- Plaques scattered but commonest sites are trunk and buttocks
- Plaques may resolve but others then appear
- Difficult at this stage to diagnose by biopsy but may be diagnosed on clinical grounds
- Differential diagnosis – may be mistaken for eczema, psoriasis or tinea.

Infiltrated plaque phase

- Plaques become more numerous and may develop bizarre shapes
- Plaques become more fixed, less likely to resolve
- Nodules may develop
- Biopsy should confirm the presence of atypical lymphocytes in the epidermis.

Tumour phase

- Nodules in or around the plaques form tumours which may break down and ulcerate
- Involvement of lymph nodes and internal organs.

The first two phases of the disease may last for many years, possibly up to 10 or 15, but once the disease reaches the tumour stage life expectancy is usually short – approximately 2–3 years (Mackie 1989a).

Not all patients present with the disease strictly within these three phases. For some patients, raised nodules may be the first clinical sign; for others, a widespread pigmentation with atrophy and some telangectasia may take the place of plaques in the first instance. Less common is an erythrodermic-type presentation. The whole body may be erythrodermic and hair loss and nail changes may be evident. This tends to be a more acute type of mycosis fungoides and the course of the disease may be shorter.

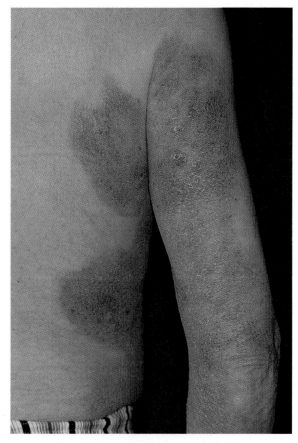

Figure 12.16 Sézary syndrome (reproduced with permission from Dr J R Corbett, Consultant Dermatologist, Department of Dermatology, Royal Group of Hospitals, Belfast).

Sézary syndrome

This is related to mycosis fungoides. Diagnosis is made on the presence of large numbers of T-helper lymphocytes, mainly in the dermis. Blood tests also reveal Sézary cells in the peripheral blood. These cells have a very large nucleus which has a distinctive hyperconvoluted style.

The patient usually presents with severe erythroderma, scaling and severe pruritus (Fig. 12.16). In the early stages, this may be compared with psoriasis, atopic eczema or a widespread unidentified contact dermatitis. However, the patient does not respond to treatments and the symptoms become more pronounced.

Diagnosis is often made on clinical judgement as skin biopsies and blood tests often fail to confirm the disease until the syndrome is well established.

Management

In the early stages, management of cutaneous T-cell lymphomas (CTCL) is based on treating the patient's symptoms as they arise. As the disease progresses, skilled and sensitive nursing will be required to help alleviate itch and pain and control body temperature, keeping the patient's skin moisturized and comfortable. The patient will require intensive nursing care and in the terminal stages, will need both psychological support and palliative care.

Treatment

Topical steroids and UVB may be enough to control the disease and symptoms of pruritus in the first phase.

As the plaques or erythroderma become more extensive and the pruritus more severe, different treatment may be considered. Much will depend on the age and physical state of the patient and how the patient reacts to the treatment of choice.

Photochemotherapy (PUVA)

Good results have been established with a regime of PUVA treatment (Mackie 1989a). It is particularly useful in controlling pruritus and has relatively few side effects. A regime of PUVA treatment is usually planned to treat the skin until lesions have cleared and then to continue with a maintenance dose. PUVA treatment is described in Chapter 4.

Long-term PUVA therapy may encourage non-melanoma skin cancers. Routine examinations of the skin should be carried out. PUVA treatment may dry the skin so patients should be encouraged to use emollients.

Interferon

Studies are being carried out into the response to interferon. There is evidence of some improvement in survival rates of patients with extensive disease (Demierre et al 1997).

Oral retinoids

Either alone or in combination with PUVA, these may be used to help control symptoms in patients with plaque mycosis fungoides. They do not appear to benefit erythrodermic patients (Demierre et al 1997).

Photophoresis

Studies have shown this form of treatment to be effective, particularly for erythrodermic patients (Duvic et al 1996).

Photophoresis is a process by which the patient's white cells are irradiated. The patient is given oral psoralen 2 hours before treatment. The treatment then consists of attaching the patient to a leucophoresis machine and a portion of blood is filtered off. The white cells are then exposed to ultraviolet light within the machine and then returned to the patient.

This treatment has been found to be particularly useful in relieving symptoms of itch, erythroderma and scaling and is usually given on two consecutive days per month. During this period, the patient's blood is carefully monitored and the patient instructed about possible side effects.

Patients responding to treatment often have a period of enhanced pruritus and erythema immediately after their treatment. This is then followed by a decrease in redness and symptoms (Demierre et al 1997). Side effects to treatment include low-grade fever, headache and nausea. Not all patients experience side effects but those who do need encouragement to continue with treatment, with appropriate analgesia, moisturizers and antihistamines to relieve symptoms.

Topical nitrogen mustard therapy

Nitrogen mustard used as a topical treatment has been found to be effective in offering long-term remission in early cutaneous T-cell lymphoma (Demierre et al 1997). However, allergic or irritant contact dermatitis is a relatively common side effect.

Nitrogen mustard is applied to the skin daily, either in an aqueous solution or an ointment base. Skin should be kept well moisturized between treatments.

Safety precautions to be taken by staff applying nitrogen mustard should include the following.

- Wearing of PVC gloves, theatre style overgarment, to prevent contamination of clothes.
- Eye protection.
- Accidentally exposed skin surfaces should be washed thoroughly and spillages cleaned with detergent and water.
- Patients' clothes, bedlinen and protective clothing worn by staff should be collected and treated appropriately in the laundry, i.e. soaked in 2.5% sodium bicarbonate solution for several hours to neutralize the mustine and then immersed in detergent to remove any emulsifying ointment. The garments/sheets may then be washed normally.
- Prolonged isolation of the patient does not seem justified but where possible, patients should have a single room.
- Pregnant staff should not be involved in the application of this treatment.

Prognosis

These rare slow-growing lymphomas may persist for many years before becoming infiltrated and fatal. Treatment depends on the stage of the disease. It may be controlled for many years with PUVA therapy and topical steroids. Infiltrated plaques and nodules will require aggressive treatments, which are continually being researched.

CONCLUSION

Research into a cure for skin cancer continues and exciting new developments are being explored. For example, vaccines are being tested whereby antigens derived from tumours are injected into patients in the hope that they will stimulate the white blood cells into attacking cancerous tissues. A diagnosis of cancer, however, is still seen as a death sentence by many patients and it is on this 'fear' that the nursing care of patients with skin cancer should be focused.

For patients with thin melanomas and non-melanoma skin cancers, the emphasis should be on the excellent prognosis expected, combined with sensible sun-care habits.

For patients with more advanced melanomas and with T-cell lymphomas, the quality of life and the psychological support of the patient are of paramount importance. This will require all the innovative nursing skills of the dermatology nurse dealing with patients and their families on an individual basis.

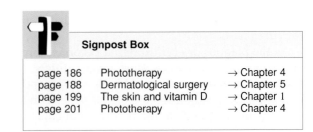

	Signpost Box	
page 186	Phototherapy	→ Chapter 4
page 188	Dermatological surgery	→ Chapter 5
page 199	The skin and vitamin D	→ Chapter 1
page 201	Phototherapy	→ Chapter 4

REFERENCES

Austoker J 1994 Melanoma prevention and early diagnosis. British Medical Journal 308: 1682–1686

Breslow A 1970 Thickness, cross sectional area and depth of invasion in the prognosis of cutaneous melanoma. Annals of Surgery 172: 902–908

Cancer Research Campaign 1991 Skin cancer, the sun and you. Your questions answered. CRC, London

Cancer Research Campaign 1995 Malignant melanoma. UK Fact Sheet 4.1. CRC, London

Champion R, Burton J, Ebling R 1992 Textbook of dermatology, vol 2. Blackwell Scientific, Oxford, pp 1687–1691

Demierre M, Foss F, Koh H 1997 Proceedings of the International Consensus Conference on Cutaneous T-Cell Lymphoma (CTCL). Treatment recommendations. Journal of the American Academy of Dermatology 36(3): 460–466

Department of Health 1992 Health of the nation. A strategy for health in England. HMSO, London

Diamandidou E, Cohen P, Kurzrock R 1996 Mycosis fungoides and Sézary syndrome. Blood 88(7): 2385–2409

Duvic M, Hester J, Lemak N 1996 Photophoresis therapy for cutaneous T cell lymphoma. Journal of the American Academy of Dermatology 35: 573–579

Gawkrodger D J 1992 Dermatology: an illustrated colour text. Churchill Livingstone, Edinburgh, p 93

Grob J J, Dreno B, de la Salmoniere P et al 1998 Randomised trial of interferon α-2a as adjutant therapy in resected primary melanoma thicker than 1.5 mm without clinically detectable node metastases. Lancet 351: 1905–1910

Johnson T, Smith J, Nelson B, Chang A 1995 Current therapy for cutaneous melanoma. Journal of the American Academy of Dermatology 32(5): 689–706

Kirkwood J M, Strawderman M H, Ernstoff M S et al 1996 Interferon alfa-2b. Adjuvant therapy of high risk resected cutaneous melanoma. Journal of Clinical Oncology 14(1): 7–17

Ley S 1997 Sunscreen for photo protection. Dermatologic Therapy 4: 59–71

Mackie R M 1983 The pathogens of cutaneous malignant melanoma. British Medical Journal 287: 1568–1569

Mackie R M 1989a Skin cancer. Martin Dunitz, London, pp 110–211

Mackie R M 1989b Malignant melanoma – a guide to early diagnosis. Pillars and Wilson Edinburgh, pp 8–47

Marks R 1992 Sun damaged skin. Martin Dunitz, London, p 62

Pedlow P, Walsh M, Patterson C, Atkinson R, Lowry W 1997 Cutaneous malignant melanoma in Northern Ireland. British Journal of Dermatology 76(1): 124–126

Walter S, Marrett L, From L, Hertzman C, Shannon H, Roy P 1990 The association of cutaneous malignant melanoma with the use of sunbeds and sun lamps. Americal Journal of Epidemiology 131(2): 232–243

FURTHER READING

Hunter J A A, Smith J A, Dahl M V 1995 Clinical dermatology. Blackwell Science, Oxford

PATIENT SUPPORT GROUPS

The Wessex Cancer Trust's Marc's Line
Marc's Line Resource Centre
Dermatology Treatment Centre
Level 3
Salisbury District Hospital
Salisbury SP2 8BJ
Tel: 01722 415 071
Web site: www.k-web.co.uk/charity/wct/wct.html
(A resource and advice centre for skin cancer patients and their families)

Cancer Research Campaign
6–10 Cambridge Terrace
Regent's Park
London NW1 4JL
Tel: 020 7317 5076
(Information about skin cancer)

13

Infections and infestations

Christine Docherty

INTRODUCTION

An intact skin is a barrier against infection, with healthy skin having a resident flora of harmless microorganisms. Destruction or penetration of this barrier permits infection and infestation. Nursing care encompasses treating the physical problem, whilst recognizing and addressing the psychological impact associated with diagnosis. Whilst improved living standards and better hygiene practices reduce the incidence of infectious skin diseases, social stigma persists. Many disorders are treated by the primary care team, with nurse prescribing and over-the-counter (OTC) preparations inherent to effective management. Educating the patient and public helps to remove the associated social stigma. Infection control measures, i.e. good handwashing technique, promote best practice in preventing transmission (Kovach 1999).

INFECTIONS

Skin infections range from minor conditions treated with OTC preparations to major life-threatening infections with a systemically unwell patient. Infections alter the appearance of the original skin condition and complicate diagnosis. Hot countries and humid conditions predispose to bacterial and fungal infections and travel is relevant to diagnosis.

Staphylococcal bacterial infections

Impetigo

Impetigo is a superficial cutaneous infection caused by *Staphylococcus aureus* or a mixture of *Staph. aureus* and beta-haemolytic streptococcus. It is common as a primary infection and can be contagious. Impetigo was associated with poor living conditions, poverty, overcrowding and poor hygiene but 20th-century improvements in social conditions have reduced its prevalence.

Clinical presentation. Cutaneous lesions are thin-roofed vesicles which rupture easily, producing a golden yellow exudate which dries to form crusts. Sites involved are face and neck but lesions can spread extensively over the body. Lesions are polycyclic and heal centrally without scarring (du Vivier 1991). Impetigo can present in bullous form with discrete bullae erupting in normal skin but without surrounding erythema. Bullae are thin-walled, containing clear yellow fluid. Bullous impetigo is implicated in staphylococcal scalded skin syndrome. Impetigo occurs as a secondary infection with excoriated lesions of skin conditions becoming impetiginized, e.g. eczema, scabies.

Treatment and management. Diagnosis is confirmed by bacteriological culture. Early-stage vesicular impetigo simulates varicella or herpes simplex. Systemic antibiotics, e.g. flucloxacillin or erythromycin, are used to treat extensive impetigo. Dilute soaks of potassium permanganate solution or saline are soothing to skin and assist in gently removing crusted lesions before applying creams. Topical antibiotic therapy, e.g. neomycin or Fucidin cream, is applied twice daily. In impetiginized eczema, topical steroid therapy is withheld until impetigo resolves. The antibacterial agent mupirocin 2% (Bactroban ointment) can be used but due to the increasing incidence of methicillin-resistant *Staph. aureus* (MRSA), infection control guidelines limit usage, reserving it to treat MRSA.

Nursing management includes explanations to the patient, parent or carer about the condition. Advice encourages basic hygiene practices to limit the contact and spread of the condition, e.g. avoidance of shared towels, face cloths, etc., and good handwashing technique after contact.

Staphylococcal infection of hair follicles

Infection affecting hair follicles is common and classification is dependent on the depth of infection.

Folliculitis (Fig 13.1) is an active pustular inflammation of superficial hair follicles caused by bacteria, e.g. *Staph. aureus*. Shaving can create folliculitis and is commonly seen in the beard area of men or the legs of women after shaving or waxing the legs. Folliculitis is triggered or exacerbated by the use of dermatological topical therapies, e.g. tar ointments, oil-based ointments and occlusive bandages (Buxton 1998). Hairs in the beard area, particularly under the jaw, grow back into the skin, creating follicular eruption resulting in keloid scarring. Scalp folliculitis caused by *Staph. aureus* is a recurrent problem, producing scarring that is very resistant to treatment and more common in Afro-Carribean people (Parish et al 1995).

A *furuncle* (boil) is a deep infection of the hair follicle caused by *Staph. aureus*. It is a tender, inflamed, hard nodule with marked inflammation and infection spreading from the hair follicle to the surrounding dermis. The overlying skin peels away until the boil ruptures, discharging its central necrotic core. Boils are common and erupt in areas subjected to sweat and friction, e.g. nose, neck, face, axillae and buttocks. Patients may be chronic *Staph. aureus* carriers. Boils can be a recurrent problem and associated with diabetes or immunosuppression.

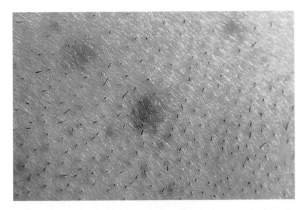

Figure 13.1 Folliculitis (reproduced with the permission of Dr G Lowe, Ninewells Hospital, Dundee).

A *carbuncle* is a deep infection in adjacent hair follicles caused by *Staph. aureus* (Graham-Brown & Burns 1997). The most common site is the nape of the neck. The lesion erupts as a dome-shaped area of erythema, developing into a deep, painful abscess. Recurrent carbuncles can be associated with diabetes. The carbuncle may rupture spontaneously, discharging pus.

Treatment and management. The infecting organism is confirmed by bacterial culture from the lesion and carrier sites, e.g. nose, axillae. Diabetes is excluded by routine urinalysis and fasting blood glucose. Systemic antibiotics, e.g. flucloxacillin and erythromcyin, are supplemented by topical antibiotics, e.g. Fucidin, mupirocin. Carbuncles rupture spontaneously but large lesions require surgical excision and drainage. Management includes encouraging the patient to complete the prescribed course of therapies and focus on preventive measures to avoid recurrence (Ritchie & Thompson 1992). Baths or showers using combined emollients and antiseptics maintain personal hygiene, e.g. Oilatum plus Ster-Zac/triclosan.

Streptococcal bacterial infections

Streptococcus pyogenes is the principal human pathogen. *Strep. pyogenes* carried in the nose or throat contaminates or colonizes damaged skin and may precede guttate psoriasis.

Erysipelas is an acute superficial infection of the dermis. The sites most commonly affected are face and legs. It presents as a unilateral, well-demarcated lesion that is erythematous, oedematous and painful with small blisters or erosions. The organism enters via a fissure or abrasion in the epidermis. Associated factors predisposing to erysipelas can be otitis externa or tinea pedis. Graham-Brown & Burns (1997) suggest that providing a separate term for this superficial infection is unnecessary as it is difficult to ascertain the depth of the tissue involved, so the term 'cellulitis' should cover streptococcal infection infiltrating superficial and subcutaneous tissue.

Cellulitis (Fig. 13.2) is infection of subcutaneous tissues by *Strep. pyogenes* and is a deeper, more extensive infection than erysipelas. The organism

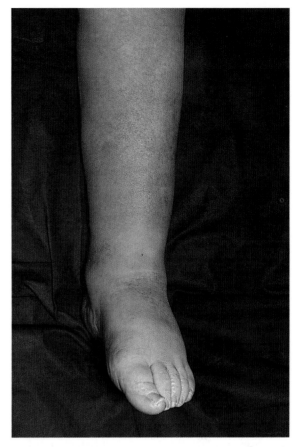

Figure 13.2 Cellulitis (reproduced with the permission of Dr G Lowe, Ninewells Hospital, Dundee).

gains entry through a fissure, i.e. tinea pedis, leg ulcer, and infection spreads due to a substance called spreading factor (hyaluronidase). This factor, produced by the causative organism, breaks down the fibrin network and other barriers that normally localize infection (Lemone & Burke 1996).

Cellulitis is a recurrent problem in leg ulcer management. Lymphangitis is common and recurrent episodes of cellulitis create lymphatic damage. The patient is systemically unwell and pyrexial. The affected area, normally the lower limbs, is erythematous and oedematous with localized pain restricting mobility. The cellulitic area produces blisters with areas of skin necrosis. Streptococcus is the commonest organism isolated but a mixed group of organisms may be identified.

Treatment and management.

- Hospitalization is essential.
- Bedrest is required if the patient is systemically unwell with oedema of the affected limb.
- Blood cultures and skin swabs determine bacteriological status.
- Skin scrapings (mycology) should be taken if associated tinea infection is exacerbating cellulitis.
- Intravenous antibiotics, e.g. benzylpenicillin (Crystapen) 1200 mg 6 hourly and flucloxacillin (Floxapen) 500 mg 6 hourly, should be used during an acute phase.
- Oral antibiotics, e.g. flucloxacillin, penicillin V, are appropriate as the condition resolves.
- Subcutaneous heparin injections prevent the long-term complications of prolonged bedrest, e.g. deep vein thrombosis.
- Monitoring of temperature during treatment therapy.
- Tracing or mapping the edges of the cellulitis site determines the spread or resolution of infection.

Topical therapy is limited to bland emollients that soothe the facial lesions of erysipelas, e.g. aqueous cream. Erosions or blisters require simple non-adherent dressings. Topical antifungals (see p. 209) treat associated tinea infections.

Cellulitis associated with a leg ulcer requires broad-spectrum antibiotics for the mixed pattern of organisms. Due to localized pain and tenderness, compression bandaging is discontinued until the infective phase resolves. Patients with recurrent cellulitis can be treated prophylactically on maintenance low-dose antibiotic therapy. Nurses should ensure the patient fully understands the rationale for this and is effectively supported to maintain therapy.

Fungal infections

Fungal infection is common in humans and mainly attributable to two groups of fungi:

- dermatophytes – multicellular filaments or hyphae
- yeasts – unicellular forms replicating by budding.

Dermatophyte (tinea) infections

These are superficial infections caused by fungi thriving in non-viable keratinized tissue, e.g. hair, nails, stratum corneum. Dermatophyte fungi reproduce by spore formation, inducing inflammation by delayed hypersensitivity or by a metabolic effect (Richardson & Warnock 1997).

There are three genera of dermatophyte:

- Trichophyton
- Microsporum
- Epidermophyton.

Among 40 species recognized, 10 are common causes of human infection. Some dermatophyte fungi are confined to man whilst others principally affect animals but occasionally infect humans. Zoophilic species, transmitted to humans from animals, produce more inflammation than anthropophilic (human only) species (Gawkrodger 1997).

Transmission of dermatophyte infections can be from three sources:

- the patient
- animals, e.g. puppy, kitten, cattle
- soil.

Contact with keratin debris carrying fungal hyphae is an indirect source, e.g. swimming pool, shower floor. Children often have scalp infections whilst adults have intertrigenous infections. Asians and Afro-Caribbeans have a lower incidence of dermatophytosis.

Clinical presentation.

- The site of infection
- The immunological response of the host
- The species of infecting fungi

Diagnosis is confirmed by skin scrapings for microscopy and culture. The presence of hyphae confirms diagnosis, whilst culture determines the species relevant to treatment and management. Fungal infections affect keratinized epidermis – hair and nails. Dermatophyte infections of the epidermis affect the trunk, groin, face and feet.

Deeper infiltration of hair follicles creates an inflammatory response with follicular inflammation, e.g. kerion.

Classification and medical management. Tinea (ringworm) is the generic term for dermatophytoses, producing annular fungal infection. Features of infection vary depending on the site. Tinea infection wrongly diagnosed and inappropriately treated with topical steroids changes its appearance. The steroid dampens the inflammatory response, removing the typically scaly annular edge. Correct diagnosis is therefore essential to management.

- *Tinea corporis* presents as single or multiple erythematous scaling plaques. Lesions affect trunk and limbs, enlarging slowly with characteristic central clearing of ringworm. Adjacent lesions fuse, becoming inflamed and pustular. Animal ringworm produces a greater inflammatory reaction. Tinea corporis is transmitted by contact with infected pets or farm animals and lesions are more extensive in immunosuppressed patients.

Tinea corporis is not uncommon in Asian patients and can be extensive (Graham-Brown & Burns 1997). Topical antifungals are the treatment of choice for localized lesions, e.g. Canesten, Daktarin. Creams are applied twice daily for 2–4 weeks and treatment maintained for 1 week after clearance. Creams are applied directly to lesions and at least 3 cm beyond lesion edges for effectiveness. Extensive lesions or failure of topical therapy require combined treatment, e.g. griseofulvin, itraconazole or terbinafine tablets for 2–4 weeks in combination with topical therapies.

- *Tinea pedis* (athlete's foot) is extremely common in adults (Fig. 13.3). Infection causes interdigital maceration and fissuring of the 4th–5th toe web space. Secondary bacterial or candidal infection creates inflammation and maceration with extensive desquamation extending to the entire sole. It is intensely itchy with an unpleasant odour. Tinea pedis responds to topical treatments, i.e. Canesten, Daktarin, applied directly to toe clefts twice daily for 2 weeks. Mixed fungal and bacterial infections are common and topical agents with combined antifungal/antibacterial action are recommended. In extensive disease, involving sole and foot, oral treatment with itraconazole or terbinafine for 2–6 weeks is effective. Recurrence rate is high and chronic infection can persist.

- *Tinea cruris* (ringworm of the groin) is a common pruritic eruption in young men, often with associated tinea pedis. It presents as rapidly spreading erythematous lesions with central clearing on the insides of the thighs. Maceration and occlusion of skin in the groin produce a moist environment encouraging development of infection. Lesions spread down the thigh but rarely involve the scrotum. It is highly contagious with minor outbreaks occurring in schools and other communities. Infection spreads via contaminated towels.

Treatment involves combined oral and systemic therapies. Topical imidazole compounds, e.g. Canesten, econazole, are applied twice daily for 2 weeks. Treatment must be continued for 2 weeks after symptoms resolve. Oral therapies include griseofulvin, itraconazole or terbinafine for 2–4 weeks in chronic recalcitrant tinea cruris.

- *Tinea manium* presents as unilateral diffuse powdery scaling of the hand. Lesions on the dorsum of hands or interdigital spaces appear, similar to tinea corporis. Hand infection arises from direct contact with an infected animal, human or soil or indirect contact with a contaminated object, e.g. shared towels. It resolves with

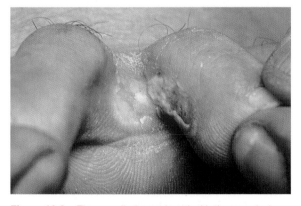

Figure 13.3 Tinea pedis (reproduced with the permission of St John's Institute of Dermatology).

local topical broad-spectrum antifungals, e.g. Canesten, Daktarin. In chronic cases oral griseofulvin or itraconazole is prescribed for 2–4 weeks.

● *Tinea unguium* affects either a single nail or all nails on feet and hands. Infection of the nail presents at the distal nail edge, spreading slowly to the whole nail. The nail thickens, becoming opaque and yellow, with associated hyperkeratosis creating onycholysis (Fig. 13.4). Tinea pedis is often present and fungal infections of toenails are common in the elderly.

This is a difficult condition to treat effectively. Local applications of topical antifungal paint to the nails, e.g. amorolfine (Loceryl), need to be maintained for 6–12 months to be effective. Oral antifungal drugs can be effective but duration of therapy depends on clinical response. Mycological investigation is repeated during therapy and before discontinuing treatment.

● *Tinea capitis* is a dermatophyte scalp and hair infection, common in children and rare in adults. Graham-Brown & Burns (1997) attribute it to changes in the fatty acid constituents of sebum at puberty as postpubertal sebum contains fatty acids which are fungistatic. The fungi involved are Microsporum and Trichophyton.

Nursing management of tinea infections. Nursing management focuses on educating patients on current therapies and preventive strategies to reduce the recurrence of infection. Simple hygiene precautions, e.g. not sharing towels, eliminate spread.

The patient with tinea pedis needs advice on:

● routine daily foot hygiene
● avoidance of occlusive footwear
● use of cotton socks
● dusting feet with antifungal powder.

The oral antifungal drug griseofulvin, whilst effective, has potential side effects, e.g. headache, nausea, gastrointestinal upset and photosensitivity, and interacts with certain drugs, e.g. warfarin, phenobarbitone and oral contraceptives. Patients should be supported in maintaining prolonged therapy and guided to understand the rationale behind continuing topical/oral therapies after the initial infection resolves. The elderly patient requires assistance to apply topical therapies so advice to carers on the management of these conditions allays fears about their contagious nature. Good infection control practice and a focus on proficient handwashing techniques help to contain the spread of infection.

Yeast infections

Candida is an opportunistic pathogen resident in the mouth and gastrointestinal tract, becoming pathogenic when situations favourable to its multiplication arise, causing infections in mucosa, skin and nails (Fig. 13.5). Candida is problematic in debilitated patients.

Classification is dependent on site.

● Oral – white plaques adherent to erythematous buccal mucosa.
● Cheilitis – infection in deep grooves at the corner of the mouth.
● Intertrigo – skinfolds where skin is in direct contact create heat and humidity, e.g. submammary, groins (Fig. 13.6)
● Genital – white plaques on foreskin and glans (candida balanitis). Creamy discharge and itchy erythema of vulva (candida vulvovaginitis).
● Paronychia – inflammation of nailfold and loss of cuticle.

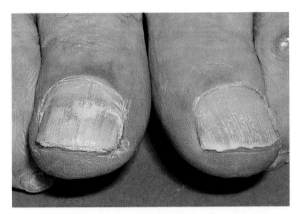

Figure 13.4 Fungal nail infection (reproduced with the permission of Dr G Lowe, Ninewells Hospital, Dundee).

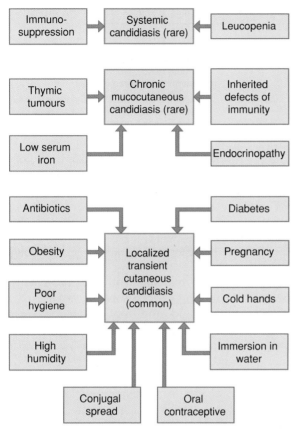

Figure 13.5 Factors predisposing to the different types of candidiasis (reproduced with permission from Hunter et al 1995 and Blackwell Science Ltd).

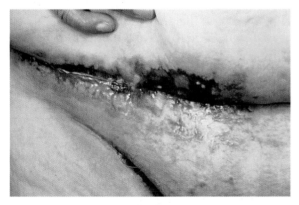

Figure 13.6 Intertrigo (reproduced with the permission of St John's Institute of Dermatology).

● Systemic candidiasis is interrelated with severe illness, leucopenia and immunosuppression.

Skin lesions are scattered, firm, red nodules containing yeasts and pseudohyphae (Hunter et al 1995).

Treatment and management. Diagnosis is confirmed by microscopy or mycology culture. Treatment is topical and oral, with antifungal agents available as tablets, suspensions, creams or pessaries (Box 13.1). Oral thrush can inhibit breastfeeding (MacDonald 1995). The mother can apply topical gel to the nipple or the baby's mouth to treat thrush and should be advised on sterilization methods for bottlefeeding to prevent recurrence. For adults, oral thrush responds to liquid suspension rinsed around the mouth and swallowed.

Improved oral hygiene and denture assessment are relevant in managing angular cheilitis and applications of a combination cream, e.g. Trimovate, to the grooves of the mouth will ease inflammation and reduce infection.

Improved personal hygiene and twice-daily applications of prescribed cream resolve intertrigo. The elderly or obese patient with recurrent intertrigo should be referred to a dietician, social worker and district nurse for full assessment to make appropriate amendments to social conditions and assist in personal hygiene.

The patient with recurrent genital thrush needs a urinalysis test to exclude diabetes. Prophylactic treatments to prevent infections and reduce intestinal and oral colonization with candida are as yet unavailable (Richardson & Warnock 1997).

Box 13.1 Examples of treatment for candidal infections (thrush)	
Oral	Nystatin, amphotericin, miconazole as lozenges, suspensions or gels
Angular cheilitis	Trimovate
Vaginal	Clotrimazole pessary 500 mg as single dose
Intertrigo	Clotrimazole cream or Trimovate cream
Systemic therapy	Itraconazole 100 mg daily Fluconazole 50 mg daily Fluconazole 150 mg single dose

Viral infections

Warts

Warts (Fig. 13.7) are benign, cutaneous tumours caused by infection of epidermal cells with human papilloma virus (HPV). The virus affects many sites and is serologically different in each area (du Vivier 1991). Warts are common in children and are a self-limiting condition whose incidence decreases in the mid-20s. HPV inoculates by direct contact – touch, sexual contact, swimming pool floors. Immunosuppressed patients are particularly susceptible. Classification is dependent on site (Table 13.1). HPV creates hyperkeratosis and thickening of the epidermis. Keratinocytes in the granular layer become vacuolated by HPV.

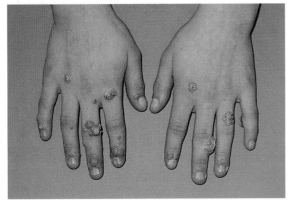

Figure 13.7 Warts (reproduced with the permission of Dr G Lowe, Ninewells Hospital, Dundee).

Table 13.1 Classification and sites affected by viral warts

Classification	Sites and those affected
Common warts	Dome-shaped papules. Single or multiple on face, hands, feet and genitalia. Common in children
Plane warts	Smooth, brown, flat-topped papules. Present on face and dorsal aspect of hands. Resolve spontaneously but can Köebnerize
Plantar warts	Painful warts growing into the dermis due to pressure. Present on sides of feet and become calloused. Affect children and adolescents
Genital warts	Female – vulva, perineum and vagina. Male – penis (anal area in homosexuals). Warts can be small but coalesce to form larger warts

Treatment and management. Thirty to fifty percent of common warts resolve spontaneously. Paring down hand and foot warts removes hyperkeratotic skin before applying topical treatment. Treatment involves combined topical therapy and cryotherapy (Table 13.2). OTC preparations, e.g. wart paints, can be tried but the patient or parent is encouraged to maintain therapies long enough to achieve effective treatment outcomes. There are no suitable antiviral agents for wart treatment so recurrent episodes require repeated therapies. Patients become distressed by unsightly warts so support and encouragement are essential during therapy. Nurse-led cryotherapy clinics are sometimes available in GP practices and dermatology units.

Table 13.2 Treatment for viral warts (reproduced with permission from Gawkrodger 1997)

Modality	Details	Indication	Contraindications/side effects
Topical	Salicylic and lactic acids (e.g. Salactol, Duofilm, Salatac)	Hand and foot warts	Facial/anogenital warts, atopic eczema
	Glutaraldehyde (e.g. Glutarol)	Hand and foot warts	Facial/anogenital warts, atopic eczema
	Formaldehyde (5% aqueous)	Foot warts	Facial/anogenital warts, atopic eczema
	Podophyllin (15%) paint	Genital warts	Pregnancy (teratogenic)
Cryotherapy	Applied every 3–4 weeks	Hand and foot, genital warts	May cause blistering
Curettage and cautery	Local anaesthetic (or general anaesthetic if large)	Solitary filiform warts, especially on face Large perineal warts	Not recommended for hand or foot warts as scars may result; warts may recur
Other	Intralesional bleomycin	Resistant hand/foot warts	Procedure can be painful
	Laser surgery	Any type of wart	Specialized treatment at present
	Interferon	Resistant (genital) warts	Systemic side effects

HPV in genital warts carries the risk of malignant change. Proctoscopy and colposcopy are treatments for rectal or cervical warts. Referral to genitourinary medicine specialists for follow-up ensures effective psychological support, counselling and screening of sexual partners, as genital warts have a significant impact on relationships.

Molluscum contagiosum

This is an infection characterized by discrete, umbilicated pearly white papules, 1–2 cm in diameter caused by a DNA pox virus. It affects children and young adults and transmission is by direct contact, sexual contact or shared towels. Multiple lesions arise on the face and neck over 2–3 months. The condition is common in HIV patients.

Treatment and management. Treatment involves expressing the centre contents of the molluscum using forceps, curettage or cryotherapy. Parents are advised to gently squeeze out the centre contents of the molluscum which is easier to do after the child has a warm bath. Supporting parents in managing the condition is more important than dermatological intervention.

Herpes simplex (Fig. 13.8)

Herpes simplex virus (HSV) penetrates the epidermis or mucous membranes to replicate within epithelial cells, causing epidermal cell destruction that produces intraepidermal vesicles (Gawkrodger 1997). HSV is contagious as the virus is shed from the local site, mucosal surfaces and in secretions. Transmission is by reinoculation on to susceptible skin.

Following primary infection, HSV remains dormant in the dorsal root ganglion until triggered to reactivate the condition, usually in the same site, e.g. cold sore. Common trigger factors causing recrudescence are colds, strong sunlight, stress and menstruation. HSV is preceded by tingling or burning in the affected area – the prodromal phase. Clusters of these vesicles arise on an erythematous background, eventually eroding to become crusted lesions. Each episode can last 10–12 days. Diagnosis is confirmed by immunofluorescence or viral cultures from vesicle fluid.

Classification. Type I HSV occurs as primary infection in childhood. It can go unrecognized or the child can be unwell with vesicles on lips, tongue and buccal mucosa. Acute gingivostomatitis is a complication causing distress and dysphagia. HSV type II occurs as primary infection due to sexual contact although 50% of patients are asymptomatic (Leppard & Ashton 1990). Recrudescence causes localized pain and burning on thighs, vulva and penis. Dysuria and vulvovaginitis with vulval erosions are common, with anal infections and proctitis presenting in both sexes. Further complications of HSV are shown in Box 13.2.

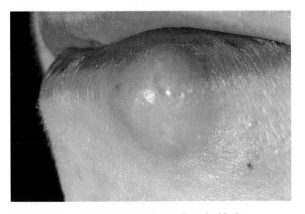

Figure 13.8 Herpes simplex (reproduced with the permission of Dr G Lowe, Ninewells Hospital, Dundee).

Box 13.2 Complications associated with herpes simplex virus (Gawkrodger 1997)	
Secondary bacterial infection	Usually *Staph. aureus*
Eczema herpeticum	Extensive herpes infection in atopic eczema patients
Disseminated herpes simplex	Widespread herpes vesicles found in immunosuppressed patients or babies
Chronic herpes simplex	Chronic condition found in HIV patients
Herpes encephalitis	Serious complication; skin lesions may be absent
Carcinoma of cervix	Common in women associated with type II herpes infection
Erytherma multiforme (EM)	Herpes simplex is a common cause of recurrent EM

Treatment and management. Aciclovir is the treatment of choice, acting by inhibiting virus DNA synthesis and reducing viral shedding to curtail infection, but treatment needs to be started within the prodromal phase to be effective. Aciclovir is available in preparations relevant to the site of infection (Table 13.3) with topical aciclovir cream now available OTC. Patients are advised to maintain supplies to ensure rapid initiation of therapy.

HSV can cause ocular keratitis. Ophthalmic aciclovir 3% five times daily, warm saline bathing and eyepads reduce discomfort and associated photophobia. Patients with eczema must discontinue topical steroids until the infection resolves. Immunocompromised patients with recurrent HSV require longer term combined oral, IV and topical therapies with dosage relevant to disease severity and the individual response to therapy.

Management of genital herpes combines the skills of dermatology and genitourinary medicine. The patient is encouraged in the basic management of their condition – regular soothing baths and use of ice packs to reduce burning in affected areas. Simple non-adherent dressings, e.g. Jelonet, Mepitel, can be applied to vulval erosions. Sex should be avoided totally during an active infective phase and advice provided on routine use of barrier methods of contraception. Regular cervical smears are encouraged. Assessment also includes excluding other sexually transmitted diseases and sexual partners should be identified and screened. Genital herpes can be dangerous to a developing fetus and during labour. Women with a history of HSV have an 8% risk of their neonate acquiring the infection even if they are asymptomatic. Midwifery management monitors HSV status and caesarean section is offered to reduce the associated risks (Dignan & Turnheim 1996).

Recurrent HSV having a significant impact on the patient's life is managed prophylactically, i.e. more than six episodes per year. Daily oral aciclovir 400 mg has been successful in reducing the frequency of recrudescence in 75% of patients. Therapy is reviewed regularly to reassess recurrence rates. Nursing management includes preventive strategies to reduce the transmission of infection.

The patient admitted to hospital with HSV is nursed in a side room. Timbury (1997) reports herpetic whitlow of the finger as an occupational hazard for professionals treating patients secreting the virus in saliva. Universal precautions and good handwashing technique minimize transmission to staff or susceptible patients.

Care also encompasses the psychological aspects involved in counselling patients (Beardsley 1993). HSV has a major impact on relationships and lifestyles so a comprehensive sexual history, thorough explanation and concerned follow-up are central in arresting herpes transmission (Andrist 1997). Support groups reinforce disease management and prevention strategies and offer peer support, with meetings and advice leaflets.

Varicella (chickenpox)

Varicella zoster virus causes chickenpox and shingles (see Fig. 13.9). Chickenpox is infectious, with an incubation period of 13–17 days and is communicable from 5 days before a rash develops until 6 days after. The patient is feverish before developing a maculopapular rash that vesicates. Treatment is non-specific although

Table 13.3 Aciclovir preparations available for management of HSV infections

Preparation	Dose	Treatment
Suspension	200 mg/5 ml	To treat the patient having difficulty in swallowing due to related gingivostomatitis
Tablets	200 mg/400 mg/ 800 mg	Dose relevant to condition taken five times daily for 5 days
Cream	5%	Applied to affected area five times daily immediately during prodromal stage
Intravenous	5 mg per kg body weight	Prescribed dosage intravenously three times daily (8 hourly)
Ophthalmic ointment	3%	Applied five times daily to affected eye

Aciclovir therapy is most effective if initiated within first 24 hours of infection

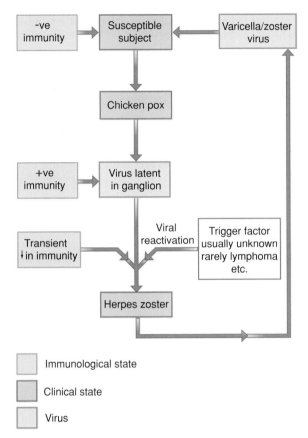

```
 -ve              Susceptible            Varicella/zoster
immunity  ──▶     subject      ◀──          virus

                     │
                     ▼

                  Chicken pox

                     │
                     ▼

 +ve              Virus latent
immunity  ──▶     in ganglion

                     │           Viral      ┌────────────────┐
                     │           reactivation│ Trigger factor │
Transient ──────────▶│◀──────────────────── │ usually unknown│
↓ in immunity        │                       │ rarely lymphoma│
                     ▼                       │      etc.      │
                  Herpes zoster              └────────────────┘
```

☐ Immunological state

☐ Clinical state

☐ Virus

Figure 13.9 Zoster/varicella relationship (reproduced with permission from Hunter et al 1995 and Blackwell Science Ltd).

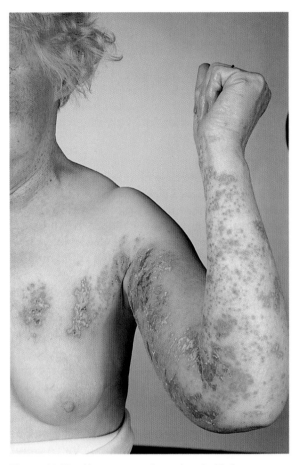

Figure 13.10 Herpes zoster (reproduced with the permission of Dr G Lowe, Ninewells Hospital, Dundee).

secondary infection requires antibiotics. The virus can be life threatening for immunocompromised patients and zoster immunoglobulin is given to those at risk. Primary infection confers long-term immunity but the virus remains dormant in the dorsal root ganglion to be reactivated as shingles. Staff nursing the patient with chickenpox should be aware of their own immune status (Stewart 1996).

Herpes zoster (shingles)

Recrudescence of the dormant varicella zoster virus causes shingles. Reactivation allows the virus to replicate and migrate along the nerve, creating the prodromal phase of pain and tenderness preceding the cutaneous eruption of erythema and vesicles. Shingles is an acute self-limiting dis-

order that occurs with dermatomal distribution and is usually unilateral (Fig. 13.10). Fifty percent of patients have involvement of the thoracic dermatome and involvement of the ophthalmic division of the trigeminal nerve is common (Gawkrodger 1997). The prodromal period precedes the vesicular eruption and the vesicles pustulate and crust, to heal leaving residual scarring. Diagnosis can be confirmed by culture.

Complications of zoster infection include:

- pain, numbness, lymphadenopathy
- secondary bacterial infection
- corneal ulcers and scarring
- disseminated zoster with haemorrhagic involvement
- postherpetic neuralgia.

Treatment and management. Management advice must clarify the infectious nature of shingles.

- Shingles cannot be caught.
- Live varicella virus is present in lesions.
- Chickenpox can be contracted from a patient suffering from shingles by anyone who has never had chickenpox.

Mild cases of shingles are treated at home, whilst hospitalization with isolation is required for extensive infection. Aciclovir used orally or intravenously, dependent on disease severity, promotes resolution and may reduce postherpetic neuralgia. Rapid referral to ophthalmology minimizes potential complications of shingles involvement of the eye.

Nursing care promotes maintenance of basic hygiene whilst local applications of dilute potassium permanganate solution soothe skin, assisting in removal of crusted lesions. Pain assessment supported by adequate analgesia during the initial stages is important. Intractable postherpetic neuralgia merits referral to specialist pain therapy teams (Hargus et al 1996). Treatment options include oral carbamazepine (Tegretol), transcutaneous electrical nerve stimulation (TENS) and topical capsaicin (Axsain) which relieves pain by inhibiting dermal nerve activity. Consideration of complementary therapies is relevant to long-term postherpetic management. In the majority of cases neuralgia does improve.

Recurrent or widespread disseminated herpes zoster merits further investigation for a systemic cause, e.g. AIDS, lymphoma. Community or hospital staff working with shingles patients must identify their own immune status. Immunocompromised patients who have never had chickenpox are at risk from the patient with shingles. Family and visitors should be restricted to those with virus immunity.

INFESTATIONS

Infestation is defined as the harbouring of insects or worm parasites in or on the body, causing diverse reactions.

Insect bites are common, presenting as itchy wheals, papules or large bullae. The cutaneous reaction of an insect bite is due to a pharmacological, irritant or allergic response to the introduced foreign material (Gawkrodger 1997). The bites can be grouped or 'track' up the affected limb.

Papular urticaria, common in childhood, consists of recurrent itchy papules occurring on limbs and trunk. Causes are many, including flea bites and mites, e.g. pets or garden insects. Secondary bacterial infection is caused by scratching.

Bedbugs survive in wooden beds, furniture and mattresses and lay eggs 3–4 times per year. Bugs bite at night, producing grouped urticarial papules on exposed sites, e.g. wrists, neck, waist and ankles.

Treatment and management

Treatment focuses on eliminating causes. Pets should be examined and treated with flea powder. Carpets and animal bedding should also be sprayed or dusted with flea powder. Bedbugs are eradicated by treatment sprayed on beds, floors and mattresses. The spray lingers for 3–4 months but to remain effective needs to be repeated regularly.

Topical applications of calamine lotion or Eurax cream soothe insect bites but secondary infection requires oral or topical antibiotic therapy.

Scabies

Scabies is a common parasitic infection caused by the mite *Sarcoptes scabei* and acquired by prolonged close physical contact. The female mite burrows 1 cm into the stratum corneum and after fertilization, lays her eggs in burrows. Four to six weeks after initial contact, due to a hypersensitive reaction to the mite, the patient describes intense itch, particularly at night. Skin examination reveals burrows commonly affecting the sides of fingers, wrists, ankles and nipples (Fig. 13.11). Genital burrows have a nodular appearance. A scabies rash may be present in

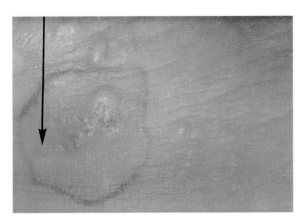

Figure 13.11 Scabies burrows (reproduced with the permission of Dr G Lowe, Ninewells Hospital, Dundee).

axillae, umbilicus or thighs. Excoriation causes burrows to become eczematized and impetiginized, confusing diagnosis.

Crusted scabies

This is a crusted variant of scabies presenting in patients who have sensory deficits where sensation of itch is absent, i.e. spinal-injured or immunosuppressed patients. Absence of scratching inhibits burrowing so large number of mites remain in crusted lesions on the skin (Elgart 1993). A normal scabies infestation involves 10–20 mites but this crusted form produces thousands of organisms and is more resistant to treatment. Mites are shed in large volume into the environment. Outbreaks tend to occur in specialist units or communities where patients are neurologically impaired or immunologically suppressed.

Treatment and management

Diagnosis can be confirmed by removing a mite from the burrow and examining it microscopically. Guidelines issued by the Department of Health advise on current treatments. Topical therapies are rotated on a 3-year basis to reduce treatment resistance. Lyclear dermal cream (permethrin 5%), lindane (Quellada) and Derbac-M are all currently used effective scabicides.

Therapeutic efficacy is achieved by correct application (Box 13.3) but these preparations cannot be used prophylactically.

Contact tracing ensures that treatments are coordinated on the same day to reduce reinfection. Contacts may be infectious asymptomatic carriers of infection but all close contacts are treated irrespective of signs and symptoms. Contact tracing should go back 6 weeks and include:

- anyone living in the household
- sexual contacts
- family or close friends who have had prolonged skin contact
- residents in homes
- staff with skin-to-skin contact during care delivery.

Box 13.3 How to apply scabicide effectively

- Read the advice leaflet before starting treatment.
- Pay special attention to these areas when you put on the lotion or cream:
  behind both ears
  both armpits
  underneath breasts
  navel
  groin and genital area between the legs
  backs of knees
  between all toes and on soles of feet.
- Skin should be cool and dry. Avoid bathing before applying the cream.
- Apply cream as prescribed from the neck down; avoid the face.
- Leave the cream on 8–12 hours as the prescription states (overnight is ideal).
- Bathe or shower at the end of the 8–12 hour period.
- Change nightwear and bed linen – normal laundering is adequate.

Additional points
- Treat all family members/contacts on the same day.
- If there is any delay in treating anyone, avoid further contact until they are treated.
- If the hands are washed during the treatment time, cream should be reapplied to the hands.
- Weaker strengths of cream are available for pregnant women or babies.
- In cases of crusted scabies, the head, scalp and neck will be treated, avoiding the eyelids (confirm with prescribing dermatologist).

Contacts with symptoms should be treated as cases and contact tracing extended to exclude their contacts. Family members of asymptomatic contacts are not treated but advised to see their GP if they develop itch. An outbreak of scabies, i.e. two or more cases, is reported as a communicable disease (Tayside Health Communicable Diseases Department 1997).

Extra precautions for crusted scabies. The patient with crusted scabies is highly infectious so additional precautions are required. Hospitals or nursing homes will have local infection control guidelines already established. Control measures include:

- isolation in a single room until treated
- contact nursing established
- use of disposable gloves and aprons
- laundry bagged as infected linen
- daily clean of room by damp dusting
- treatment of staff, residents, family, visitors.

Throughout diagnosis and treatment, reassurance and psychological support are relevant to management. Staff should recognize and address the distress that infestation produces in those involved. Sensitive, caring, practical support encourages the successful outcome of therapies and alleviates emotional distress. Many patients are merely relieved to have the condition diagnosed and effectively treated. Follow-up can include referral to the social work team if social circumstances are counterproductive to preventing recurrence.

Lice

Lice are flattened, wingless creatures producing eggs (nits) that attach to hair or clothing. The two species are body/head lice and pubic lice. Infestation produces severe itch of the affected area with scratching and secondary infection.

Head lice (pediculosis capitis) are transmitted by close contact. The adult female louse lays eggs cemented to the hair about 0.5 cm from the root. Nits are easily identified as the empty larvae cases left after hatching. Itch and irritation are common and the nape of the neck is characteristically excoriated and impetiginized. Head lice is

an emotive topic, endemic among school children and having a significant psychological impact on parent and child that must be addressed as part of treatment management.

Body lice infestation tends to be associated with poverty and poor social hygiene. The skin is excoriated and infestation spreads via infested bedding and clothing with lice found in the seams of clothing.

Pubic lice (crabs) cause pruritus, with secondary infection and eczema. Spread is by sexual contact and in extreme cases can involve the eyelashes.

Treatment and management

Head lice (see Chapter 7).

Body lice can be eradicated from clothing and bedding by laundering, dry cleaning or tumble drying at high temperatures. Applications of topical lindane or permethrin lotions will treat skin infestation. Topical steroid or antibiotic therapy will be required to treat secondary eczema or impetigo. Full assessment of social circumstances by a care manager from the social work team will be necessary to address the social issues associated with the infestation.

Pubic lice can be eradicated by applications of malathion or lindane to the body. Sexual partners should also be treated.

METHICILLIN-RESISTANT *STAPHYLOCOCCUS AUREUS* (MRSA)

Staphylococcus aureus is a group of Gram-positive bacteria resident on skin with the ability to either colonize a person or cause infection. This group of bacteria spreads easily on the hands of healthcare workers and has the ability to develop resistance to commonly used antibiotics, including methicillin. This has become a major challenge to the provision of care and its prevalence has initiated numerous policies and guidelines to control MRSA.

MRSA is a significant pathogen for vulnerable patients, e.g. intensive care, burns units. The range of antibiotics available to treat MRSA is limited (Sheff 1999) and costs are escalating with its increasing prevalence. Infection control guidelines have been established based on risk assessment dictated by local circumstances and clinical experience (Working Party Report 1998).

The principles of management include:

- general infection control policies (Box 13.4)
- clinical pathway action once diagnosis confirmed, i.e. isolation, cleaning and disinfection
- screening protocol for patients and staff
- treatment guidelines for carriers (Box 13.5).

Sceening involves taking swabs for bacteriology from:

- the nose, perineum/groin and axillae

- umbilicus in infants
- open wounds/excoriated skin, e.g. eczema, leg ulcers
- nose and throat of medical and nursing staff.

Admission screening and isolation of known or suspected carriers is now good practice in hospitals. Treatment, screening and decolonization programmes vary depending on risk factors but the priority is to prevent crossinfection to the most susceptible high-risk groups (Griffiths-Jones 1999).

CONCLUSION

It should be apparent from this chapter that rapid diagnosis, correct treatment and preventive advice will combat many commonly encountered infections and infestations. The emphasis on infection control measures to prevent recurrence or spread of infection needs to be seamless across the primary and secondary care interface. It must include infection prevention advice to the general public that dispels the social myths and stigma associated with these conditions. Handwashing technique is the simplest and cheapest everyday infection control measure, effectively interrupting and limiting the spread of infection in the hospital, home or community setting.

Box 13.4 Basic infection control guidelines for MRSA

- Clean ward/home environment
- Use of protective clothing – gloves and aprons
- Staff levels/skill mix appropriate for isolation nursing
- Ongoing audit and surveillance of infection control policies and their efficacy
- Isolation policy
- Adherence to disposal of clinical waste/laundry
- Minimal movement of patients between wards

Box 13.5 Treatment protocol for MRSA

Nasal carrier	*Skin carrier*
Mupirocin nasal ointment 2% applied three times daily for 5 days	Daily bath with antiseptic detergent, e.g. triclosan 2%, chlorhexidine 4% Use antiseptic shampoo
If mupirocin-resistant strain, use neomycin 0.5%/chlorhexidine cream 0.1%	Infected/colonized skin lesions – use antiseptic wash but observe for skin irritation
Or consider systemic vancomycin	Small lesions – apply mupirocin 0.5% in glycol base Large lesions – apply mupirocin in paraffin base
	Systemic antibiotics if the patient is clinically unwell

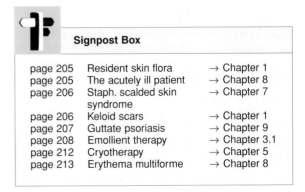

REFERENCES

Andrist L C 1997 Genital herpes: overcoming barriers to diagnosis and treatment. American Journal of Nursing 10: 16

Beardsley J 1993 Understanding herpes simplex. Professional Nursing 8(5): 322–328

Buxton P K 1998 ABC of dermatology. BMJ Publishing Group, London, pp 54–55

Dignan K, Turnheim R 1996 Sexually transmitted diseases: genital herpes. Professional Nurse 12: 801–802

Du Vivier A 1991 Atlas of infections of the skin. Gower Medical, London

Elgart M L 1993 Scabies: diagnosis and treatment. Dermatology Nursing 5(6): 464–467

Gawkrodger D J 1997 Dermatology: an illustrated colour text, 2nd edn. Churchill Livingstone, Edinburgh

Graham-Brown R, Burns T 1997 Lecture notes on dermatology, 7th edn. Blackwell Science, Oxford

Griffiths-Jones A 1999 Taking the strain. Nursing Times 13(95): 260–261

Hargus E P, Clark J, Gadbaw J, Paige D 1996 Post herpetic neuralgia: treatment and reminder. Journal of Pain and Symptom Management 12(3): 149

Hunter J, Savin J, Dahl M 1995 Clinical dermatology, 2nd edn. Blackwell Science, Oxford

Kovach T L 1999 Freedom from the septic flow: handwashing in infection control. Journal of Practical Nursing 49(1): 34–45

Lemone P, Burke K 1996 Medical surgical nursing. Critical thinking in client care – assessing clients with skin disorder. Addison Wesley, California, ch 16

Leppard B, Ashton L J 1990 Differential diagnosis in dermatology. Lippincott Williams and Wilkins, Philadelphia

MacDonald H 1995 Candida: the hidden deterrent to breast feeding. Canadian Nurse 91(9): 27–30

Parish L, Witkowski J A, Vassileva S 1995 Colour atlas of cutaneous infections. Blackwell Science, Oxford

Richardson M, Warnock D 1997 Fungal infection: diagnosis and management, 2nd edn. Blackwell Science, Oxford

Ritchie S R, Thompson P J 1992 Primary bacterial skin infections. Dermatology Nursing 4(4): 261–268

Sheff B 1999 VRE & MRSA: putting bad bugs out of business. Nursing Management 30(6): 42–50

Stewart M 1996 The immune system and infectious disease. In: Alexander M, Fawcett J, Runciman P (eds) Nursing practice hospital and home: the adult. Churchill Livingstone, Edinburgh, pp 569–570

Tayside Health Communicable Diseases Department 1997 Guidelines for the control of scabies infections. Dundee, Scotland

Timbury M C 1997 Notes on medical virology, 11th edn. Churchill Livingstone, Edinburgh, pp 93–109

Working Party Report 1998 Revised guidelines on the control of methicillin-resistant *Staphylococcus aureus* infection in hospitals. Journal of Hospital Infection 39(4): 25–28

FURTHER READING

Adler M A 1998 ABC of sexually transmitted diseases, 4th edn. BMJ Publishing Group, London

Cerio R, Archer C B 1998 Clinical investigations of skin disorders. Chapman and Hall Medical, London

Khan R M, Goldstein E J C 1993 Common bacterial skin infections: diagnostic clues and therapeutic options. Postgraduate Medicine 93(6) 175–182, 195–197

Perry C 1998 Infection control competition: three major issues in infection control. Community Nurse 7(16): 946–950

Sugar A M, Lyman C A 1997 A practical guide to medically important fungi and the diseases they cause. Lippincott-Raven, Philadelphia

Windsor A 1998 Tinea capitis – a growing headcount. British Journal of Dermatology Nursing 2(3): 10–12

PATIENT SUPPORT GROUPS

The Herpes Association
41 North Road
London N7 9DP

Herpes Viruses Association and Shingles Support Group (SPHERE)
41 North Road
London N7 9DP
Tel: 020 7609 9661 (24 hour helpline)

Women's Health and Reproductive Rights Information Centre
52–54 Featherstone Street
London EC1Y 8RT

14

Epidermolysis bullosa and bullous diseases

Jacqueline Denyer   Esther Hughes

EPIDERMOLYSIS BULLOSA

Introduction

Epidermolysis bullosa is the name for a group of genetically determined skin disorders in which the skin and other epithelia are liable to separate following minimal everyday friction and trauma.

The most severe of these diseases (junctional epidermolysis bullosa) often results in death in infancy. In most types, however, the patient survives into adulthood but frequently has an impaired quality of life.

There are many different types of epidermolysis bullosa, the three main ones being simplex, dystrophic and junctional (Priestley et al 1990).

There is tremendous variation in severity in each of the three types.

At birth, the presentation may vary from minimal blistering to large areas of denuded skin. Due to the rarity of the condition, epidermolysis bullosa is not always suspected immediately, with alternatives such as sepsis or amniotic bands being suggested as the initial diagnosis. This leads to a delay in instigation of correct handling and management and may lead to the infant receiving unnecessary treatment such as insertion of nasogastric tubes and intravenous cannulae, these being secured with adhesive tape which damages the skin on removal.

Diagnosis is made from a skin biopsy to determine the type of epidermolysis bullosa and analysis of DNA from blood samples from the affected child and his parents may enable identification of the specific mutation.

Epidermolysis bullosa simplex is a defect of keratin and affects the structure of the tonal filaments within the skin structure. It is almost exclusively a dominantly inherited condition, one parent being affected, and in many cases there is extensive family history. However, infants with a severe type of epidermolysis bullosa simplex are sometimes seen to have a new mutation of the disorder.

The blisters may be limited to the hands and feet (Weber–Cockayne type) or occur at all sites of friction (Köebner type) (Fig. 14.1).

The most severe form of epidermolysis bullosa simplex is the Dowling Meara type in which blistering is exceptionally severe in the neonatal period. There is a significant neonatal mortality rate in this group, death commonly resulting from sepsis and/or respiratory distress from internal blistering (Fig. 14.2).

However, if the infant survives the early difficulties, the blistering reduces as the child grows older. Indeed, many adult sufferers may have minimal blistering, the only residual sign being a covering of hard skin over the palms and soles.

Junctional epidermolysis bullosa is a defect of laminin and the genetic fault lies within the basement membrane. It is a recessively inherited condition, both parents being healthy carriers. The most severe form (Herlitz junctional epidermolysis bullosa) inevitably results in death in infancy or childhood. Death results from internal blistering leading to a combination of failure to thrive and respiratory distress (Fig. 14.3).

Even those with the Herlitz form may appear to be only mildly affected at birth, but blisters appear rapidly when the infant is handled. Infants with junctional epidermolysis bullosa

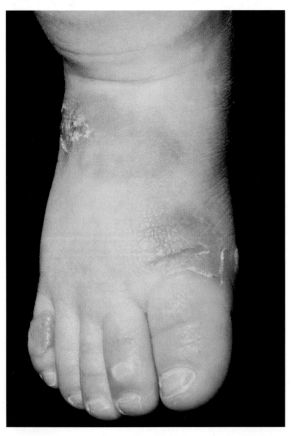

Figure 14.1   Epidermolysis bullosa simplex.

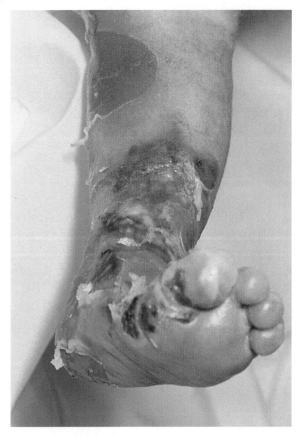

Figure 14.2   Dowling Meara type.

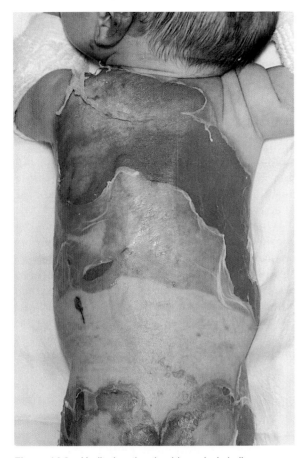

Figure 14.3 Herlitz junctional epidermolysis bullosa.

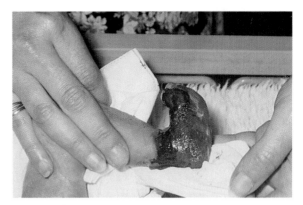

Figure 14.4 Dystrophic epidermolysis bullosa.

have a characteristic hoarse cry which develops within the first few days of life.

Other types of junctional epidermolysis bullosa can be very mild, the affected individual experiencing minimal blistering and little or no disability. In others, blistering may be widespread but the absence of internal blistering makes the disease less severe than the Herlitz form.

Dystrophic epidermolysis bullosa is a defect of collagen which affects the anchoring fibrils. It may be either dominantly or recessively inherited. In common with many other genetic conditions, the dominant form is often the more mild. There is, however, tremendous variation in severity within those with the recessive form.

There is a tendency for blisters and wounds to heal with a contracting scar, leading to permanent and progressive disability in those with a severe form of recessive dystrophic epidermolysis bullosa.

Neonates commonly present at birth with large areas of denuded skin over the feet and legs, a result of the infant kicking in utero and further aggravated by the trauma of the delivery. Despite a careful dressing technique, the toes may fuse together during the healing process (Fig. 14.4).

Older children may require plastic surgery to separate digital fusion of the hands and to release contractures in order to restore function (Mullett et al 1996).

Scarring leads to strictures within the oesophagus and the resulting dysphagia impairs nutrition.

A later complication of severe recessive dystrophic epidermolysis bullosa is the development of squamous cell carcinoma, often presenting in young adults, but vigilant inspection of the skin for sinister changes should begin in the teenage years.

The importance of a multidisciplinary approach to care

This applies to sufferers with all types of epidermolysis bullosa but is particularly relevant to those with the dystrophic form.

Children within this group have multiple problems and require input from a wide range of specialists. Those involved include:

- dermatologist
- paediatrician

- dietician
- physiotherapist
- clinical nurse specialist
- ophthalmologist
- psychologist
- occupational therapist.

In order to avoid multiple trips to the outpatient department, it is less disruptive to the family to attend multidisciplinary clinics to which all the relevant professionals are invited (Dunnill & Eady 1995).

Care of the skin

Blisters are not self-limiting and must be lanced with a sterile needle or scissors to prevent them from enlarging. The fluid is gently expelled and the roof left on the blister wherever possible.

Wounds are dressed with a non-adherent dressing and secondary dressings used to absorb exudate and to add padding for protection from further injury in vulnerable sites. There are no dressings manufactured specifically for use in those with epidermolysis bullosa, the design of the majority of dressings being orientated towards short-term indications, such as the management of burns.

Care must be taken in the choice of dressing as many advertised as 'non-adherent' behave differently on skin affected by epidermolysis bullosa. Where possible, the dressing should be allowed to remain in place for several days in order to reduce pain and trauma at dressing changes and allow epithelialization to take place.

Other important factors in the selection of dressings include social acceptability, cost and availability in the community.

A complication in those with a severe form of dystrophic epidermolysis bullosa is the development of joint contractures at sites of recurrent blistering and ulceration. Poor dressing techniques can accelerate this process and lead to premature loss of mobility.

Tips on handling

- Never use adhesive tape.
- Avoid throat swabs unless medically indicated.
- Use commercial transparent foodwrap as a temporary dressing after bathing.
- Never lift from underneath the arms.
- Check clothes have not adhered to wounds prior to undressing.

Nutritional management

Nutritional problems commonly occur in severe recessive dystrophic epidermolysis bullosa but they are also seen in Herlitz and non-Herlitz junctional forms and the Dowling Meara subtype of epidermolysis bullosa simplex.

Wherever possible, oral feeding should be encouraged in the neonatal period. Large blisters on the tongue may need to be lanced prior to feeding. If the mouth is very sore, teething gel can be applied to the teat immediately prior to feeding, otherwise the teat should be dipped into sterile or cooled boiled water to prevent it from adhering to raw areas. White soft paraffin applied to the lips minimizes damage from contact with the teat.

Sadly, breastfeeding is rarely successful in those severely affected, as the positioning of the infant and rubbing of the skin of the face against the breast when rooting causes blistering.

When oral feeding is not possible, nasogastric tubes must be used with caution and secured with soft tubular bandage rather than adhesive tape. Tubes designed for long-term use should be chosen, as passing the tube risks damage to the oesophagus and may encourage formation of strictures in those with dystrophic epidermolysis bullosa.

Additional calories are often required as a portion of the nutritional value of the feed is diverted towards wound healing and the remainder may prove insufficient for growth. Initially a low birthweight formula may be used.

Gastrooesophageal reflux is a common problem in all types of epidermolysis bullosa. In the dystrophic form refluxed acid can encourage blistering and subsequent stricture formation within the oesophagus. Medical treatment is instigated as soon as reflux is suspected in order to protect against these complications.

Older children with a severe form of dystrophic epidermolysis bullosa commonly develop nutritional problems as a result of scarring and contractures, leading to a restricted mouth opening, immobile tongue and oesophageal strictures. These problems cause a reduction in nutritional intake and, in combination with the increased nutritional requirements, mean aggressive management is required.

Many children in this group benefit from gastrostomy feeding (Haynes et al 1996). A button gastrostomy is inserted as an open procedure via a laparotomy, rather than the conventional method using a gastroscope, which may cause further damage to the oesophagus.

Personal choice dictates whether the child receives the enteral feed overnight, delivered via a feeding pump, or divided into bolus feeds by day.

Nutritional problems in dystrophic epidermolysis bullosa

These include:

- reduction of nutritional intake due to discomfort from gastrooesophageal reflux and oral and oesophageal blistering
- oesophageal strictures
- scarring leading to restricted opening of the mouth and tethering of the tongue
- dental caries and gross dental overcrowding.

Constipation caused by perianal blistering leads to retention of faeces as a result of avoidance of painful defaecation, resulting in loss of appetite.

Nutritional requirements are raised as a result of loss of blood and plasma and continual wound healing.

Anaesthesia

Although there are concerns regarding the fragility of the mucous membranes and problems due to the limited mouth opening in those with dystrophic epidermolysis bullosa, administration of general anaesthesia has proved relatively straightforward in this group of patients.

In order for minimal trauma to occur, all personnel involved must have prior instruction with regard to handling. The unconscious patient should be lifted in a sheet to avoid shearing forces and the trolley and operating table padded to reduce pressure.

A layer of Clingfilm under the patient avoids any fresh wounds from adhering to the sheet and so reduces the risk of any further tears to the skin.

Adhesive tapes should be avoided and cannulae and electrodes secured with silicone dressings or bandages.

The eyes should be closed and protected or corneal blistering or erosions may occur (Atherton & Denyer 1997).

Analgesia

Management of pain for those with epidermolysis bullosa can be divided into two categories: relief of chronic pain which reduces mobility and reduction of pain experienced during dressing changes.

A small dose of the drug amitriptyline given daily has proved effective in reduction of background pain, resulting in improved quality of movement.

Pain at dressing changes can to an extent be relieved by use of the appropriate non-adherent dressing. Drugs such as paracetamol, morphine, midazolam or codeine are helpful prior to dressing changes but the possible sedative effect can be inconvenient to those going on to school or work. In this group of patients, provision of Entonox for home use is often more appropriate.

Physiotherapy

Physiotherapy is mainly indicated for those with dystrophic epidermolysis bullosa in an attempt to avoid contractures in those severely affected.

Gross motor milestones and abilities are frequently delayed in those with all types of epidermolysis bullosa, due to the protective environment created by those caring for them and hesitance demonstrated by the children themselves.

Management and treatment

Management is by regular assessment to tailor exercise programmes in order to encourage motor development. Treatment may include hydrotherapy, active exercises and passive stretches and splintage.

At present, management of epidermolysis bullosa is by treatment of the symptoms and prevention of avoidable damage.

Research is progressing towards gene therapy which will hopefully provide an effective treatment.

Prenatal testing

It is now possible to offer prenatal testing to parents following the birth of an affected child. This is in the form of analysis of a fetal skin biopsy or, if specific mutation has been identified, by analysis of a chorionic villus sample.

BULLOUS DISEASES

The aetiology of the autoimmune bullous diseases remains unknown. Genetic factors may have a role to play, which would make some families more likely to develop these diseases (Kirtschig et al 1999). However, although their aetiology remains a mystery, they can have devastating effects on affected individuals. As nurses, we must be aware of these conditions and have some understanding of them, particularly as, due to their rarity, they may not immediately be diagnosed and it may well be the community nurse who is the first contact with the affected individual.

We will deal with three important autoimmune diseases and their nursing management: bullous pemphigoid, pemphigus and dermatitis herpetiformis.

Bullous pemphigoid

This is the most common of the autoimmune blistering disorders. It occurs most frequently within the elderly, commonly in the seventh and eighth decades, and affects both sexes equally. With an increase in the elderly population, those nursing this age group should be aware of the clinical presentation of bullous pemphigoid as the diagnosis may be unrecognized. It is rare in infancy and childhood although there have been reported cases (Nemeth et al 1991). The condition is autoimmune and two bullous pemphigoid antigens have been identified. It has been associated with certain drugs such as diuretics (spironolactone, frusemide and bumetanide) and neuroleptics. Other drugs, including penicillamine, captopril and ampicillin, may also be causative agents (Vassileva 1998). As recently as 1999, in France, bullous pemphigoid was diagnosed following the use of fluoxetine (Rault et al 1999).

Clinical presentation

The clinical presentation is of large, tense, intact bullae which are predominantly situated on the limbs but may also present on the trunk. It may also appear at the sites of previous trauma, e.g. surgical scars or amputation stumps (McFarlane & Verbov 1989). Itchy, erythematous patches surround the blisters (Fig. 14.5). Mucous membrane involvement is less common than in pemphigus and usually restricted to the mouth although a rarer type of scarring (cicatricial) pemphigoid can occur with lesions mainly affecting the mucous membranes.

The blister in bullous pemphigoid is subepidermal, between the dermis and the epidermis. Due to this deeper position (than in pemphigus), these bullae often stay intact for long periods of time. Biopsy of a fresh bulla and adjacent skin should be sent for histological examination and immunofluorescence. Immunofluorescence shows linear

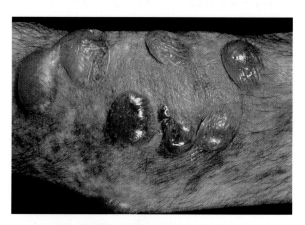

Figure 14.5 Pemphigoid (reproduced with the permission of St John's Institute of Dermatology).

IgG or C3 antibodies at the basement membrane zone.

Clinical management

Systemic steroids are usually required to bring the disease under control and the patient will require a maintenance dose for several years. Other immunosuppressive drugs may also be required. The condition usually remits within 3–6 years. Morbidity is lower than that of pemphigus but although the disease is not usually fatal in itself, mortality may relate to secondary effects of systemic treatments.

Nursing advice and skin care

- Make an accurate skin assessment as a baseline which can be used to effectively monitor the progress of the disease. Chart the amount and site of new blisters.
- Swab any eroded areas of the skin and send skin swab to bacteriology for culture and sensitivity to allow appropriate antibiotic therapy of any secondary bacterial skin infection.
- Daily bath/shower with antiseptics such as a weak solution of potassium permanganate (in bath) and soothing emollients. Pat the skin to prevent excess friction.
- Check for any new blisters and aspirate fluid contained within (see Nursing management of blisters, p. 231).
- Apply emollients prior to application of topical steroid.
- Apply any prescribed topical steroid using the fingertip measurement. A potent steroid, e.g. Dermovate cream, or steroid–antibiotic combination, e.g. Dermovate NN cream, is often the treatment of choice and may be sufficient in localized disease.
- Protective paraffin gauze and non-adherent dressings should be applied to infected and open skin lesions and fixed with appropriate bandaging.
- Daily monitoring of blood pressure and urinalysis whilst on high-dose systemic steroid therapy. Observe for side effects of steroid treatment.

- Observe for signs of dehydration and protein loss as a result of fluid loss from skin. Encourage oral fluids or monitor the administration of IV fluids if necessary. Record input and output accurately.

Pemphigus

This is a chronic bullous disorder, affecting both sexes equally and usually occurring in middle age. It is an important blistering condition to recognize because it carries a high mortality rate if left undiagnosed. Prior to the use of systemic steroids the condition would certainly have proved fatal, with a 75% mortality rate within the first year (Harman & Black 1997) but the number of deaths has reduced significantly with their introduction. There are four types of pemphigus.

Pemphigus vulgaris is the most common of the group and presents with flaccid blisters of the skin but particularly affects the mucous membranes, including mouth and genital areas. The oral cavity is the initial affected site in 70% of patients (Meurer et al 1977). Other stratified squamous epithelial sites can be affected, including the larynx, pharynx, oesophagus, conjunctivae and anus (Korman 1990). It can often go unrecognized if it presents in a localized area only, such as the mouth or vulva. Most patients develop skin lesions particularly affecting the scalp, face and axillae. The blisters are easily ruptured and leave very painful erosions. It is more common in the

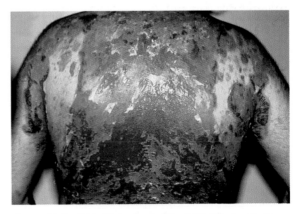

Figure 14.6 Pemphigus (reproduced with the permission of St John's Institute of Dermatology).

Jewish population but studies have also shown that compared with any other ethnic group, Indians of Malaysian origin are also more likely to develop this type of pemphigus (Adam 1992).

Pemphigus foliaceus is less common (10–20% of cases of pemphigus) and less severe than pemphigus vulgaris. It can affect a younger age group, although it is rare in childhood. Drugs such as penicillamine, captopril and gold can induce a pemphigus reaction similar to that of pemphigus foliaceus. The blistering is more superficial in pemphigus foliaceus such that it may not actually be obvious, with only scaly crusted erosions seen. Commonly affected areas include the back, chest, face and scalp. Mouth lesions are uncommon.

The rarer *pemphigus erythematosus* has a similar presentation to pemphigus foliaceus but the affected area may be much more localized. There may be a 'butterfly distribution' on the face (cheeks and nose) which must be distinguished from that of systemic lupus erythematosus.

Pemphigus vegetans is another rare presentation of pemphigus and is usually restricted to flexural areas and the oral mucosa. The presentation is similar to that of pemphigus vulgaris but differs in that, as the lesions are healing, they leave behind a hypertrophic, vegetating, warty mass.

Clinical presentation

The blisters are intraepidermal, which accounts for their fragility and finding of erosions rather than intact blisters. Itch is unusual, unlike bullous pemphigoid, although lesions are often painful. Nikolsky's sign is present: when firm sliding pressure is applied to normal skin, the epidermis separates off as a result of its poor attachment to the dermis underneath.

The diagnosis is made from a biopsy of an affected area sent to pathology for histology and immunofluorescence. Immunofluorescence will reveal antibodies to the epidermal intercellular material. Blood taken at the same time will also show circulating antibodies of the same nature.

Clinical management

High-dose systemic steroids are the treatment of choice; their effectiveness is well established (Bystryn 1984) at the expense of potential side effects. The patient will require a maintenance treatment for life to prevent relapses. Azathioprine and other immunosuppressive agents, including ciclosporin, methotrexate and cyclophosphamide, may be required for their steroid-sparing effect, so that lower doses of steroid are required to control the disease.

Nursing advice and skin care

- Make an accurate skin assessment as a baseline to effectively monitor the progress/deterioration of the disease.
- Pay special attention to washing of the skin with soothing emollients. Avoid unnecessary handling of the patient which may traumatize normal skin, inducing more blistering. A special pressure-relieving mattress/bed may be required for the patient who has generalized disease.
- Apply protective non-adherent dressings such as paraffin gauze or silicone-based dressings, e.g. Mepitel. Topical steroids may be prescribed to relieve some discomfort.
- Regularly swab eroded skin to screen for secondary bacterial infection which may require treatment with topical or systemic antibiotic therapy.
- Pay careful attention to fluid input and output. IV hydration may be necessary in the patient with severe oral involvement, although IV sites introduce the potential risk of infection, particularly whilst on high-dose steroids. Encourage oral fluids in the patient who is able to drink without too much discomfort.
- Pay careful attention to oral hygiene. Encourage the patient to rinse their mouth with regular mild antiseptic mouthwashes. There is an added risk of oral candidal infection whilst on high-dose corticosteroids.
- Liaise with the dietician for a soft, puréed diet if there is oral involvement and the patient requires a soft diet. For the patient nursed at home, encourage regular, small meals of favourite foodstuffs that are soft in nature.

- Daily monitoring of blood pressure and urinalysis whilst on high-dose systemic steroid therapy. Observe for side effects of steroid treatment.

Dermatitis herpetiformis (Table 14.1)

This is a chronic, recurrent, intensely pruritic condition which affects all age groups but especially the young and middle-aged population. It is rare, affecting only 110 per million in Scotland and Finland and 588 per million in Ireland (Fry 1990). A familial history is seen in about a tenth of all patients (Reunala 1996). Its name is misleading as it bears no relation to the herpes virus (other than the grouping of lesions) and is not infectious. This is important to stress to the individual receiving their diagnosis. It is also not a dermatitis, although

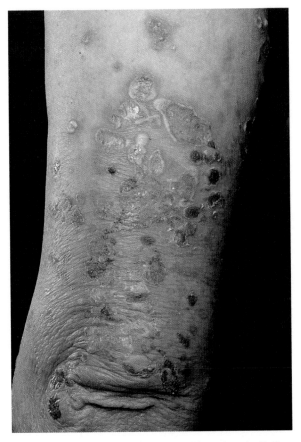

Figure 14.7 Dermatitis herpetiformis (reproduced with the permission of St John's Institute of Dermatology).

some patients can show eczematous changes around the affected areas. Autoantibodies such as antithyroid antibodies and antigluten antibodies may be found. It is also linked to other autoimmune disorders including coeliac disease and pernicious anaemia (Setterfield et al 1997).

Clinical presentation

Classically, lesions consist of groups of erythematous papules, urticarial weals or small vesicles which are often so quickly excoriated by the patient due to extreme itch that it is rare to see blisters in the intact form. They are usually lying on an erythematous base and have a symmetrical distribution. Commonly affected areas include the knees, elbows, buttocks, axillary folds, shoulders, trunk, face and scalp. Oral lesions are often present but are asymptomatic (Fraser et al 1973). The distribution of lesions and associated intense itch may lead to a misdiagnosis of scabies but on clinical examination, there are no burrows present and on questioning the patient there is no history of contact with scabies. The itch is often described by the patient as a 'stinging' or 'burning' sensation. Indeed, some patients can predict where new lesions will appear, because they experience this sensation several hours before the newly affected area appears (Hall 1987).

Dermatitis herpetiformis should be suspected in patients who demonstrate a pruritic, grouped eruption in symmetrical distribution of the above areas, which fails to respond to topical treatments. An underlying gluten-sensitive enteropathy is present in about 60–75% of patients and may or may not be symptomatic (Marks et al 1966). Often the gluten sensitivity is only discovered if jejunal biopsy is performed, which shows changes similar to coeliac disease. Histology of a skin biopsy of an affected area shows IgA deposits in the dermal papillae. It is known that gluten causes the IgA to be deposited here, although the mechanism for this is still unknown.

Clinical management

The disease does not respond to corticosteroids, unlike the other two conditions discussed.

Table 14.1 Bullous pemphigoid, pemphigus and dermatitis herpetiformis

	Age group	Presentation	Affected areas	Pruritus	Topical treatment	Systemic treatment
Bullous pemphigoid	Usually the over-60s Rare occurrences in infancy and childhood Sexes equally affected	Large, tense, resilient blisters which can remain intact for days Usually found on an erythematous base, sometimes blood filled	Primarily limbs and trunk	Commonly present	Topical steroid or steroid + antibiotic combination Potassium permanganate soaks/bath Liberal emollients Protective dressings	High-dose systemic steroids to bring disease under control Reduced as condition improves Immunosuppressive agents as adjuvant therapy Self-limiting disease within 3–6 years
Pemphigus vulgaris	Middle-aged predominantly although can occur in any age group	Superficial flaccid blisters containing clear fluid Burst easily to leave painful erosions Nikolsky sign positive	Initial lesions occur in the mouth Commonly other mucosal surfaces include conjuctiva, pharynx, larynx, oesophagus and vulva The scalp, face, groins and axillae can also be involved	No itch but severe pain is common	Protective dressings (paraffin gauze and non-adherent dressings) Topical steroids may be used	High doses of systemic steroids to bring the disease under control Low maintenance dose is essential for life, to prevent relapse Immunosuppressive
agents						may also be used as adjuvant therapy
Dermatitis herpetiformis	Young and middle-aged Male predominance Familial history	Crops of tense, small vesicles on erythematous plaques Symmetrical distribution Large blisters occur rarely	Buttocks, elbows, knees, axillary folds, shoulders, scalp and face	Severe, usually the affected area is so excoriated the blisters are not intact	Topical steroids may lessen symptoms Calamine soaks may relieve pruritus	Dapsone is the drug of choice A gluten-free diet, if adhered to, may remove the need for dapsone therapy

Dapsone, used in the treatment of leprosy, is the drug of choice, although it too must be monitored carefully for side effects. These include severe rashes, anaemia, motor neuropathy, glucose-6-dehydrogenase deficiency and hepatitis. Patients are advised to commence a gluten-free diet and should be referred to a dietician for the appropriate advice. Patients who manage to keep to a gluten-free diet often cease to require dapsone (Garioch et al 1994) although it can be a difficult diet to adhere to.

There is a small increase in the number of intestinal lymphomas in patients who suffer from a gluten-sensitive enteropathy but there is some protection from this if the patient remains on a gluten-free diet (Lewis et al 1996).

Nursing advice and skin care

- Take an accurate skin assessment. Observe for signs of improvement or deterioration.
- Broken skin should be swabbed for infection. If infection is present it may require treatment.
- A mild solution of potassium permanganate will help to dry up any broken areas.
- Apply emollients and prescribed topical treatments. Topical steroids may help to lessen symptoms.
- Calamine soaks may help to soothe skin and relieve pruritus.
- Regular sedating antihistamines will also relieve pruritus in the acute stages of the disease.
- Avoid using iodine preparations and dressings as these can exacerbate the disease.
- Full blood count should be checked on a regular basis if the patient is taking dapsone, to detect anaemia early.
- Refer to the dietician for appropriate advice on gluten-free diet.
- Offer support and encouragement at all times, particularly in adhering to a gluten-free diet.

NURSING MANAGEMENT OF BLISTERS

Tense, fluid-filled bullae are uncomfortable and painful for the patient who develops them. It is not enough, however, to merely 'pop' or burst the blisters. Likewise, blisters should never be deroofed; this only leaves raw open areas which are more likely to become infected and are also much more uncomfortable and painful for the individual.

The blister should be aspirated using a reasonable-sized needle (Fig. 14.8). It should not be so large that it traumatizes the blister more than is necessary. Similarly, it should not be so small that the blister is allowed to refill with fluid shortly after the procedure. The roof of the blister aids in the reepithelialization of the area and it is therefore important that it should be traumatized as little as possible.

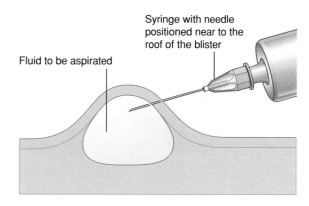

Figure 14.8   Correct technique for aspirating a blister.

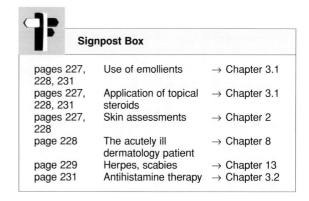

Signpost Box		
pages 227, 228, 231	Use of emollients	→ Chapter 3.1
pages 227, 228, 231	Application of topical steroids	→ Chapter 3.1
pages 227, 228	Skin assessments	→ Chapter 2
page 228	The acutely ill dermatology patient	→ Chapter 8
page 229	Herpes, scabies	→ Chapter 13
page 231	Antihistamine therapy	→ Chapter 3.2

REFERENCES

Adam B A 1992 Bullous disease in Malaysia: epidemiology and natural history. International Journal of Dermatology 31(1): 42–45

Atherton D J, Denyer J 1997 Epidermolysis bullosa: an outline for professionals. DEBRA, Crowthorne

Bystryn J C 1984 Adjuvant therapy of pemphigus. Archives of Dermatology 120: 941–951

Dunnill M G S, Eady R A J 1995 The management of dystrophic epidermolysis bullosa. Clinical and Experimental Dermatology 20: 179–188

Fraser N G, Kerr N W, Donald D 1973 Oral lesions in dermatitis herpetiformis. British Journal of Dermatology 89: 439–450

Fry L 1990 Dermatitis herpetiformis. Chapman and Hall, London

Garioch J J, Lewis H M, Sargent S A et al 1994 25 years experience of a gluten-free diet in the treatment of dermatitis herpetiformis. British Journal of Dermatology 131(4): 541–545

Hall R P 1987 The pathogenesis of dermatitis herpetiformis: recent advances. Journal of the American Academy of Dermatology 16(6): 1129–1144

Harman K, Black M 1997 Managing pemphigus vulgaris. Dermatology in Practice 5(5): 12–14

Haynes L, Atherton D J A, Ade-Ajayi N et al 1996 Gastrostomy and growth in dystrophic epidermolysis bullosa. British Journal of Dermatology 134: 872–879

Kirtschig G, Mittag H, Wolf M, Gorski A, Happle R 1999 Three different autoimmune bullous diseases in one family: is there a common genetic base? British Journal of Dermatology 140(2): 322–327

Korman N J 1990 Pemphigus. Dermatology Clinics 8: 689–700

Lewis H M, Reunala T L, Garioch J J et al 1996 Protective effect of gluten-free diet against development of lymphoma in dermatitis herpetiformis. British Journal of Dermatology 135(3): 363–367

McFarlane A W, Verbov J L 1989 Trauma induced bullous pemphigoid. Clinical and Experimental Dermatology 14: 254–259

Marks J, Shuster S, Watson A J 1966 Small bowel changes in dermatitis herpetiformis. Lancet 2: 1280–1282

Meurer M, Millns J L, Rogers R S, Jordan R E 1977 Oral pemphigus vulgaris. Archives of Dermatology 113: 1520–1524

Mullett F, Smith P, Wade A 1996 Dystrophic epidermolysis bullosa. A survey of predisposing factors and the development of the hand deformity in children with dystrophic epidermolysis bullosa. British Journal of Hand Therapy 2(4): 18–21

Nemeth A J, Klein D, Gould E W, Schachner L A 1991 Childhood bullous pemphigoid. Archives of Dermatology 127: 378–386

Priestley G C, Tidman M J, Weiss J B, Eady R A J 1990 Epidermolysis bullosa: a comprehensive review of classification, management and laboratory studies. DEBRA, Crowthorne

Rault S, Grosieux-Dauger C, Verraes S et al 1999 Bullous pemphigoid induced by fluoxetine. British Journal of Dermatology 141(4): 755–756

Reunala T 1996 Incidence of familial dermatitis herpetiformis. British Journal of Dermatology 134: 394–398

Setterfield J, Bhogal B, Black M M, McGibbon D H 1997 Dermatitis herpetiformis and bullous pemphigoid: a developing association confirmed by immunoelectronmicroscopy. British Journal of Dermatology 136(2): 253–256

Vassileva S 1998 Drug induced pemphigoid: bullous and cicatricial. Clinical Dermatology 16: 379–387

FURTHER READING

DEBRA publications:
  Care and management of children with dystrophic epidermolysis bullosa
  The management of junctional epidermolysis bullosa
  Epidermolysis bullosa simplex, Dowling Meara
  Epidermolysis bullosa: an outline for professionals
DEBRA publications are available from DEBRA House (see Patient Support Groups, below).

Du Vivier A 1993 Atlas of clinical dermatology, 2nd edn. Gower Medical Publishing, London.

Lin A N, Carter D M 1992 Epidermolysis bullosa. Basic and clinical aspects. Springer-Verlag, New York

Mackie R M 1991 Clinical dermatology, 3rd edn. Oxford Medical Publications, Oxford, ch 11, pp 244–254

PATIENT SUPPORT GROUPS

Bullous Pemphigoid Support Group
17 Barley Mount
Redhills
Exeter EX4 1RP

Coeliac Society
PO Box 220
High Wycombe
Bucks HP11 2HY
Tel: 01494 437278

DEBRA (International Patient Support Group)
Debra House, Wellington Business Park
Duke's Ride, Crowthorne, Berks RG45 6LS
Tel: 01344 771961, Fax: 01344 762661
Web site: www.debra.org.uk

Pemphigus Vulgaris Network
Flat C, 26 St German Road, London SE 23 1RJ
(s.a.e. required for information)
Shared web site with National Pemphigus Foundation:
www.Pemphigus.org

APPENDIX – PATIENT INFORMATION LEAFLETS

◆ PatientWise
Medical and Health Information for Patients

1.20 PEMPHIGUS

◆ What is it?

Pemphigus is a blistering skin condition which occurs in people between the ages of 20 and 50. It starts as an itchy red rash, and the skin becomes slightly swollen in well-defined areas. Following this, blisters develop in the skin, which are of variable size. These blisters readily burst to leave erosions on the skin. The erosions tend to increase in size with time. In one variety of pemphigus, blisters may be absent and are replaced by surface skin loss. The eruption can occur on any part of the body, and the insides of the mouth are frequently affected.

◆ How does it occur?

Pemphigus is regarded as an autoimmune disease. That is, the body's defence or immune system regards part of the skin as being foreign and mounts a destructive response against it. The part of the skin to which the response is mounted is the 'cement' that sticks the cells of the skin together. The inflammation initially creates itching of the skin. It then causes the cells of the skin to separate from each other, producing the blistering.

◆ Why does it occur?

Nobody knows why pemphigus occurs. It may be associated with other auto-immune diseases affecting other organs of the body. Certain drugs which are used for arthritis or tuberculosis may induce a rash very similar to pemphigus.

◆ What does treatment/management involve?

It is important that the correct diagnosis is established. This is done by taking a small piece of skin under local anaesthetic and examining it under the microscope. Using special tests, the 'immune response' against the skin can be identified, which proves the diagnosis. Treatment of pemphigus relies on the use of steroid (cortisone-like) drugs. Steroid tablets are usually started at quite a high dosage. As the skin eruption is brought under control, the dosage is gradually reduced. In some people, the pemphigus flares up once the steroid tablets have been reduced below a certain level. If this occurs, another medicine (called azathioprine) can be used. This works also by suppressing the body's abnormal immune response. Use of this drug allows the steroid tablets to be reduced further. You may require low doses of steroid tablets for months or even years to prevent recurrences of the disease.

◆ What to watch out for during treatment

Response to steroid tablets is rapid in pemphigus. The blisters and erosions quickly heal and irritation is relieved. Steroid tablets do have side-effects and can cause a variety of noticeable changes in the body. A common side-effect is fluid retention, with an increase in weight. Very often the face becomes rounded. If steroid tablets are used for long periods of time, they may cause thinning of the bones, resulting in pain in the spine. Diabetes may also develop. Some patients get peptic ulcers or high blood pressure as a result of the steroids. If you notice any new symptoms whilst on steroids, you should let your doctor know straight away. Steroid tablets can also cause problems within the skin itself, producing a rash like acne on the face, chest, and back, together with stretch marks. For these reasons, the dose of steroid tablets is kept at the lowest possible level. Drugs such as azathioprine are used to enable the doctor to reduce the steroid tablets to the lowest possible dose. However, this type of drug can affect bone marrow, stopping the formation of red and white blood cells. This can produce anaemia and a proneness to infections. Regular blood tests are therefore needed for patients taking this drug.

◆ What to watch out for after treatment

Eventually the disease resolves and the tablets can be withdrawn. After this it is unlikely that the pemphigus will recur, but this is always a possibility.

◆ What would happen if the condition was not treated?

Pemphigus tends to be a progressive disease. If not adequately treated, the rash would become widespread. Because the skin breaks down into erosions, fluid and protein would be lost from the body, and infection could get into the body through the broken skin. This can be extremely dangerous. Before the discovery of steroids and effective treatment of pemphigus, there was a high mortality associated with pemphigus.

◆ What is involved for family and friends?

Pemphigus is a chronic disabling condition and although effective treatment is available, the treatment does carry side-effects which can profoundly affect the individual. Considerable support is needed by family and friends to be able to help the patient cope with the disease.

1.20 This sheet describes a medical condition or surgical procedure. It has been given to you because it relates to your condition and may help you understand it better. It does not necessarily describe your problem exactly. If you have any questions, please ask your doctor.
Copyright © 1997 John Wiley & Sons, Ltd (Reproduced by permission of John Wiley & Sons Limited.)

Pemphigoid

Pemphigoid is an uncommon but well-recognized blistering skin disorder which usually occurs in later life. In some cases blisters can develop in the mouth and can affect the eyes. However, pemphigoid is not usually associated with internal disease.

Nobody fully understands the cause of the disease. For an unknown reason antibodies (natural substances important in your body's defence) form in the blood and then attack the border between the top layer of the skin (epidermis) and the bottom layer (dermis). This leads to splitting of the skin and hence blisters. Pemphigoid is not infectious.

Treatment to prevent the blisters usually consists of steroid tablets. Steroid creams can also be helpful. Other drugs such as azathioprine can be used in addition to help suppress the antibodies.

The disease is not affected by diet or lifestyle. Some patients can gradually come off treatment usually after a few months, others may need to continue with a lower dose of treatment long-term.

(Reproduced with permission from the British Association of Dermatologists)

Dermatitis herpetiformis

This is a rare but well-recognized intensely itchy rash which in many patients is associated with a bowel disorder similar to mild coeliac disease. Patients are sensitive to gluten, a protein found in wheat and rye flour.

The name dermatitis herpetiformis is misleading as the condition is in no way related to herpes infection and is not infectious.

The rash can be confused with scabies, eczema and other very itchy skin disorders. A skin biopsy taken by a dermatologist is usually essential to confirm the diagnosis.

Dermatitis herpetiformis occurs mainly in young and middle-aged adults but is occasionally seen in children. Itching is the first and main symptom. The rash consists of small red spots, blisters and weals. The commonest sites affected are the elbows, knees, scalp, bottom and back.

The condition usually runs a very prolonged course, over many years, sometimes improving, sometimes getting worse. However, it may eventually burn itself out.

Treatment

Dermatitis herpetiformis usually improves with a drug called dapsone and patients may also improve on a gluten-free diet. In some patients the diet removes the need to take tablets.

(Reproduced with permission from the British Association of Dermatologists)

15

Other common skin conditions

Una Donaldson   Maxine Whitton

LICHEN PLANUS

Lichen planus is a disorder seen in 0.2–0.8% of patients attending a dermatology centre. It is a disorder of unknown cause but it presents with intensely itchy, flat-topped, red to lilac-coloured papular lesions, a few millimetres in diameter (Fig. 15.1). They tend to start on the limbs and initially spread quite rapidly and the patient can present with a wide distribution of papules covering forearms and wrists, thighs and legs, palms and soles, occasionally including the genitalia and mucous membrane of the mouth but rarely found on the scalp.

Box 15.1 Features of lichen planus

- Sometimes related to stress
- Well-defined raised lesions
- Flexor surfaces
- Köebner phenomenon
- Nails affected in 10% of patients
- Oral mucosa affected with white spongy lesions on inner cheeks which are commonly asymptomatic

---

Widespread lesions can occur within 4 weeks. The pattern of distribution tends to be symmetrical.

The rash can last for a period of 3 months up to 2 years and as the lesions resolve, they become flatter and darker in colour.

Histopathology, sent for immunofluorescent study, confirms the diagnosis. In 50–70% of patients the white lace-like pattern in the buccal mucosa can be diagnostic, as can the shiny white

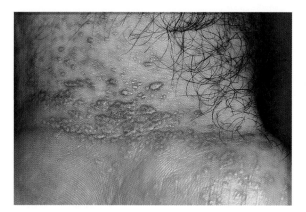

Figure 15.1 Lichen planus.

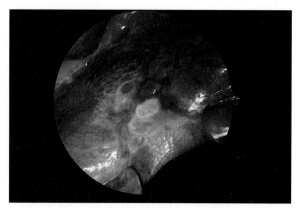

Figure 15.2 Wickham's striae.

lace pattern seen on the other lesions when studied carefully, known as Wickham's striae (Fig. 15.2). The Köebner phenomenon may also be present.

Lichen planus is a self-limiting disorder, burning itself out in most cases. The patient can be reassured that it is not serious or contagious. Unfortunately, approximately one in six patients may have a recurrence and a drug-related eruption should be excluded before initiating treatment. The drugs most likely to cause this are beta blockers, antimalarials and gold (injections used for arthritis).

After eliminating possible causes, the treatment of symptoms is important, the most likely being severe itch. This can be controlled by using antihistamines and topical emollients or a preparation of 1% menthol in aqueous cream. Where the rash is very extensive, a potent to moderately potent steroid may be effective in relieving the itch.

If there are widespread lesions becoming ulcerated, it may be necessary to introduce a short course of oral steroids. Systemic retinoids or Ciclosporin A have been used successfully in recalcitrant cases.

Nursing advice and skin care

- Application of topical emollients.
- Safe adminstration of topical steroids, documenting skin changes.
- Care of mouth lesions with Corlan pellets or Orabase cream. Difflam mouthwashes may also give symptomatic relief.

- Reassurance and support.
- Supply written information (Fig. 15.3).

LICHEN SCLEROSUS

Lichen sclerosus is an uncommon disorder presenting with white lichenified atrophic macular lesions commonly on the genitalia, but they may occur at any site. This disorder is 10 times more common in women than men and usually presents in middle age with an intractable vulval or perianal itch. On examination there are ivory-coloured lesions surrounding the vulva and anus (Fig. 15.4). These lesions atrophy and may result in purpura and small telangiectases. Occasionally the lesions may become ulcerated, causing further itch and pain. At this stage women may experience dysuria. In the long term, this condition can cause shrinkage of the genitalial tissue and in rare cases may develop into vulval carcinoma.

In men, lichen sclerosus may cause phimosis (a constriction of the prepuce). It can also cause adhesions of the foreskin and the glans penis, leading to recurrent balanitis (inflammation of the prepuce and the glans penis) and ulcerations of the glands. The atrophy this produces can lead to squamous cell carcinoma.

Unfortunately, lichen sclerosus in adults is a chronic problem that is usually permanent, relapsing and remitting (Marren et al 1997). However, it may be helped by topical steroids. For a confirmed clinical diagnosis, a biopsy is essential. Although the cause is unknown it may

LICHEN PLANUS

Lichen planus is a well-recognized itchy, non-infectious skin disease, usually occurring in adults. It develops slowly and can take up to eighteen months to clear. In a small number of patients the condition can persist beyond this time.

The rash consists of small, flat topped, purplish spots, most commonly found around the wrists, ankles and lower back. The spots, however, can be more widespread. There may also be associated changes in the lining of the mouth, causing white streaks. Occasionally these can be very sore and require special treatment.

Lichen planus can affect the scalp and nails. If the attack is a severe one this can lead to lasting nail damage, but such cases are uncommon.

The cause of the condition is unknown. Fortunately it does not influence the sufferer's general health.

In most cases the condition slowly burns itself out without any special treatment. Itching can be a problem and moisturising creams, or steroid creams, may provide some relief.

In the more aggressive cases the dermatologist may recommend steroids in tablet form for a limited period.

FL:\PATIENT LEAFLETS
MF-DOCS\SHARED\ORIGINAL\LEAFLETS

Registered Charity No 258474

Figure 15.3   Information sheet for lichen planus (reproduced with permission from the British Association of Dermatologists).

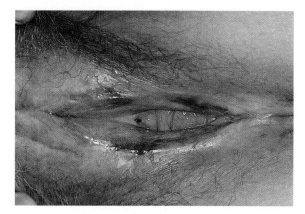

Figure 15.4   Lichen sclerosus.

be associated with autoimmune disease (Marren et al 1995).

Lichen sclerosus can occur in children who complain of genital discomfort and bleeding. It is very important for nurses to be aware of this, as some children have been inappropriately suspected of being victims of childhood sexual abuse (Mackie 1996).

Nursing advice and skin care

- Reassurance and counselling.
- Advice on sexual activity. As lichen sclerosus is non-contagious, sexual contact need not be curtailed.
- Pregnancy and childbirth remain unaffected.
- Application of topical steroids, e.g. Trimovate. In the prepurbertal child, 1% hydrocortisone may be used.
- Current treatment is a potent steroid, e.g. Dermovate ointment, applied very specifically, e.g. twice daily for first month, daily for second month, 2–3 times weekly for third month, depending on symptoms. Thereafter used PRN, 30 g tube, for a minimum of 3 months or as long as necessary. Further atrophy from itch or steroid use will increase the likelihood of developing squamous cell carcinoma in the atrophic skin.
- Men should be treated with a weak steroid unless symptomatic. With stenosis of the urethra, a potent steroid can be used until symptoms are under control.

Box 15.2	Treatment for lichen sclerosus
Prepuberty	1% hydrocortisone
Men	Asymptomatic – mild steroid Symptomatic – potent steroid
Women	In remission – no treatment or mild steroid In acute phase – potent steroid, or topical oestrogens (Dinoestrol cream)

PRURITUS

Pruritus is the medical term for an itchy skin. This is a common symptom and therefore much easier to treat if the specific cause is discovered. To do this, we must exclude a number of conditions and take a very detailed history.

First, the patient often feels dirty and imagines something crawling under their skin, so it is useful to exclude body lice and scabies. Other more obvious skin conditions can also be easily excluded, e.g. eczema and lichen planus.

During the history taking it can also be established if the patient has been in contact with fibreglass or with any substances they may be allergic to. It may be useful to take a contact history.

Once possible causes have been excluded it may be necessary for the patient to undergo more rigorous investigation and rule out any systemic diseases which can cause pruritus. These include diabetes, liver disease, underlying malignancy, neurological disorders, polycythaemia, renal failure and thyroid dysfunction.

Systemic causes

- Endocrine disease – diabetes, myxoedema, hyperthyroidism
- Metabolic disease – hepatic failure, chronic renal failure
- Blood disorders – polycythaemia, haemachromatosis
- Malignancy – lymphoma, reticulosis, carcinomatosis, Hodgkin's disease
- Psychological – anxiety, parasitophobia
- Tropical infections – filariasis, hookworm
- Drugs – alkaloids, drug addiction and abuse

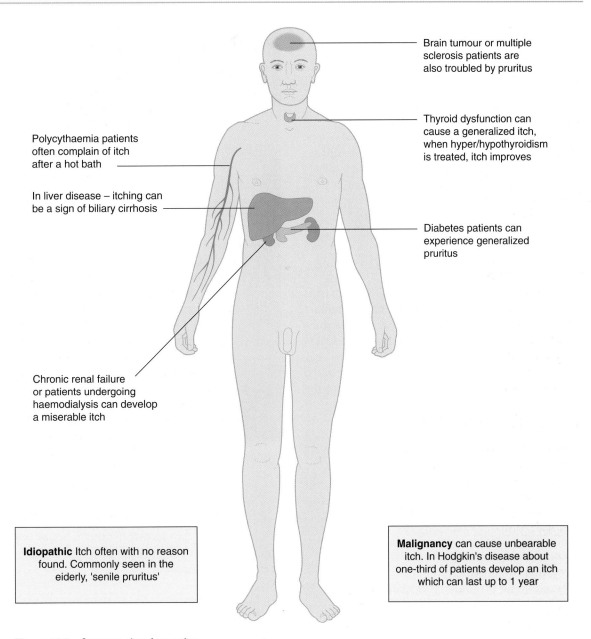

Brain tumour or multiple sclerosis patients are also troubled by pruritus

Thyroid dysfunction can cause a generalized itch, when hyper/hypothyroidism is treated, itch improves

Polycythaemia patients often complain of itch after a hot bath

In liver disease – itching can be a sign of biliary cirrhosis

Diabetes patients can experience generalized pruritus

Chronic renal failure or patients undergoing haemodialysis can develop a miserable itch

Idiopathic Itch often with no reason found. Commonly seen in the eiderly, 'senile pruritus'

Malignancy can cause unbearable itch. In Hodgkin's disease about one-third of patients develop an itch which can last up to 1 year

Figure 15.5 Common sites for pruritus.

Investigations

- Skin scraping for fungal culture
- Patch testing to exclude allergic reactions
- Full blood haematology and biochemistry, which may indicate systemic disease
- Urinalysis to eliminate diabetes, liver disease and renal disease
- Stool for culture (parasites)
- Stool for faecal occult blood

The management and treatment of the patient will depend on the results of the investigations.

Nursing advice and skin care

- Bathe with soap substitute.
- Encourage patient to pat skin dry.
- Use frequent emollient of choice.
- 1% menthol in aqueous cream may relieve itch.
- Explanation of itch–scratch–itch cycle, encouraging patient to rub skin and not scratch when itchy. Habit reversal techniques.
- Mild or moderate steroids may be necessary.
- If patient persists in scratching, occlusive bandaging may be necessary.
- Possible prescription of antihistamine, especially at bedtime.

PRURITUS ANI

This is a localized itch causing irritation often exacerbated by defaecation. This can be an embarrassing, socially unacceptable and very disabling condition. Any obvious cause, e.g. fissure, flexural psoriasis, contact dermatitis, threadworms and infections, e.g. candidosis, trichomenal vaginitis, should be treated but often no precipitating factor can be found.

Pruritus ani often arises for psychogenic reasons and patients suffering this condition are often obsessive and extremely anxious. Their behaviour often makes the problem worse as they become obsessive about washing the anal area, causing irritation.

Nursing advice and skin care

- Avoid excessive soap and water and highly coloured toilet paper.
- Avoid using proprietary local anaesthetic preparations.
- Advise patient to use olive oil and cotton wool to cleanse after defaecation.
- Weak steroids or topical antibiotic combinations may be necessary to reduce the inflammation and then a protective cream around the anal area, e.g. Sudocream or Zinc and castor oil cream.

URTICARIA

Urticaria is an eruption of extremely itchy, erythematous papules, plaques or wheals. It can last

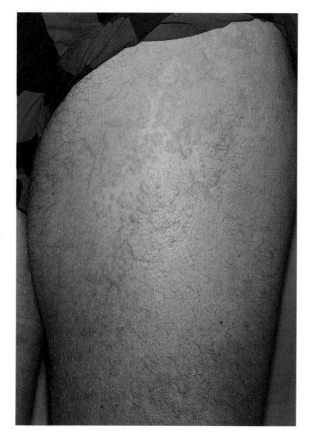

Figure 15.6 Urticaria.

from hours (an acute attack) to many days (a repeated or chronic attack). Urticaria is also known as hives or nettle rash.

Lesions can be multiple and appear very quickly; each type requires different investigations and treatment.

Angiooedema

The most potentially dangerous type of urticaria, angiooedema, which is hereditary or in response to an allergy, affects the subcutaneous tissue and appears as swelling around the eyes and often the mouth. It may be associated with swelling of the tongue or laryngeal mucosa. The swelling may become gross and can develop into a full anaphylactic shock reaction, which is very alarming for the patient.

In severe cases with respiratory obstruction, a tracheostomy may be required. Adrenaline given intramuscularly and repeated at 10-minute intervals usually relieves symptoms. Antihistamines can also be given which have a longer lasting effect. Systemic steroids may also be a treatment option but should be monitored carefully, due to adverse side effects (Monroe 1997).

Causes

- Wasp and bee stings
- Severe drug reaction – histamine-liberating drugs, e.g. salicylates, codeine, morphine and indomethacin
- Food allergy, often to shellfish and tartrazine group of food dyes in yellow/orange drinks/sweets
- Contact urticaria, e.g. to animal fur, especially in atopics
- Physical urticaria caused by pressure, heat or cold
- Related to general medical problems, e.g. lupus erythematosus, thyrotoxicosis
- No known or identifiable cause

Nursing advice and skin care

- Watch for signs of airway obstruction. Acute cases will require subcutaneous adrenaline.
- Refer to a dietician if a food allergy is suspected. The dietician may promote a salicylates-free diet.
- Avoid aspirin and codeine as these contain salicylates. Foods containing tartrazine colouring and food preservatives should also be avoided.
- Alert patient and document drug allergy.
- Treat itch with antihistimine, giving instructions to avoid driving or operating machinery.
- Treat established lesions with a moderately potent topical steroid for symptomatic relief.

Cholinergic urticaria

This manifests in the form of a papular rash, often apparent around the blush area and neck. It is usually connected with anxiety, strenuous exercise or a rise in body temperature. It often affects teenagers and young adults.

Nursing advice and skin care

- High necklines can conceal this in stressful situations. Wear cool clothing when exercising.
- Concealer make-up may also be useful.

Cold-induced urticaria

This is, as the name suggests, a condition where the patient develops wheals if exposed to the cold. They appear within minutes of exposure and last up to 24 hours.

Nursing advice and skin care

- Treatment is an antihistamine taken prior to the activity, e.g. if skiing for the day, an antihistamine should be taken the night before.

Solar urticaria

This is similar to the above, as the small pinhead wheals appear within minutes after exposure to the sun.

Nursing advice and skin care

- Treatment again would include an antihistamine or perhaps a desensitizing programme of UVB before holiday.

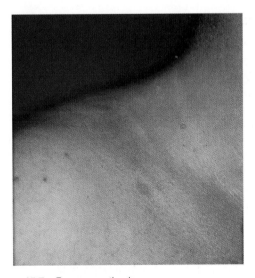

Figure 15.7 Pressure urticaria.

Pressure or delayed pressure

This type of urticaria results from the pressure of tight-fitting clothes which can produce wheals. Equally, delayed pressure can induce this type of reaction. After clapping for a long time, hands may develop an urticaria as sustained pressure can cause oedema in the underlying subcutaneous tissue. Similarly, a reaction in the feet may develop a few hours after a long walk.

Nursing advice and skin care

- Soaking hands and feet in lukewarm emollient can be soothing.

Dermographism

This is a traumatically induced form of urticaria; wheals can be produced on the skin by physical stimuli. It occurs in about 5% of the population and is often only noted by dermatologists. As discussed in Chapter 2, it can be a useful diagnostic tool.

ALOPECIA

Hair grows everywhere on the body except the palms, soles, glans penis, nipples and lips. The hair follicle is an invagination of the epidermis into the dermis and it terminates around a richly vascular dermal papilla. The part of the follicle around the papilla actively divides and is called the hair root.

There are three main types of human hair, shown in Table 15.1.

Terminal hair follicles undergo a regular cycle of growth activity. The length of the cycle is variable depending on the body site, e.g. a few months for the growth of eyelashes and a few years for the growth of hair on the scalp.

There are three phases of hair growth (Fig. 15.8).

1. *Anagen* – this is the growing phase. Approximately 85–90% of hairs are in this phase at any given time.
2. *Catagen* – this is the involutional phase lasting only a short period of time. The metabolic processes associated with hair

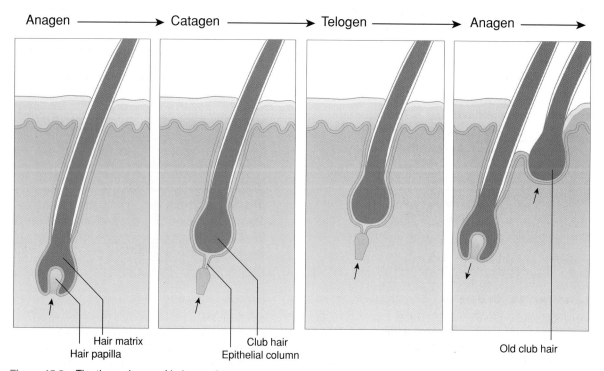

Anagen ⟶ Catagen ⟶ Telogen ⟶ Anagen ⟶

Hair matrix
Hair papilla
Club hair
Epithelial column
Old club hair

Figure 15.8 The three phases of hair growth.

Table 15.1 Types of human hair

Type	Body site	Appearance and consistency
Lanugo hair	Covers the fetal skin whilst the fetus is in utero	Soft, fine hair with light pigmentation
Vellus hair	Covers the body (excluding palms, soles, parts of genitalia, lips, nipples) of child and adult female	Short hair of fine consistency, has little pigmentation
Terminal hair	Scalp, eyebrows in all ages. Present in the axillary, pubic, beard (males) regions following puberty. This is under hormonal influences	Longer hair, coarser in texture

growth gradually decrease and the hair follicle regresses.

3. *Telogen* – this is the resting phase. Existing hair will cease to grow and hairs will be shed from the follicle.

Hair is continually falling and being replaced. Scalp hair grows about 1 cm ($\frac{1}{2}$ inch) per month and a normal scalp sheds approximately 50–100 hairs daily. Hair is said to be one's 'crowning glory' and is also seen as a fashion asset. It is also associated with sexual attraction, so alopecia in young men and women can be socially very unacceptable and can cause considerable distress.

Understanding the psychosocial effect alopecia may have must be paramount when dealing with a patient suffering from this condition.

Alopecia can be diffuse or localized and can be either scarring or non-scarring.

Androgenic alopecia

The onset and severity of baldness is gene dependent. Women, especially postmenopausal, may also be affected by this type of alopecia although it can occur in premenopausal women also. These women, unlike men, have diffuse thinning, often worse centrally. The scalp may become visible and there may be accentuation of the M-shaped frontal temporal hairline. In men, the pattern varies, as shown in Hamilton's classification table (Table 15.2; see also Fig. 15.9).

Androgen-dependent loss of scalp hair, otherwise known as common baldness, is extremely common in men and increases with age. It can begin in the teens, 20s and 30s and is often established by the 40s. Over a period of time the terminal follicles change to vellus-like follicles which

Table 15.2 Hamilton's classification of male androgenic alopecia (from Hordinsky 1996)

Type	Clinical features
I	Normal frontoparietal hairline.
II	Symmetrical triangular areas of recession in the frontoparietal regions.
III	Borderline cases.
IV	Deep frontotemporal recession in association with hair loss along the midfrontal border of the scalp.
V	Extensive frontoparietal and frontal recession in association with sparse hair growth on the vertex.
VI	Vertex region of alopecia is separated from the anterior area of hair loss by a region of sparse scalp hair density.
VII	Area dividing the crown region with the anterior area of hair loss begins to disappear.
VIII	Complete baldness.

then produce shorter and finer hairs called miniaturized hairs. These hairs vary in diameter and length.

Nursing advice and skin care

Male

- Reassure patients that this condition is so common it is considered the norm.
- Referral can be made at the patient's request for a hairpiece or wig.
- Supply information regarding Hairline support group

Female

- Advise patients to consult hairdresser on styling techniques and products available, e.g. mousse to volumize the remaining hair.
- Supply addresses of companies specializing in camouflage make-up.

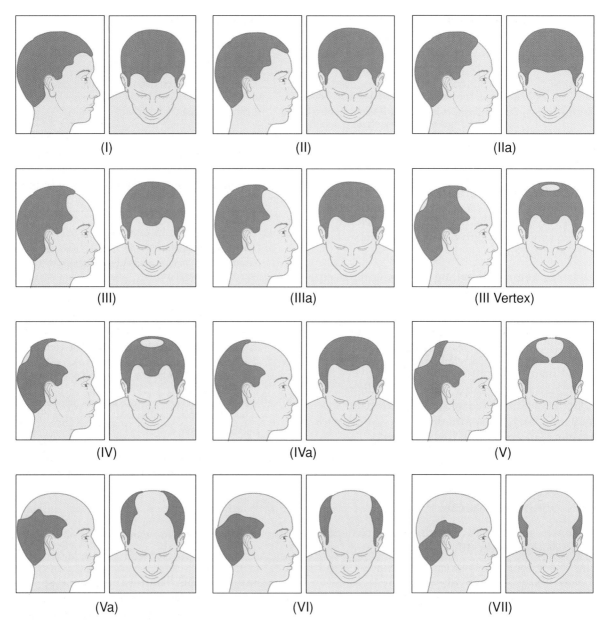

(I)   (II)   (IIa)

(III)   (IIIa)   (III Vertex)

(IV)   (IVa)   (V)

(Va)   (VI)   (VII)

Figure 15.9 Hamilton's classification of male androgenic alopecia (reproduced with permission from Olsen E A 1994 Disorders of hair growth: diagnosis and treatment. McGraw Hill, New York).

Endocrine changes and nutritional factors

Patients with either hypo- or hyperthyroidism, hypopituitarism and diabetes mellitus may have poor hair growth and diffuse thinning of the hair which can lead to alopecia. Protein is also required for hair growth, so alopecia is seen in Third World countries. These people suffer from kwashiorkor, which is a result of a diet low in protein. Interestingly, they also have a change in pigmentation, causing the hair to become a rust colour. This is very apparent in negroid hair; the hair becomes very brittle and breaks off.

Zinc or iron deficiency (through diet or other related conditions) can also result in this type of hair loss.

Nursing advice and skin care

- A detailed history including weight loss/gain, constipation/diarrhoea, lethargy or hyperactivity, goitre or exophthalmos, excessive thirst, frequency of micturition, blood present in stool.
- Specific blood tests related to history, including serum ferritin, iron, blood glucose, thyroid function tests, etc.
- Referral to a dietician.
- Reassurance that hair loss will resolve when the condition is treated.

Telogen effluvium

Telogen effluvium is the name given to the alopecia that occurs after an episode of stress. It is common after childbirth, severe febrile illness, shock or surgery. The hair becomes diffusely thin and falls out rapidly. This happens because most of the hairs pass suddenly from the anagen to the telogen (or resting) phase. A new hair bulb is formed and the hair that arises from this pushes out the old hair. The damage is done long before the hair is lost and the loss of the hair itself can be seen as the first sign of recovery. After 3–4 months, hair follicles resume to their normal cycle.

Nursing advice and skin care

- Reassure the patient that this is only a temporary loss and hair growth will resume.
- Refer to previously mentioned cosmetic techniques.

Drugs

Drugs can also cause this type of hair loss, most commonly certain types of cytotoxic drugs. Anticoagulants like warfarin and heparin occasionally cause alopecia. Acetretin, the vitamin A derivative used for inflammatory skin conditions, can be a causative agent. Antithyroid drugs, e.g. carbimazole, can also have the same effect.

Nursing advice and skin care

- If informed of drug side effects, patients will be more tolerant of hair loss.

Alopecia areata

This condition occurs in both sexes and at all ages and is characterized by either generalized or localized sudden hair loss from the scalp or other body sites, leaving a completely smooth scalp with visible hair follicles. The condition is more common amongst patients with Down's syndrome, diabetes, thyroid disorders and other autoimmune conditions, e.g. vitiligo.

Alopecia areata can account for approximately 2% of new cases seen in dermatology units. Most cases are children or young adults who often present with one or more well-demarcated bald areas. The hair follicle is in the telogen phase and there may be broken hairs looking like exclamation marks around the edge of the bald area. This aids diagnosis.

If there is complete loss of scalp hair, the condition is known as alopecia totalis. Alopecia universalis is the term used when all body hair is lost.

In many cases spontaneous regrowth of the hair takes place in a few months' time, although some patients remain affected for a number of years. If atopy is present, the prognosis is poorer.

Trauma

Trauma can cause localized areas of alopecia without scarring. This can occur in children who pull, twist or tug at their hair. This type is often seen in people with learning disabilities. This hair loss has no real pattern and the visible broken hairs can be suggestive of this diagnosis.

Some hairdressing techniques can result in this type of alopecia, such as prolonged traction caused by rollers, excessive use of hair dyes or perming lotions. Tight ponytails have also been known to cause localized hair loss and broken hairs.

Nursing advice and skin care

- This condition resolves once the trauma ceases.

Fungal infections

Fungal infections can cause patchy, scaly alopecia. Some types of fungus can cause an inflammatory reaction which forms a 'boggy' lesion with hair loss known as a kerion, e.g. in tinea capitis, and a malodorous discharge from the follicles. When the infection has cleared, hair grows normally except when the lesions cause scarring.

Nursing advice and skin care

● Treat underlying fungal infection (tinea capitis) with systemic antifungal agents.

Scarring alopecia

Causes of scarring alopecia include burns or irradiation. As mentioned earlier, fungal, viral or bacteriological infections can cause scarring in the scalp which also may result in permanent damage.

Patients with lesions of chronic discoid lupus erythematosus in the scalp will also experience permanent alopecia. Occasionally, morphea and lichen planus occur in the scalp with the same result.

VITILIGO

Definition

Vitiligo is a common depigmenting disorder of the skin which affects an estimated 2% of the population worldwide regardless of race, ethnic background or sex (Halder & Young 2000). It is characterized by discrete, amelanotic macules resulting from the absence of melanocytes. The skin, though remaining smooth in texture, develops white patches which may be large or small, may affect all areas of the body either in a symmetrical or unilateral pattern. The course of the disease is unpredictable but lesions can spread to cover the whole body. Rarely, the pigment in the eyes, and hair may also be affected. In a recent paper investigators proposed that the definition of vitiligo should be 'an acquired, progressive depigmentation with unpredictable course … which involves the integument and probably affects the pigmen-

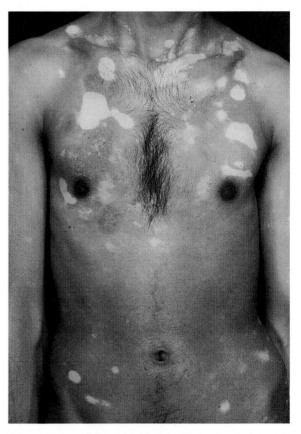

Figure 15.10 Vitiligo (reproduced with the permission of St John's Institute of Dermatology).

tary system of other organs' (Hann & Nordlund 2000).

Aetiology

Vitiligo is not contagious and can appear at any age with a mean age of onset of 19 years in males and 24 years in females (Majumder et al 1993). The aetiology of vitiligo is still unknown though there are many theories to explain the depigmentary processes involved. These include neurological, cytological, environmental and immunological factors which may destroy or damage melanocytes. These may all be precipitating factors but it has become increasingly clear that a genetic predisposition is the basis for the disease (Bhatia et al 1992). Roughly a third of patients have close family members with the disease and studies suggest that vitiligo is probably not caused by a single gene but is multigenetic, which may explain the contradictions in the presentation of the disease by patients. Vitiligo has also been linked to autoimmune diseases such as thyroid disorders and diabetes mellitus and many patients with polyglandular dysfunction have vitiligo (Bloch & Sowers 1985). Antibodies to melanocytes have been found in the sera of some patients. These factors combine to suggest that there may be an autoimmune form of vitiligo.

Triggers

Many patients report that their vitiligo was triggered or exacerbated by specific events including stress, hormonal changes, bereavement, contact with certain chemicals, particularly phenols, sunburn, PUVA, and damage of any kind to the skin. The latter is known as the Köebner phenomenon.

Psychosocial factors

Although the general health of people with vitiligo is not affected the psychosocial effects may be devastating. On tanned or dark skin the white patches on face, neck and arms can be disfiguring (Lessage 1997). In some individuals vitiligo can be a social and psychological handicap causing great distress to sufferers and their families. Most people with vitiligo feel isolated, have a poor body image and lack self-confidence and self-esteem. Some become depressed and withdrawn. Children, teenagers and women are particularly vulnerable groups. Indians and Pakistanis who develop the disease are often ostracised due to the stigma associated with it, a legacy of the ancient but mistaken belief that vitiligo is a form of leprosy. Young girls with vitiligo can be condemned to loneliness as marriages for them are difficult to arrange.

Coping

People cope with vitiligo in varying ways. Strong support from friends and family and an understanding family practitioner make a difference. Joining a support group, such as the Vitiligo Society, can help by providing information and an opportunity to share experiences with others. Some patients can benefit from psychological counselling which helps to put the disease into perspective and can improve body image and self-confidence and build self-esteem.

Treatments

Treatment for vitiligo aims to restore pigmentation to the skin. Occasionally vitiligo patches regain their colour spontaneously but this is never complete and tends to occur mainly in children. Unfortunately, there is no single, specific, licensed treatment for vitiligo and those that are used are often difficult and lengthy with a risk of relapse as they only treat the symptoms not the underlying cause of the disease.

Topical steroids

Potent or very potent topical steroids applied once daily can be effective for small patches of recent onset. They are reported to halt the spread in some cases and may even restore colour to the white patches. Topical steroids may stimulate the melanocytes (Fitzpatrick et al 1997) but use should be closely monitored to avoid steroid atrophy. If there is no response after three months they should be discontinued though they can be used on new patches.

Phototherapy

PUVA (psoralen and ultra violet A) has been used for vitiligo for many years with varying degrees of success. Psoralens, which occur naturally in more than 30 common plants, are now synthesized and given orally as capsules or applied topically to the affected areas only. They are photosensitizers and used in conjunction with ultraviolet A light. Patients attend a dermatology clinic twice a week and need to wear protective sunglasses for 24 hours after taking the capsules. This treatment needs careful monitoring and may take several months before any improvement is seen. This requires commitment from the patient and encouragement by the dermatology staff. Adverse effects include itching, redness, nausea and in rare cases, skin cancer. Those patients who do respond may regain some or all of their pigment. However, there is evidence that most patients subsequently relapse after a few years.

Depigmentation

This is a permanent treatment using monobenzylether of hydroquinone which destroys remaining melanocytes. It is rarely used and usually only when more than 70% of the body is affected. Patients need to be counselled carefully as the treatment increases photosensitivity and should any repigmentation occur the bleached areas may not repigment. It is not recommended for children and long-term effects are unknown.

Sun screens

All patients with vitiligo are advised to use high factor sun screens (SPF25) on affected, exposed areas before going out. Vitiligo patches lack protection from the sun, putting patients at risk of sun damage including photoaging, skin cancer and sunburn which can cause the patches to spread. Sun screens can be obtained on prescription.

Cosmetic camouflage and fake tanning preparations

In the absence of effective treatment patients may be prescribed special cover creams to be applied to the white patches on exposed areas such as the face. Referral by the doctor or dermatologist can be made to the Red Cross Skin Camouflage Service whose trained volunteers can instruct the patient in how to find the correct shade for their skin and apply the cream correctly. The result can be cosmetically effective and may help some patients, including men, to regain their self-confidence. However, the creams may rub off on clothing, are time consuming to apply and need to be applied daily.

Fake tans on the other hand last for 3–5 days but it is difficult to find a suitable match for all skin types. They are widely available over the counter at most pharmacists. Patients should also be reminded to apply sun screens as these preparations offer no protection from the sun.

New and emerging treatments

These include skin grafting, melanocyte transplantation, narrow band UVB (311 nm) monotherapy, pseudocatalase with narrow band UVB and psychological counselling.

It was recently discovered that the skin of patients with vitiligo has high levels of hydrogen peroxide, a natural by-product of melanin production, and low levels of the enzyme, catalase, which neutralizes it. This has led to the development of a topical laboratory analogue of catalase, pseudocatalase, as a replacement therapy in the form of a cream used in conjunction with narrow band UVB (311 nm). Results so far in a case study of 33 patients have been encouraging. (Schallreuter et al 1995). Further studies are now underway.

Narrow band UVB monotherapy has also been shown to give encouraging results. In the Netherlands studies have been conducted comparing this treatment with topical PUVA and using it with children. It had a response rate of 67% compared with 46 % with PUVA (Westerhof & Nieweboer-Krobotova 1997). The advantages of this treatment include less erythema, fewer cytotoxic effects, no hyperkeratosis after long-term use, less contrast between normal and white skin and no need to use sunglasses after treatment.

The strong psychological element in vitiligo has led to studies of the use of cognitive behavioural therapy which not only helps patients to live with the disease but may also influence the progression of it (Papadopoulos et al 1999).

The role of the nurse

Nurses can help patients by increasing their understanding of vitiligo, by providing information on sun screens and camouflage creams, being the link between the dermatologist and the patient and by supporting and encouraging them through their treatments which may last for many months. Most importantly, nurses can find time to listen and talk.

Signpost Box

page 236	Systemic treatments	→ Chapter 3.2
pages 236, 238, 240, 241	Topical steroids	→ Chapter 3.1
page 246	Fungal infections	→ Chapter 13
page 239	Skin scraping	→ Chapter 2
page 242	Hair growth	→ Chapter 2
page 246	Tinea capitis	→ Chapter 7

REFERENCES

Bhatia P S, Mohan L, Pandy O N, Singh K K, Arona S K, Mukhija R D 1992 Genetic nature of vitiligo. Journal of Dermatological Science 4: 180–184

Bloch M H, Sowers J R 1985 Vitiligo and polyglandular autoimmune endocrinopathy. Cutis 36: pp 417–419, 421

Fitzpatrick T B, Johnson R A, Wolff K, Polano M K, Suurmond D 1997 Colour atlas and synopsis of clinical dermatology. McGraw-Hill, New York, pp 287–295

Hann S-K, Nordlund J J (eds) 2000 Vitiligo. Blackwell Science, p 5

Halder R M, Young C M 2000 New and emerging therapies for vitiligo. Dermatologic Clinics 18: pp 79–89

Hordinsky M K 1996 Hair. In: Sans W M, Lynch P J (eds) Principles and practice of dermatology. Churchill Livingstone, New York, pp 779–800

Lessage M 1997 Vitiligo: understanding the loss of skin colour. Vitiligo Society, London.

Majumder P P, Nordlund J J, Swapan K 1993 Pattern of familial aggregation of vitiligo. Archives of Dermatology 129: 994–998

Majumder P P, Nordlund J J, Swapan K 1993 Pattern of familial aggregation of vitiligo. Archives of Dermatology 994–998

Marren P, Yell J, Charnock F M, Bruce M, Welsh K, Wojnarowska F 1995 The association between lichen sclerosus and antigens of the HLA system. British Journal of Dermatology 132: 197–203

Marren P, Millard P R, Wojnarowska F 1997 Vulval lichen sclerosus – lack of correlation between duration of clinical symptoms and histological appearances. Journal of the European Academy of Dermatology and Venereology 8(3): 212–216

Monroe E 1997 Therapy of acute and chronic urticaria. Journal of the European Academy of Dermatology and Venereology 8(supplement 1): 511–517

Papadopoulos L, Bor R, Legg C 1999 Coping with the disfiguring effects of vitiligo. A preliminary investigation into the effects of cognitive-behavioural therapy. British Journal of Medical Psychology 72: 385–396

Schallreuter K U, Wood J M, Lemke K R, Levenig C 1995 Treatment of vitiligo with a topical application of pseudocatalase and calcium in combination with short-term UVB exposure: a case study on 33 patients. Dermatology 190: 223–229

Westerhof W, Nieweboer-Krobotova L 1997 Treatment of vitiligo with narrowband UVB versus topical psoralen plus UVA. Archives of Dermatology 133: 1525–1528

FURTHER READING

Buxton P K 1998 ABC of dermatology, 3rd edn. BMJ Publishing Group, London, pp 25, 26, 70, 73, 99

Gawkrodger D J 1997 Dermatology: an illustrated colour text, 2nd edn. Churchill Livingstone, Edinburgh

Hunter J A A, Savin J A, Dahl M V 1994 Clinical dermatology. Blackwell Science, Oxford, pp 55–57, 60–65, 110, 212–216

PATIENT SUPPORT GROUPS

Hairline International – The Alopecia Patients' Society
Lyon's Court
1668 High Street
Knowle
West Midlands B93 0LY
Tel: 01564 775281
Fax: 01564 782270

National Lichen Sclerosus Support Group
2 Ivy House
Wantage Road
Great Shefford
Berkshire RG17 7DA
(Enclose s.a.e.)
Web site: www.hiway.co.uk/lichensclerosus

Vitiligo Society
125 Kennington Road
London SE11 6SF
Tel: 0800 018 2631 (Freephone)
Fax: 020 7840 0866
Web site: www.vitiligosociety.org.uk

16

Dermatology nursing

Lynette Stone

INTRODUCTION

Dermatology care in the UK has been affected by the various health-care reforms during recent years. The government White Paper *Working for patients* (DoH 1989) was followed by the introduction of the internal market with its purchaser–provider split, the establishment of commissioning authorities with responsibility to purchase health care for their local area (NHSME 1990) and the development of hospital and community health services into self-governing trusts to become providers of health care. Additionally, with the higher profile role of general practitioners as providers of primary medical care and purchasers of secondary care and the advent of fundholding GPs, a review of dermatology services has continued.

The contribution of nursing to the provision and shaping of health care services in all areas has steadily increased. The government White Paper *The new NHS: modern, dependable* (DoH 1997) proposed the establishment of primary care groups (PCGs) to replace GP fundholding. PCGs will have a major responsibility in commissioning services for the local community and membership of the PCG will include GPs and nurses (NHSE 1998). Community nurses as well as nurses working in specialist dermatology units will therefore need to prepare themselves for dealing with the dermatology issues which affect up to 30% of the population at any one time (Rea et al 1976, Williams 1997).

Inevitably, all these developments have had major implications for the role of the dermatology nurse. Issues that need to be addressed include identifying who provides the patient care, whether it should be a nurse or a doctor, whether its focus should be in the primary or secondary care sector and where it should be provided – in the hospital, GP surgery or in the home – or a mixture of all these options, depending on the patient's condition and needs. Wherever patient care is provided, the role of the nurse in dermatology will have the same remit.

THE ROLE OF THE NURSE IN DERMATOLOGY

The role of the nurse in the skin-care team was described by Stone (1983) and is equally relevant to all areas wherever dermatology patients receive their care. The main facets of the role are to:

- help patients in maintaining a healthy skin and in controlling their skin condition by carrying out prescribed treatments as well as encouraging them to manage their own skin care independently
- provide education for the patient, their families and carers about the skin condition and its treatments. Education of clinical colleagues is important so that skin disease sufferers receive appropriate skin care when being treated for other medical conditions in other areas. Nurses can contribute to the education of all people about the need for routine skin care to help them maintain a healthy skin and prevent skin failure. They can help raise the awareness of the public generally to reduce the social isolation experienced by many skin disease sufferers
- coordinate the various aspects of care needed by working with patients and all members of the professional team involved in the patient care programme
- support the patient by giving emotional and psychological help and advising about patient support groups and the availability of other self-help opportunities.

More recently, the scope of dermatology nursing practice has been described as including an emphasis on assessment, accountability, health promotion, education, infection control, safety and psychosocial support (Dermatology Nurses Association 1992).

EDUCATION AND TRAINING IN DERMATOLOGY NURSING

As dermatology services have been established in the primary care area and nursing roles introduced in local district hospitals, there has been a resulting increase in demand for dermatology nurse training and education. An increasing awareness of the needs of people with skin disorders and a recognition of the unmet need for dermatology services in primary care have highlighted the need for more trained specialist dermatology nurses and this has occurred in parallel with changes in nurse education, the introduction of Project 2000 and the move towards a degree-based profession. The report of the All-Party Parliamentary Group on Skin (APPGS 1998) identified the lack of dermatology nurse training and education at both pre- and postregistration levels. Its recommendations included compulsory basic training in dermatology nursing care in the undergraduate curriculum and commissioning of appropriate educational programmes in dermatology for qualified nurses.

In the undergraduate nurse programme there is a need to include the subject of dermatology and skin care in the curriculum so that all nurses gain the basic knowledge and skills to provide care for people with skin disorders. When patients with skin disease attend other clinical areas for treatment, e.g. during admission to hospital for surgery, they still need to receive appropriate skin care. Practical experience and acquisition of clinical skills should be an essential element of the education programme. This experience depends on the availability of clinical placements. Students should be given the opportunity to work in any area providing dermatological care – hospitals, outpatient clinics, day-care units and community-based clinics.

Allocation to a dermatology outpatient clinic as part of community/hospital interface experience or to a dermatology ward as part of medical nursing experience provides an ideal opportunity to gain insight into the needs of people with skin disease. Formal postregistration dermatology education courses have to date included Developments in Dermatological Nursing (London and Southampton), Dermatological Nursing (Sheffield) and Diploma in Practical Dermatology Nursing (Cardiff). New courses are being developed with the higher education institutions to prepare nurses at degree and higher degree level for specialist roles.

Specialist skills courses

Dermatology nurses must develop their specialist clinical skills, be able to assess the patient's skin and the response to treatment programmes, advise on health promotion, teach their patients about their condition and how best to manage it themselves. Other important areas of education for the specialist trained dermatology nurse should include:

- pharmacology of topical medications and preparation for the responsibilities of nurse prescribing
- development of counselling skills.

Preparation for nurse prescribing is needed to equip specialist nurses as this is expanded into dermatology. The benefits of trained dermatology nurses prescribing for their patients have already been identified by Bowman & Walton (1996) and in a survey of specialist dermatology nurses, Jackson (1998) found that many were already involved in prescribing through agreed treatment protocols.

Recommendations of the Crown Report (DoH 1999) for the introduction of two new categories of prescriber – independent and dependent – create further opportunities for dermatology nurses to expand the services they offer their patients. As Gooch (1999) says, it should also help ensure patient safety, improve adherence to treatment, reduce the burden on carers and make better use of human resources in the health-care professions. Crown also requires that suitable training programmes, including a period of supervised practice, are developed to ensure practitioners have the required prescribing competencies.

The psychological and emotional effects of a chronic skin disease such as psoriasis have been identified by Ramsay & O'Reagan (1988) and confirm the need for nurses to have the skills to help their patients to cope with their disease.

Additionally, specialist skills courses in the subspecialties, such as phototherapy, must be developed. These courses should include basic theory, have clear aims and objectives and will need to look at nursing responsibility in practice. The *Standards of care for dermatology nursing* (RCN 1995) provide an established requirement on which to base specialist practice. There is also a need to develop programmes that include supervised practice with assessment of competence and to have some accreditation level attached. Similarly, there is an urgent need to develop higher degree programmes for specialist dermatology nursing.

Other training and education is available through locally organized study days, the Skin Information Days run by the patient support group, the Skin Care Campaign and national conferences. In recognition of the need to promote dermatology nursing and support nurses working with patients with skin diseases, the RCN Dermatology Nurse Forum and the British Dermatological Nursing Group (BDNG) (which is affiliated to the British Association of Dermatologists) were formed in 1989. Educational initiatives of both groups include holding an annual national conference in addition to local study days. The BDNG annual conference includes a day of core educational modules in dermatology and they launched their quarterly publication, the *British Journal of Dermatology Nursing*, in May 1997.

A recent initiative to support nurse education and evidence-based practice has been the publication of an annotated bibliography of nursing literature in conjunction with the Department of Health (Ersser 1997, 1998).

PRIMARY CARE-LED SERVICE

The change in focus from secondary to primary care has been emphasized by the government and the Department of Health with the future strategy for the health service to be a primary care-led service. This was formalized in *Primary care: the future* (NHSE 1996) and emphasized again in *Establishing primary care groups* (NHSE 1998). In this plan for the future, most health care should be provided and organized by a primary care team. It has been recognized that there is an important role for the practice nurse in dermatology care (Edwards 1997) and it is vital that nurses are prepared to provide these patient services.

SHARED CARE

In order to benefit dermatology patients, shared care programmes must be developed. These should involve the multidisciplinary team: the liaison between community and hospital is strengthened and the expanded role of the nurse is developed. This allows shared care between doctors, nurses and health visitors to become more effective and provides a seamless care programme for patients. The Chief Medical Officer and the Chief Nursing Officer referred to this when looking at the interface between junior doctors and nurses (Calman et al 1994).

Developments in multidisciplinary shared care and nurse-led clinics place increasing demands on nurses. All nurses registered within the United Kingdom have to practise within the UKCC guidelines (UKCC 1992a, b). In the Code, it is stated quite clearly that nurses are personally accountable for their practice and for maintaining and improving their professional knowledge and competence. They must acknowledge any limitations in their knowledge and competence and not undertake anything unless they are able to perform it in a safe and skilled manner. Within *The scope of professional practice*, nurses are required to honestly acknowledge any limits of personal knowledge or skill and do whatever is necessary to equip themselves to care safely and effectively for patients. In developing new roles and expanding nursing practice, nurses have to identify innovations to help achieve the objectives of shared care.

CARE TRANSFER

The expanded role of the nurse and the aim to provide continuity of care should be combined to develop a process of 'care transfer' – a two-directional movement between the hospital and the community. The partnership across the primary and secondary care interface could be helped further by implementing a system of direct referrals to nursing services and nurse-to-nurse referrals. Support and back-up for nurse specialists need to be identified so that clear guidelines are in place for fast-tracking patients who need access to specialist nursing or medical care. The specialist nurses could also assist in:

- developing nurse-led clinics
- looking at the provision of dermatology care services
- continuing care programmes
- developing integrated care pathways for patients with chronic skin diseases
- assessment and screening opportunities.

SPECIALIST DERMATOLOGY NURSING

Patients with chronic skin disease value the role of the specialist trained dermatology nurse and the benefits of individualized nursing care (Jobling 1978, APPGS 1997).

Proposals were outlined in PREP (UKCC 1994) for nurses to develop as specialists and advanced practitioners. More recently, the UKCC (1998) has suggested that these be replaced by two levels of nursing practice. The specialist dermatology nurses have a real role in the future within the domain of higher level practice. They would include senior clinical nurses who are also expert specialist nurses (Castledine 1998). Nurses specializing in dermatology at a higher level in both primary and secondary care could have several levels of responsibility, which might be identified as follows:

- The general nurse with specialist knowledge and training in dermatology: perhaps somebody similar to a general medical practitioner with a specialist interest in dermatology.
- The dermatology specialist clinical nurse who is a general trained nurse and who has specialized both in dermatology and a particular area of dermatology practice, for example phototherapy.
- The advanced dermatology nurse practitioner who would be comparable with the consultant dermatologist. These nurses would have a highly developed knowledge of complex nursing care, dermatology and dermatology nursing practice. They would also be able to 'act' as consultants and specialist dermatology nursing resources for all members of the multidisciplinary team, both in the primary and secondary care sectors. It would be expected that these nurses should be educated to Master's or doctorate level.

INNOVATIONS IN DERMATOLOGY NURSING

During the past few years there have been various innovations in dermatology where nurses have set up and developed clinics or services which they lead (Box 16.1).

In phototherapy, nurses are trained to manage the care of patients undergoing ultraviolet light (UVL) treatments such as UVB or photochemotherapy (PUVA) (Stone et al 1989) (see Chapter 4).

In most units, day treatment programmes have replaced inpatient care for psoriasis patients. Day treatment patients, having been referred by a doctor for a programme of care, make a contract with the nurses to attend for their course of treat-

ment. This will involve the nurses ensuring that the patient receives the topical treatments, learns about their condition and how to care for their skin during and after the course of treatment. Patient education programmes play a major role in helping patients deal with their condition and developing positive coping strategies (Burr & Gradwell 1996).

In the minor surgery field, in order to provide an all-female team, nurses have been specially trained and have taken on the responsibilities of doing biopsies in special clinics for vulval disorders.

Nurses are carrying out laser therapy for treatment of port wine stains in addition to pre- and postoperative care and advice.

INITIATIVES IN DERMATOLOGY NURSING

Many people with skin diseases can be treated effectively in the community and nurses in the primary care setting have a major role to play. The health-care needs of people with skin disease are frequently unmet and when one considers that some 15% of the population consult their GP annually with a skin disease (Carmichael 1995), it gives some measure of the size of the problem.

The main reason for the demand for treatment in skin disease is its high prevalence. The rising incidence of some skin diseases such as skin cancer can be related to more frequent sunny holidays, atopic eczema, especially in children, and venous leg ulcers due to the increasing ageing population. Additionally, publicity and development of better treatments for conditions such as acne and psoriasis and education about moles and other skin growths have led to the general public becoming more aware and having increased expectations.

With the emphasis on care in the community and a primary care-led health service, more is being done to raise awareness of the needs of patients with skin conditions. Specialist hospital-based dermatology nurses have been developing community liaison roles (Perkins 1994, Ruane Morris et al 1995, Venables et al 1995) and some practice and district nurses have taken a special

---

Box 16.1 Innovations

Leg ulcer clinics	Patient education programmes
Phototherapy	Wart clinics
Camouflage	Day treatment clinics
Photopheresis	Laser therapy
Minor surgery	Nurse counselling
Complementary therapies	

interest in patients with skin problems, particularly families where children have eczema (Edwards 1997).

If people with skin diseases are to have access to dermatological nursing care, nurses must:

- know how to examine and assess the patient's skin
- be aware of common skin problems
- know how to prevent them or limit the likelihood of a flare-up
- know about the treatments which are commonly prescribed and how to apply them.

Through working with patients and their families or carers to teach them about these issues, nurses can help them to develop greater understanding of their disease and become more independent. Nurses may facilitate such activities by establishing nurse-led clinics that offer such services as:

- skin assessment/screening
- patient teaching and advice about therapy
- application of topical treatments
- promotion of healthy skin care and prevention of disease
- development of local support/self-help groups (Burr & Gradwell 1996)
- occupational health advice (Clare 1997)
- chronic disease management, particularly for patients with eczema and psoriasis.

These initiatives should be expanded or developed. A positive and valuable development has already been achieved with the emergence of the dermatology community liaison nurse roles (Perkins 1994, Venables et al 1995). Specialist dermatology nurse practitioners can participate in multidisciplinary clinics and services (e.g. for patients with epidermolysis bullosa) and establish more dermatology nurse-led clinics (e.g. healthy skin promotion, sun awareness, skin assessment). These nurses have been shown to be effective in prescribing compared with junior medical staff (Cox et al 1995). Most patients with a well-established history of a chronic condition such as psoriasis or eczema do know what treatments are appropriate for them so emollient therapies and routine treatments could readily be prescribed by the specialist trained dermatology nurse. Such initiatives help to improve the access to care for these patients, especially when their condition relapses.

Dermatology nurses need to be working in and with the local community to assess local need for continuing care and build on previous strategies for developing patient partnerships (NHSE 1996). As with all other clinical services, it is necessary to look at developing nursing contracts and arranging for direct referrals to specialist dermatology nursing services. With care transfer between primary and secondary care and between members of the various disciplines of the health-care team, patients should benefit from continuity in their care programmes.

Opportunities for groups of nurses to join together to provide direct care for patients with chronic diseases should be explored. Dermatology nurses are in an advantageous position to work with their patients, particularly as many patients with chronic disorders such as psoriasis or eczema have a very clear idea about what is required to manage their condition. Dermatology nurses work closely with their patients and should be involved in the commissioning and coordinating of multidisciplinary care. They are in an ideal situation to identify the needs of dermatology patients, as well as providing appropriate care for them.

Education and advice are vital in helping patients and their families or carers to understand about the disorder and how to look after and protect their skin. Dermatology nurses can provide emotional and psychological support and make patients aware of the available social services. They have an invaluable role in contributing to the activities of local patient support groups and the umbrella patient group, the Skin Care Campaign.

DERMATOLOGY NURSING RESEARCH

Research in dermatology nursing is in its infancy and the first step was to recognize the situation by producing the annotated bibliography mentioned above (Ersser 1998). In 1998 the BDNG awarded its first two dermatology nursing research fellowships. It is essential that nursing in dermatology progresses so that nursing care keeps up to date with and complements medical developments in dermatology.

There are a number of research issues that dermatology nurses need to consider and the following are some suggested fields.

There is a need for systematic reviews in dermatology. A systematic review is an up-to-date, unbiased and accurate assessment of the evidence supporting the efficacy of an intervention in health care. The Cochrane Skin Group is a voluntary international organization committed to producing and updating systematic reviews in dermatology. These reviews are intended for all professionals and consumers in the health service and therefore nurses have a particular role in helping with work for this group (Williams 1998). Opportunities to contribute to this work should be pursued.

Evaluative studies of dermatology nursing services need to be undertaken to build on the work done in Oxford (Ersser et al 1998). Investigations into the effectiveness of clinical nursing practice in dermatology generally and its specialist areas will contribute to improvements in the provision of patient care.

There is a need to clarify the roles of nurses in the provision of dermatology care – what aspects of care should be expected from each level of clinician? Established procedures and practices should be reviewed with reference to supporting evidence for their efficacy. Where is the care best provided for the benefit of the patient? Should it be in the primary or secondary care area or a combination of both?

The value of the counselling and support elements of care in dermatology nursing is well recognized and evidence to support developments in this aspect of nursing care will help in planning future services.

VISION FOR THE FUTURE

Nurse-led initiatives have a major role to play in the future of dermatological care. As more care transfers into the community, dermatological services provided by community and practice nurses will increase. Dermatology community liaison nurses will become key professionals, coordinating patient care between the primary and secondary areas, health and social services and the multidisciplinary clinical teams. Joint appointments of specialist dermatology nurses to the hospital and local PCGs will strengthen their links as well as facilitating continuity of patient care. Creation of these posts would also enable specialist dermatology nursing expertise to be more easily accessible for advice, education and training in the community.

Specialist trained groups of dermatology nurses might form independent clinics to provide all types of treatment for skin disease. Primary care groups could access such a resource for skin care for their local community.

The need for improving skin care throughout the world has been recognized (Grossman 1995, Ong & Ryan 1998). Dermatology nursing has been gaining a higher profile in many countries, with specialist groups such as the BDNG and the American Dermatology Nurses' Association becoming increasingly active and starting to network with each other and their medical colleagues.

In 1998 a networking group, the International Skin Care Nursing Group (ISCNG), was established and it was launched at the VIII International Congress of Dermatology in Cairo in 1999. The ISCNG will lead the way, together with an established steering group, to the launch of an International Skin Care Nursing Development Committee (ISCNDC) by 2001. It is proposed that the ISCNG will work with the International Committee of Dermatology and the International Council of Nurses to advise on specific international skin care projects requiring the input of nursing expertise. The ISCNDC, drawn from the international group as an expert panel, would provide an advisory service and assist in developing standards and policies for clinical practice, education and research related to skin-care nursing. It is envisaged that the ISCNG will be a forum for facilitating communication between nurses working in the skin-care field throughout the world with an overall objective of improving the standards of skin-care services for all communities.

CONCLUSION

As care needs are identified, nurses must be prepared to undertake and expand their role as they work with the multidisciplinary team of patients, colleagues and commissioners in developing future plans. Continuity is essential so that the interface between primary and secondary care becomes more blurred and a seamless programme of care is available for people with skin disorders.

Nurses have a responsibility to acquire the education and training to prepare themselves for the specialist dermatology nursing role. Research into dermatological nursing and nursing care must be promoted so that patients benefit from practice and education based on the most up-to-date evidence.

Dermatology nursing has a sound base of proven traditional methods of training, education and care provision on which to build for the future. Dermatology nurses must ensure that they are always open to the new needs and developments in the care of patients with skin problems.

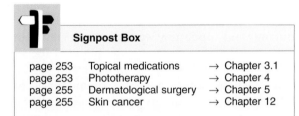

Signpost Box

page 253	Topical medications	→ Chapter 3.1
page 253	Phototherapy	→ Chapter 4
page 255	Dermatological surgery	→ Chapter 5
page 255	Skin cancer	→ Chapter 12

REFERENCES

All Party Parliamentary Group on Skin 1997 An investigation into the adequacy of service provision and treatments for patients with skin diseases in the UK. All Party Parliamentary Group on Skin, London

All Party Parliamentary Group on Skin 1998 Enquiry into the training of healthcare professionals who come into contact with skin diseases. All Party Parliamentary Group on Skin, London

Bowman J, Walton Y 1996 Development of specialist dermatology nurse prescribing. Nursing Standard 10(42): 34–36

Burr S, Gradwell C 1996 The psychosocial effects of skin diseases: need for support groups. British Journal of Nursing 5(19): 1177–1182

Calman K, Moores Y, Jarrold K 1994 The Greenhalgh Report: the interface between junior doctors and nurses. EL(94)75. NHSE, Leeds

Carmichael A J 1995 Achieving an accessible dermatology service. Dermatology in Practice 3(5): 13–16

Castledine G 1998 From specialist practice role to level of practice. British Journal of Nursing 7(11): 682

Clare M 1997 My advice to patients with hand dermatitis. British Journal of Dermatology Nursing 1(4): 6–7

Cox N, Walton Y, Bowman K 1995 Evaluation of nurse prescribing in a dermatology unit. British Journal of Dermatology 133: 340–341

DoH 1989 Working for patients. Cm555. HMSO, London

DoH 1997 The new NHS: modern, dependable. The Stationery Office, London

DoH 1999 Review of prescribing, supply and administration of medicines. Department of Health, London

Dermatology Nurses Association 1992 Dermatology nursing: scope of practice. Dermatology Nursing 4(6): B–D

Edwards V 1997 Dermatology care and the practice nurse – a primary role. British Journal of Dermatology Nursing 1(2): 5–7

Ersser S J 1997 Dermatology nursing literature and the future of dermatology nursing. British Journal of Dermatology Nursing 1(4): 4–5

Ersser S J (ed) 1998 Annotated bibliography of the dermatological nursing literature. Oxford Brookes University, Oxford

Ersser S J, Newton J N, Taylor H R et al 1998 A descriptive and evaluative study of a dermatology nursing service. Oxford Centre for Health Care Research and Development, Oxford Brookes University, Oxford

Gooch S 1999 Nurse prescribing and the Crown review. Professional Nurse 14(10): 678–680

Grossman H 1995 Community dermatology – a response and challenge of dermatological health for all. European Conference on Tropical Medicine, Hamburg, Germany

Jackson K 1998 Nurse prescribing in dermatology. British Journal of Dermatology Nursing 2(1): 10–12

Jobling R 1978 With and without professional nurses – the case for dermatology. In: Dingwall R, Macintosh J (eds) Readings in the sociology of nursing. Churchill Livingstone, Edinburgh, pp 181–195

NHS Executive 1996 Primary care: the future. NHSE, Leeds

NHS Executive 1998 Establishing primary care groups. HSC 1998/065. NHSE, Leeds

NHS Management Executive 1990 NHS trusts: a working guide. HMSO, London

Ong C-K, Ryan T J 1998 Healthy skin for all: a multi-faceted approach. Keith Williams, London

Perkins P 1994 Caring for skin in the community. Practice Nurse 7(2): 96–99

Ramsay B, O'Reagan M 1988 A survey of the social and psychological effects of psoriasis. British Journal of Dermatology 118: 195–201

RCN 1995 Standards of care for dermatology nursing. Royal College of Nursing, London

Rea J, Newhouse M, Halil T 1976 Skin disease in Lambeth. A community study of prevalence and use of medical care. British Journal of Preventative and Social Medicine 30: 107–114

Ruane Morris M, Thompson G, Lawton S 1995 Community liaison in dermatology. Professional Nurse 10(11): 687–688

Stone L A 1983 The role of the nurse in the skin care team. Nursing 2(9): 244–245

Stone L A, Lindfield E M, Robertson S 1989 A colour atlas of nursing procedures in skin disorders. Wolfe Medical, London

UKCC 1992a The code of professional conduct for the nurse, midwife and health visitor, 3rd edn. UKCC, London

UKCC 1992b The scope of professional practice. UKCC, London

UKCC 1994 The future of professional practice: Council's standards for education and practice following registration. UKCC, London

UKCC 1998 Report of the higher level practice (specialist practice project – phase II). UKCC, London

Venables J, Ersser S, Vineer K 1995 Report of the work of a dermatology liaison service: (1) analytical description of role, its development and evaluative research strategy (Nov 1993–Oct 1994). Unpublished report. National Institute for Nursing and Department of Dermatology, Oxford Department of Dermatology, Oxford

Williams H C 1997 Dermatology health care needs assessment: the epidemiologically based needs assessment reviews, 2nd series. Stevens A, Raftery J (eds). Radcliffe Medical Press, Oxford

Williams H C 1998 The need for systematic reviews in dermatology. Dermatology Core Educational Module, British Dermatological Nursing Group, London

USEFUL ADDRESSES

American Dermatology Nurses' Association (DNA)
East Holly Avenue
Box 56
Pitman
New Jersey 08071-0056
USA
Web site: dna.inurse.com

British Dermatological Nursing Group (BDNG)
BAD House
19 Fitzroy Square
London
W1P 5HQ
Tel: 020 7383 0266
Fax: 020 7388 5263

International Skin Care Nursing Group (ISCNG)
c/o Rebecca Penzer – international skin care nurse
co-ordinator / Dr Steve Ersser – Head of Nursing
Development
School of Nursing & Midwifery
University of Southampton
Level B(11) South Block
Southampton General Hospital
Tremona Road
Southampton
SO16 6YD
02380 79 6579: reception
02380 79 5115: direct
02380 79 6922: fax

RCN Dermatology Nurses' Forum
Royal College of Nursing
20 Cavendish Square
London
W1M AB
Tel: 020 7109 3333

Index